Spiritual Wellness and the Built Environment

I0797859

Imagine a world where buildings and cities actively nurture our well-being, not just physically but spiritually. There is a growing awareness of the need for a more inclusive and comprehensive approach to wellness strategies in everyday life. This book explores spiritual wellness as a foundational attribute of urban planning and design with the hope of influencing a more flourishing trajectory of development with the built environment. Chapters reflect the beginning of this evolving movement in home and community design that tackles our uniquely modern problems of sedentary lives, unhealthy diets, stress, social isolation, pollution, nature deprivation, and inaccessibility to spiritually nurturing places. The attributes of spiritual wellness are presented as defining characteristics informing design strategies. These specific planning and design strategies are presented through case studies from around the globe that highlight the importance of spiritual wellness considerations at all scales of the built environment, from rooms to cities. This book is essential to help architects, planners, designers, engineers, healthcare providers, project stakeholders, and graduate students embrace and implement a successful wellness design approach.

"Phillip Tabb's work on *Spiritual Wellness and the Built Environment* is deeply rooted in unity, sustainability, and transcendence. Driven by a keen sense of purpose, he shares insights into spiritual placemaking and well-being. Tabb outlines a path to holistic harmony, exploring how values and beliefs in designing with nature contribute to universal balance. His approach reveals the intricate relationship between humanity and the cosmos, emphasizing our connections to forces greater than ourselves. Tabb's vision illustrates a wide range of liminal human experiences, from intimate spaces like a tea ceremony to grand awe-inspiring natural spaces. Tabb's message subtly emphasizes that achieving true well-being requires heightened awareness and personal growth on all levels. His work not only guides but invites us to join him in exploring the profound connection between the built environment, spirituality and wellness. Through this journey, Tabb offers a unique perspective on our place in the universe and the role of mindful design enhancing our lives."

Nader Ardalan, *Architect and Board of Directors, Architecture, Culture, and Spirituality Forum*

"There are so many aspects to sacred geometry. When I first learned of it in England in 1996, I was taken with using the relationship between Earth and the Heavens to design structures. So when we were creating Serenbe, we knew that sacred geometry must be included. And synchronistically, Phill Tabb appeared. What we didn't know then but makes total sense now, is that when you work with sacred geometry, you are aligning all the energy points of the land and buildings, much like the meridian points in the body, to make a whole and balanced project. And when this is executed consciously, you are creating an environment of Well of Being where all can prosper. Dr. Tabb has expertly studied places that have done just that. And in so doing, he makes a great case for including sacred geometry in a multitude of designs."

Marie L. Nygren, *Co-Founder, Serenbe Community, Georgia*

Spiritual Wellness and the Built Environment

Phillip James Tabb

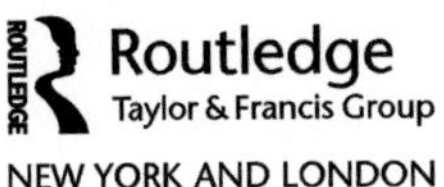

NEW YORK AND LONDON

Designed cover image: Getty Images

First published 2026
by Routledge
605 Third Avenue, New York, NY 10158

and by Routledge
4 Park Square, Milton Park, Abingdon, Oxon, OX14 4RN

Routledge is an imprint of the Taylor & Francis Group, an informa business

Library of Congress Cataloging-in-Publication Data
Names: Tabb, Phillip, author.
Title: Spiritual wellness in the built environment / Phillip James Tabb.
Description: New York, NY : Routledge, 2026. |
Includes bibliographical references and index.
Identifiers: LCCN 2025005288 (print) | LCCN 2025005289 (ebook) |
ISBN 9781032900780 (hardback) | ISBN 9781032895567 (paperback) |
ISBN 9781003546085 (ebook)
Subjects: LCSH: Architecture–Psychological aspects. |
Spirituality in architecture. | Built environment–Health aspects.
Classification: LCC NA2540 .T325 2026 (print) | LCC NA2540 (ebook) |
DDC 720.1/9–dc23/eng/20250611
LC record available at https://lccn.loc.gov/2025005288
LC ebook record available at https://lccn.loc.gov/2025005289

ISBN: 9781032900780 (hbk)
ISBN: 9781032895567 (pbk)
ISBN: 9781003546085 (ebk)

DOI: 10.4324/9781003546085

Typeset in Univers
by Newgen Publishing UK

This work is dedicated to my youngest grandson, Jack Ronan Tabb, who was one year old when I began writing this book. My hope is that the world becomes a healthier place as he and my other three grandsons grow older.

Contents

Figures

Tables

About the Author

Phillip James Tabb is Emeritus Professor of Architecture at Texas A&M University and was the Liz and Nelson Mitchell Professor of Residential Design. He served as head of the department from 2001 to 2005 and was director of the School of Architecture and Construction Management at Washington State University from 1998 to 2001. In 1990, he completed a PhD dissertation on *The Solar Village Archetype: A Study of English Village Form Applicable to Energy Integrated Planning Principles for Satellite Settlements in Temperate Climates*. His publications include *Solar Energy Planning*, published by McGraw-Hill in 1984; he co-authored *The Greening of Architecture: A Critical History and Survey of Contemporary Sustainable Architecture and Urban Design*, published by Ashgate in 2014; and he co-edited *Architecture, Culture and Spirituality*, also published by Ashgate, in 2015. He is the author of *Serene Urbanism: A Biophilic Theory and Practice of Sustainable Placemaking*, published in 2017; *Elemental Architecture: Temperaments of Sustainability*, published in 2019; *Biophilic Urbanism: Designing Resilient Communities for the Future*, published in 2021; *Thin Place Design: Architecture of the Numinous*, published in 2023; and co-author of *Wellness Architecture and Urban Design* in 2025, all published by Routledge. Since 2001, Tabb has been the master plan architect for Serenbe Community – an award-winning sustainable, biophilic, and wellness community being realized near Atlanta, Georgia, and the architect of his solar residence in Serenbe. He is a board member of the Biophilic Institute and an editor and author of the Wellness Architecture & Design Initiative for the Global Wellness Institute. He received his Bachelor of Science in Architecture from the University of Cincinnati, Master of Architecture from the University of Colorado, and PhD in the Energy and Environment Programme from the Architectural Association in London. He has been a design educator for 20 years and a practicing urban designer and licensed architect for 30 years; he is a member of the American Institute of Architects and holds a NCARB Certificate.

Foreword

Phillip James Tabb has done it again. He captivates us in a deeper knowing and understanding of why our spaces matter, especially on a spiritual level. Why we *feel* places and spaces more so than others. In a time when the relentless pace of modern life pulls us away from the core of what it means to be whole, it is easy to overlook the essence of spiritual wellness. Yet, it is precisely this overlooked element – our spiritual connection to ourselves, others, and the world around us – that holds the key to our well-being, our communities, and perhaps even the future of our planet.

This book, *Spiritual Wellness and the Built Environment*, is a powerful reminder that true wellness extends far beyond physical health, beyond productivity and efficiency, beyond the mere appearance of success. It delves into the deeply interconnected dimensions of our spiritual existence, grounded in the environments we inhabit and the spaces we create. It challenges us to reconsider how we live, work, and design the world around us – inviting us to foster environments that support not only our physical needs but also our deeper, spiritual selves. Phill has the ability to put you at ease while exploring deep connections in the spiritual realm and place making.

At the heart of this work is a profound call to action: to recognize that our built environments are not merely backdrops to our lives but active participants in shaping our experiences, our emotions, and our spiritual well-being. From the smallest room to the largest city, the spaces we inhabit influence the rhythms of our daily lives and the quality of our connections – both with ourselves and with the world. The idea of spiritual wellness, while ancient, is more relevant today than ever before. As we face the crises of climate change, social division, and escalating global tensions, we are also confronting a crisis of meaning. Many of us feel disconnected – disconnected from nature, from each other, and even from ourselves. This disconnection manifests in the way we treat the world, how we design our cities, and how we live our lives.

This book offers a path forward by drawing on ancient wisdom and contemporary design principles, presenting practical strategies to integrate spiritual wellness into our built environments. The author, through thoughtful research and a deep understanding of architecture, urban planning, and wellness, reminds us that we are not separate from nature, nor from each other. Instead, we are inextricably linked, and it is through this interconnectedness that we can find healing, purpose, and resilience. Several chapters in this book particularly resonate with me, given my work in biophilia, nature, and the brain. The attribute on "Healing Environments" in Chapter 2 feels like a direct echo of my mission. Nature can transform mental and physical well-being. Phill's insights into healing landscapes not only validate but also enrich a deeper understanding of biophilic design as a tool for personal and communal health.

The chapter on "Place-Based Attributes of Spiritual Wellness" explores concepts such as "thin places" and sanctuary spaces – areas that evoke a deep sense of calm and transcendence. This chapter aligns with my belief that spaces designed with intention and beauty can foster profound human connection. Dr. Tabb's exploration of these spiritual places underscores the importance of creating spaces that allow people to reconnect with the essence of being human, something I actively champion and deeply believe in. The chapter on "Spiritual Wellness at the Urban Design Scale" is particularly powerful as it addresses the integration of nature within city planning. This chapter's strategies provide a compelling blueprint for how cities can embrace beauty, wellness, and biophilic elements not just for aesthetic enhancement but for the holistic well-being of their communities.

The four "Narrative Vignette" chapters at the end of the book are particularly interesting as they represent deep dives into Dr. Tabb's personal experiences of spiritual wellness. The vignettes focus on the significance of solar energy, the role of sacred geometry, the value of mythic landscapes, and the importance of pilgrimages. The projects and drawings recount and emphasize his attributes of spiritual wellness. Dr. Tabb's stories reveal certain spiritual wellness concepts and detail specific attributes discussed earlier in the book. They are intended to give voice to firsthand, insightful, and accessible spiritual wellness design strategies in more anecdotal ways.

This book is more than a guide for architects, urban planners, or designers. It is an invitation to all of us to reconsider how we interact with the spaces around us. It is an invitation to pause, to reflect, and to ask ourselves how we can create environments – whether in our homes, workplaces, or communities – that support not only our physical well-being but also our spiritual growth. It is a reminder that we each have the power to shape the world around us, to create spaces that nurture connection, kindness, and a sense of belonging.

The challenges we face today – climate change, resource depletion, social fragmentation – are daunting, but they are not insurmountable. At the core of each of these challenges is a deeper, spiritual disconnection, one that can be healed by reimagining our relationship with the world around us. As Dr. Tabb so eloquently argues, the solution lies not only in technological advancements or policy changes but in a fundamental shift in how we see and engage with the world. By designing spaces that honor our spiritual needs, we can create a future where both people and the planet can thrive.

As you read this book, I encourage you to open your mind and heart to the possibilities it presents. Whether you are an architect, a city planner, a healer, or simply someone seeking greater meaning in life, you will find inspiration in these pages. The strategies outlined here are not just theoretical – they are actionable, practical, and grounded in a deep understanding of what it means to be human in an increasingly complex world.

At its core, *Spiritual Wellness and the Built Environment* is about hope. It is about envisioning a future where we live in harmony with our surroundings, where the spaces we create reflect our highest values, and where spiritual wellness is seen not as a luxury but as an essential component of a thriving society. It is a call to embrace the sacred in the everyday, to find beauty in the spaces we inhabit, and to recognize that, in doing so, we are not only enhancing our own well-being but also contributing to the healing of the world.

This book is a gift, offering us the tools and insights we need to create a more spiritually attuned world. It is a reminder that, in the end, wellness is not just about the absence of illness – it is about living in balance, with ourselves, each other, and the planet. As you embark on this journey, may you be inspired to create spaces that reflect the best of who we are and the world we want to create. May you find, in the words and ideas shared here, a deep connection to the sacred and a renewed sense of purpose in shaping a more holistic, spiritually vibrant future for all.

Jennifer Walsh
Founder and Creative Director,
LABH Lab and Institute

Preface

This preface presents a series of events and experiences in autobiographical form that have led to my interest in wellness, spirituality, and the built environment. Key takeaways have contributed to my evolving understanding of the world. I was born in the village of Richland, Washington, in the summer of 1945. Nearby Richland, the Hanford Site was the location of the Manhattan Project that constructed and operated the world's first nuclear production reactor, the B Reactor. It produced full-scale plutonium used in the Trinity Test and the atomic bomb dropped on Nagasaki, Japan, on August 9, 1945 (see the contrast between a Golden Sunset and the B Reactor, Figures 0.1a and 0.1b). My father was an engineer working for Dupont at this time. The site was considered the Manhattan Project's signature facility and has been designated a National Historic Landmark by the National Park Service. The site was selected because of its proximity to an abundant supply of cold Columbia River water needed to cool nuclear reactors, ample available hydroelectric power, mild climate, excellent transportation facilities, and distance from major population centers.[1] My dad, mom, sister, and I lived about a block from the Columbia River, a dangerous river but full of adventures and access to nature. It wasn't until I was older that I learned about Richland's history and its relationship to nuclear energy. I always wondered why I was born in this place and at that time, and this led me to a lifelong journey that, over time and many experiences, fed a curiosity about my direction and purpose in life.

In 1953, our family moved to Idaho Falls, Idaho, the site of the Experimental Breeder Reactor and the world's first power plant to produce electricity (see Figure 0.1b). In 1961, this was America's only nuclear reactor fatality, and my father was one involved in the cleanup. Despite the closeness to the reactor, my sister and I thoroughly loved growing up in Idaho. At that time, Idaho Falls was the second largest city in the state, with a population of around 35,000 people. The Snake River flows directly through the middle of the city, and its presence is very much felt. We lived in a new subdivision at the end of town. At the edge of the subdivision was an irrigation canal that ran for miles and miles and, for us, served as a source of adventure in both summer and winter. Also, next door was Tautphaus Park, a place of great adventures and fun. There were an amusement park, zoo, ice arena, baseball and softball fields, basketball courts, tennis courts, playground equipment, and picnic shelters. For young, free-range kids, this was heaven.

In sharp contrast to the Arco desert and Experimental Breeder Reactor site, Idaho is beautiful and has seven parks that are a part of the National Parks System.

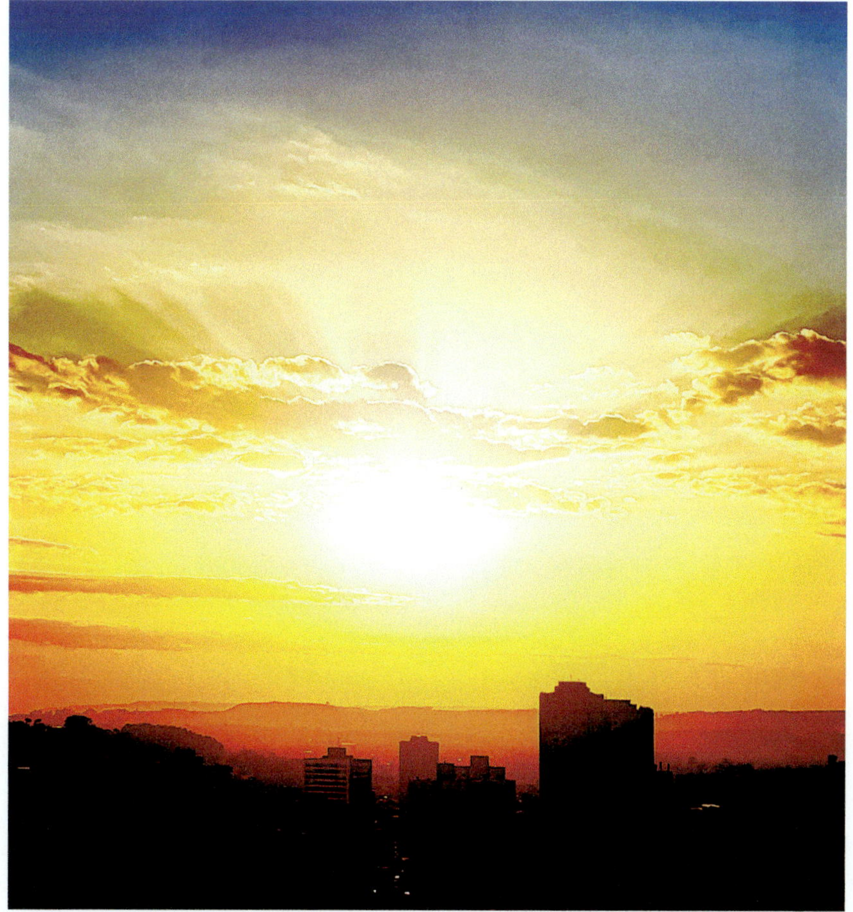

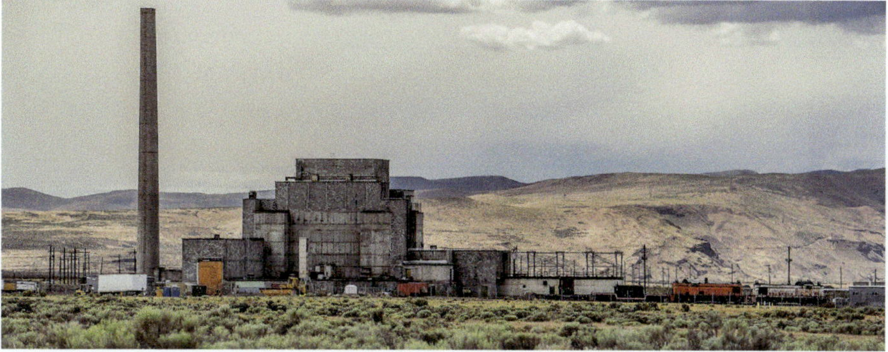

0.1
Contrasting images (a) Golden Sunset, (b) Hanford Nuclear Reactor Richland, Washington

Our family spent summer vacations traveling to these parks and especially a place called Island Park, which is directly west of Yellowstone Park. Each summer we spent a week or so in Island Park, living in a cabin next to the incredibly beautiful Buffalo River. In our 1959 Bonneville Pontiac, we visited most national parks in the West. The only cities we experienced were Denver, where my parents grew up, Boise, and Las Vegas. While I loved growing up near nature, I had a longing to experience larger cities and to have broader cultural experiences.

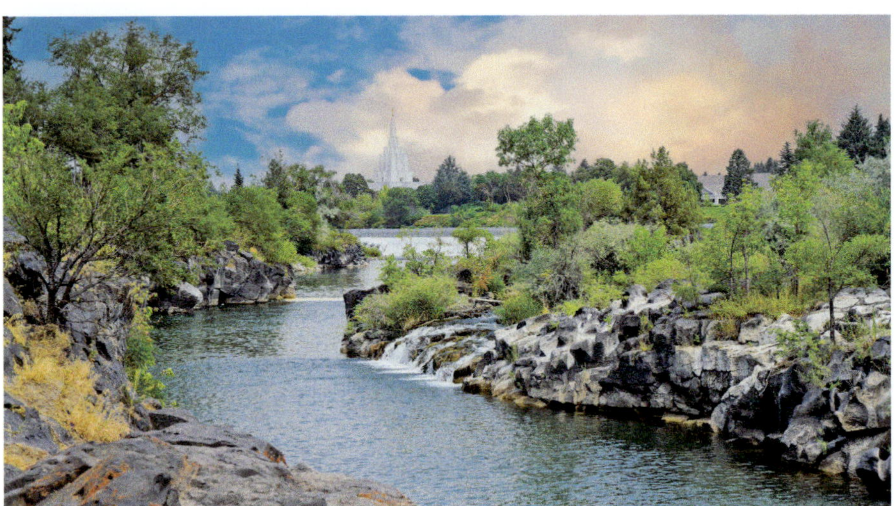

0.2
Snake River in Idaho Falls, Idaho

In 1961, we moved to Cincinnati, Ohio, where I finished high school and later attended the University of Cincinnati in its work-study program in architecture. I suppose this was my first real experience of a city. The architecture program led me to work in Dayton, Indianapolis, and Chicago. By this time, my rural Western upbringing was being eclipsed by city living. I particularly was influenced by working for Skidmore, Owings and Merrill in Chicago, where I was exposed to large-scale buildings and urban design work. I worked for the principal, Walter Netsch, who at that time had developed a new design approach and language involving the rotated square geometric system. After graduation, I moved to Boston and worked in Cambridge and, in the early 1970s, I left Boston and moved to Boulder, Colorado, where I lived for nearly 30 years. Boulder had an interesting influence, especially in the first couple of decades. While developing a practice in architecture, our firm became deeply involved in solar energy and its applications to architecture and counter-culture projects. This led to a lifelong interest in solar energy and its application to planning and design and, finally, to my retirement home in Georgia. Figure 0.3 shows the spring equinox at Sunset Point, my photovoltaic array and residence, eventually realized in Serenbe in 2017.

For me, the 1970s were a blend of professional development and continuing education in solar energy applications and research as well as esoteric and spiritual areas of study. As a university student in the 1960s, I was highly influenced by social change and interested in the ways that architecture contributed to such change. So, the 1973 oil embargo was a harbinger of change for me and influenced the next ten years of my practice and teaching. Our firm won five national solar energy demonstration grants from AIA/RC, HUD, and DOE. With this support, we were able to realize the concept in bricks and mortar. I was involved in the realization of approximately three dozen or more solar-related projects. We added a solar greenhouse to my home in Boulder, but I always dreamed of living in an off-grid house fully capable of functioning on its own.

0.3
Solar
Energy: (a) Sunset
Point,Serenbe,Georgia;
(b) Photovoltaic
Array; (c) Tabb
Residence (2017)

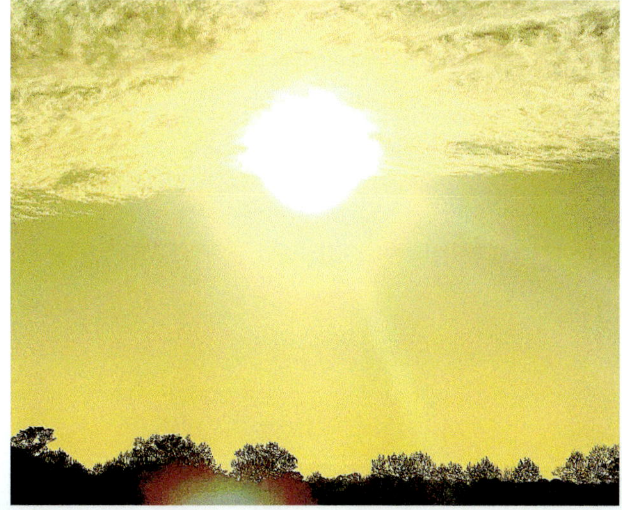

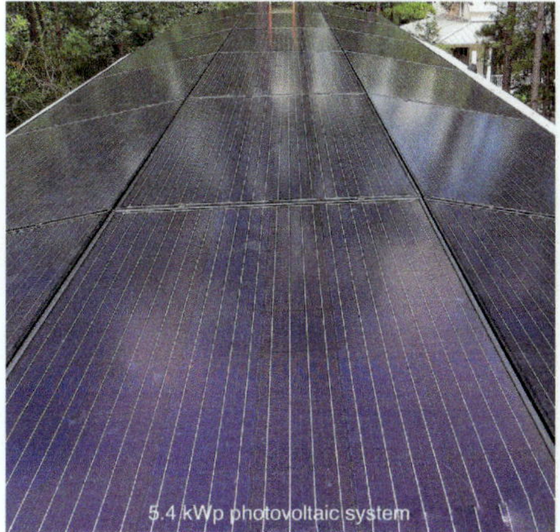

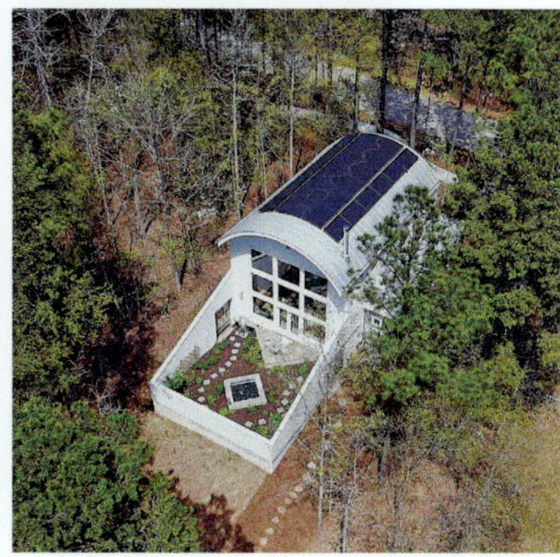

Later in 1990, one of my clients, David Tresemer, commissioned me to design the StarHouse, a community structure in the foothills of the Rocky Mountains designed with sacred geometry and constructed with non-toxic building materials. Its primary mission was to provide a sanctuary and meeting place for sacred studies and celebration of the changing seasons (see Figure 0.4a). This project offered me an opportunity to work with sacred geometry but also to observe sacred intentions throughout the entire process, from design conception through construction and use. Another project was Nancy Stetson's art therapy studio, located in Boulder, that offered the opportunity to design a structure based on golden mean geometry.

Later in the mid-1990s, I was given a graph-paper drawing and commissioned to create the design and construction documents for the 42-foot-high (12.8-meter) Tashi Gomang Stupa located in Crestone, Colorado. It was created to commemorate the 16th Karmapa, Rangjung Rigpa Dorje, who escaped Tibet after the Chinese invasion (see Figure 0.4b).[2] The Tashi Gomang Stupa was designed as the "*Stupa of Many Auspicious Doors*."[3] The site was located close to the Sand Dunes National Park and, therefore, was highly sandy, posing structural foundation challenges for

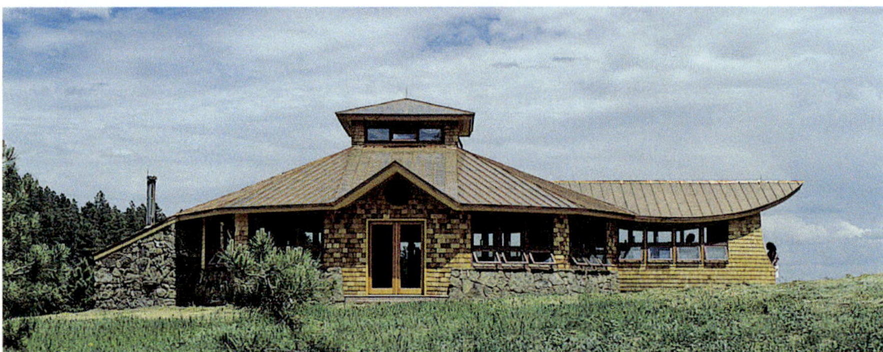

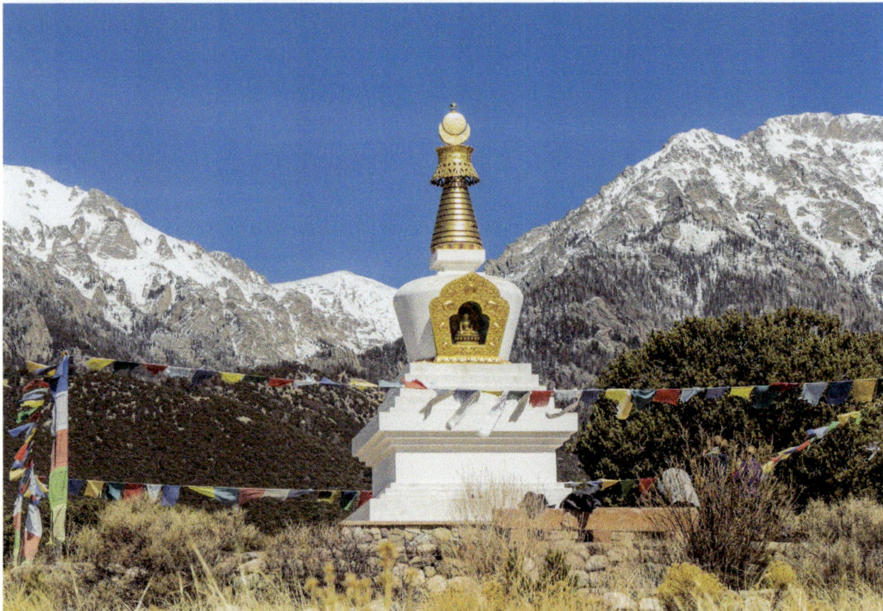

0.4
Sacred Architecture: (a) StarHouse (1991), (b) Tashi Gomang Stupa (1995)

support of the heavy stupa. The solution was a reinforced concrete table foundation upon which the stupa was then constructed. In creating the final drawings for the stupa, we had to be extremely careful in dimensioning the various geometric shapes making up the form and proportions. The erection of this stupa was part of a Native American myth that the San Louis Valley would be replenished with its ancient Pleistocene waters, Lake Alamosa, after a number of spiritual structures were built.[4]

As my professional career progressed, I became involved in wellness and spiritual pursuits offered in Boulder. In the mid-1980s, I attended a series of workshops led by Dr. Keith Critchlow, who was a leader in the field of sacred geometry. These workshops were held primarily in Crestone, Colorado, in a pristine natural environment at the base of the Sangre di Cristo Mountains and the Sand Dunes National Park. The course wove together Pythagorean, Platonic, Buddhist, Christian, Islamic, mathematical, and esoteric notions of sacred geometry with a particular focus on the "*quadrivium*." Number, geometry, music, and astronomy were seen as contexts

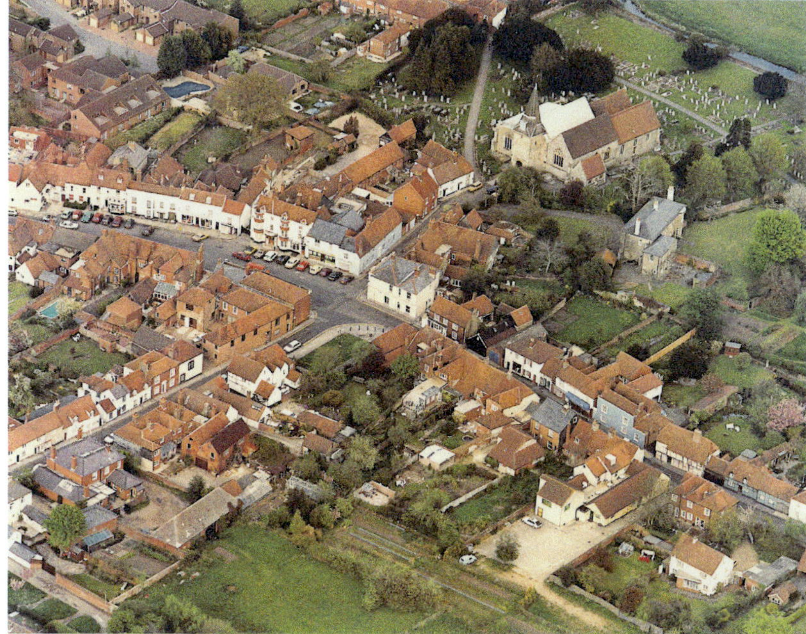

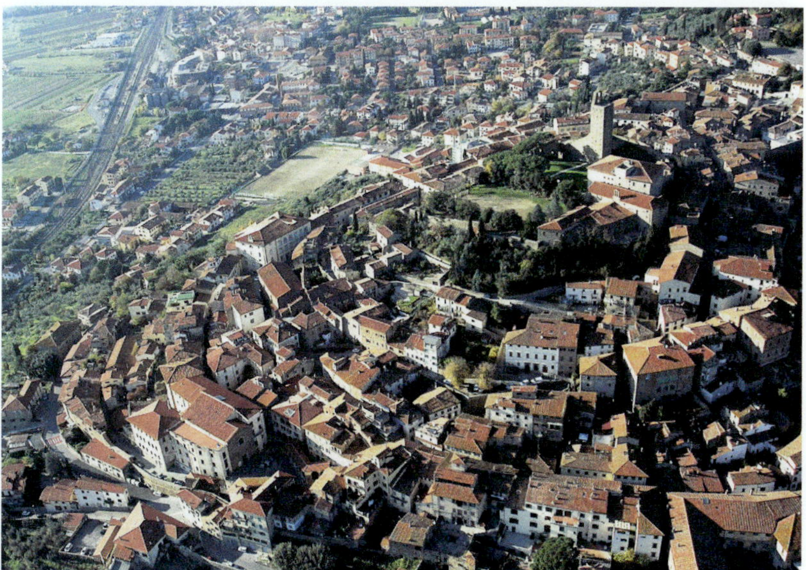

0.5
European Places Where I Lived: (a) Titchfield, UK; (b) Castiglion Fiorentino, Italy

for the embodiment of significant or sacred sensibilities. I was blown away by the historic nature of the pursuit of existential questions and their connections to the evolution of our understanding of geometry.

In the mid-1980s, my family and I moved to England, where I further studied and worked with Dr. Critchlow and pursued a PhD in village planning. I attended the Architectural Association Graduate School in the center of London. My doctoral work shifted from single buildings to an interest in communities, with a focus on the relationship between energy and village form. I worked with the village of Titchfield

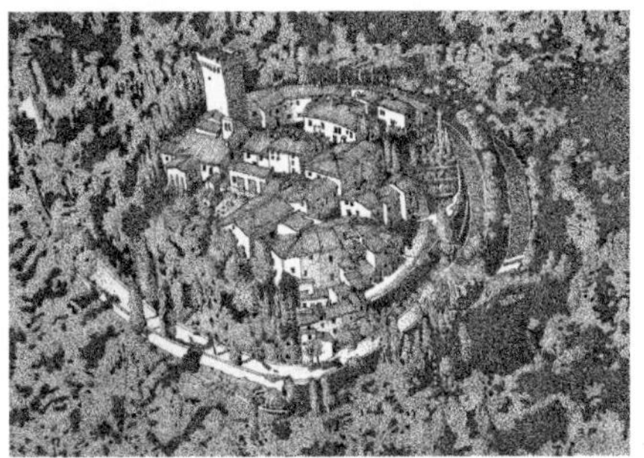

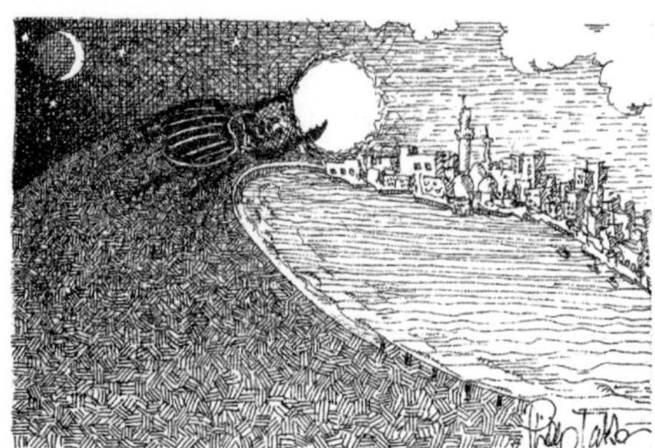

0.6
Freehand Drawings: (a) Aerial View of Castello di Gargonza, Italy; (b) the Scarab and Alexandria, Egypt

for over a year, gathering data, taking photographs, and performing research analysis (see Figure 0.5a). On weekends, my family and I traveled to sacred sites including Glastonbury Tor; the stone circles of Avebury, Stonehenge, and Carnac; the cathedrals of Westminster, Notre Dame in Paris, and Chartres; the Parthenon in Athens; the Pantheon in Rome; and the chapel in Ronchamp, France. My doctorate led to conference presentations and keynote presentations in places such as Cambridge, London, Istanbul, Alexandria, Cairo, Seoul, Tokyo, Rome, Milan, Traini, and Venice.

Far from my isolated youth in Washington and Idaho, I was finally experiencing the broader world. From 2005 to 2013, I was fortunate to participate in a faculty-led study abroad program in Tuscany, Italy through, my teaching career at Texas A&M University. Every other fall semester I lived in Castiglion Fiorentino and traveled extensively while there. One of my favorite adventures was flying and photographing with the director of our program, Paolo Barucchieri, over the Tuscany landscape in a small Cessna (Figure 0.5b). As it has for many architects before me, Italy left a lasting impression that informs my work even today.

In high school, geometry, biology, and art were my best subjects, and so it is fitting that I became an architect with an interest in biophilia and sacred geometry. As a high school student, I attended a summer art program at the University of Kansas and further honed my drawing skills. Further, as an architecture student, I took many drawing and painting courses. When I entered the discipline of architecture, drawing was considered a necessary requirement. What I did not know was the magic that came along with it. Later, throughout the 2000s and largely inspired by travel throughout Europe, I began drawing again. The work was primarily a combination of pen-and-ink drawings of architectural and urban scenes in Greece, Italy, Egypt, and Turkey and re-creations of myths, including Plato's allegory of the cave, Prometheus stealing fire from the sun, Pegasus creating a healing spring, and the labors of Hercules. The four sacred beasts of ancient China are the *green dragon* (east), *red phoenix* (south), *white tiger* (west), and *black tortoise* (north) and are said to have aided in the creation of the world in Feng Shui. Figure 0.6 is a drawing of Castello di Gargonza, drawn from one of my photographs taken from a Cessna airplane, and a view of the scarab beetle pushing the sun across the sky over Alexandria, Egypt. My mythic landscapes were a drawing process, where the mythic realms coexisted with the natural or human-made elements of the places in which I was drawing.

As wonderful as these places were, they seemed to be missing something that lingered from my youth, which later I was able to realize in my work in the 2000s at Serenbe Community and my solar home outside of Atlanta, Georgia. Serenbe is located in the heart of Chattahoochee Hill Country, which lies near the end of the Blue Ridge Mountain range. Most of the surrounding land encircling Atlanta has been developed, except for a southwestern strip that includes most of South Fulton County. Serenbe is planned for 3,500 residents on 2,000 acres of land. While Serenbe shares some of the tenets of the New Urbanism, it stands apart from this movement in some important ways as it has created its own unique qualities and brand of authenticity. Serenbe reflects my doctoral work in England. It is in harmony with the land, is farm-to-table, is sustainable and authentic, supports active living, attracts a diverse population, and creates a permanent, vital, and alive sense of community. I began design work in Serenbe in 2001 and continue today. Pictured in Figure 0.7a is one of several neighborhoods, Mado, that comprise Serenbe Community.

I retired from teaching in 2017 and moved to Georgia. My home is in the center of Serenbe in a small cluster of 24 homes called "The Crossroads." My home is a modest size of 1,650 square feet (153 square meters), with three bedrooms, an office studio, living room, dining room, kitchen, and three bathrooms. Most interesting is the vaulted roof with 35 photovoltaic panels, Tesla Powerwall, the large south-facing passive solar glazing and thermal mass, and the walled-in garden (Figure 0.7b). I am surrounded by woods on three sides and with geothermal heating and cooling, where it is extremely quiet and peaceful. Living in this community and in my solar home has renewed my faith that there are better ways to live.

Recalling David Attenborough's reference to the Holocene epoch that is becoming more acutely in decline, human behaviors, lifestyles, and pursuits are in need of change.[5] The Holocene epoch, which started roughly 11,700 years ago, represents change after the fifth mass extinction, and a period of relative stability in which biodiversity has flourished, climate has been predictable, and the human race emerged as the dominant species on the planet. According to the United Nations, the world population in 2050 is projected to be 9.7 billion people.[6] If we continue to function as we have, we will exact heavy tolls on critical planetary resources, food supplies, species extinction, carbon sequestering, and climate behavior, affecting biodiversity, pollution levels, poverty, migrations, and planetary health.[7] Further, religious differences, racism, natural disasters, human conflicts, military build-ups, and continual war threaten our very existence. The concept of spiritual wellness is designed to recall and elicit biospheric values and the beneficial qualities of interconnectedness, planetary stewardship, and resilience of restorative environments. Further, it helps to serve in informing a survival advantage by ensuring wellness for future generations. A problem is that few planners and architects are aggressively addressing the necessary changes. According to Sarah Ichioka and Michael Pawyln, "with the exception of a few small practices, it is our understanding that even the most environmentally progressive architecture and engineering companies are designing, at best, a small minority of their projects that respect planetary limits."[8] Further, both *greenwashing*, the deceptive marketing of a product or practice as

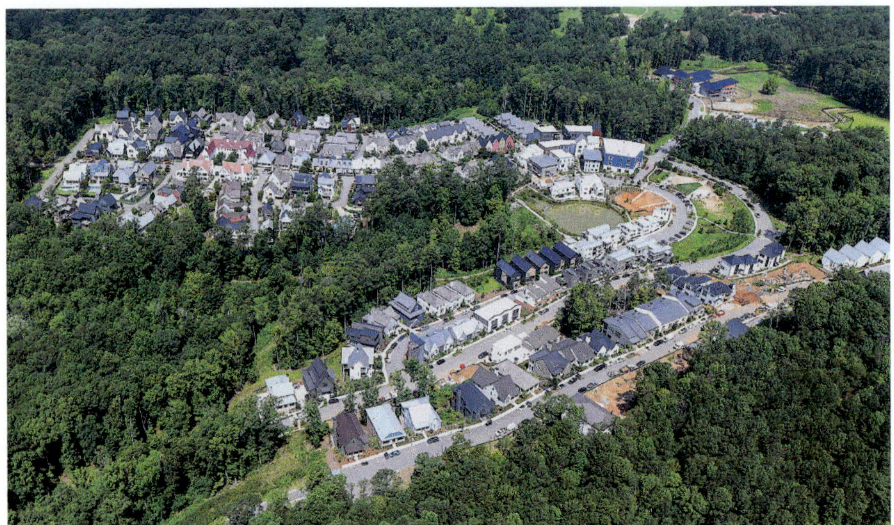

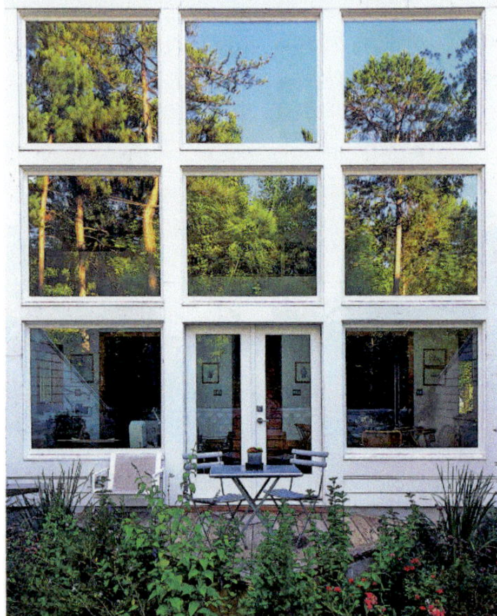

0.7 Design Work: (a) Serenbe Community, Georgia; (b) My Solar Residence, Serenbe, Georgia

environmentally friendly, and *well-washing*, the superficial promotion of user well-being without evidence and substantive action, erode trust and hinder genuine progress toward sustainability, wellness, and spiritually oriented environments.

Other challenges to our survival exist. Nine countries possess nuclear weapons worldwide. Currently, the worldwide number of nuclear warheads is 12,121.[9] It appears that stabilizing "global peace" is a function of "global weapons buildup." This escalation creates uncertainty and risks potential disasters causing death and destruction, and displacement and long-term harm for those who happen to escape.[10] Is this really the best path forward? We seem focused on symptoms and are increasingly inept at addressing the problems and finding effective solutions.

This brings me back to climate change and nuclear energy, both of which pose serious threats. Do we choose death and destruction, or do we choose life and flourishing vitality? The spiritual dimension of wellness needs to be an acceptable universalizing catalyst. Something everyone buys into. This awakening is not necessarily religious, but rather secular spirituality focused on principles, values, ethics, the numinous, and moral and civic responsibilities. And, importantly, it moves us to action. Its wellness outcomes are to be applied to all scales of the planet, primarily directed to the built environment. Otherwise, I am afraid we may be too late and accelerating into the sixth mass extinction. What is the strategy and survival advantage to help us avoid extinction?

As for my personal purpose in life, I see it as an evolving process accumulating certain key insights. These insights include the health effects and energy conservation of solar energy, regenerative design, biophilia and nature, and the role of sacred geometry. They also include a balance between rural and urban environments, a focus on societal critical life-support functions, and the making of the necessary physical and cultural changes in the ways in which we behave and live. So, what would this look like? The images in Figure 0.8 may depict the harbinger of things to come – nuclear destruction or a world like the Amazon biome. It is our choice to make changes as we move to the decades ahead.

This work on spiritual wellness as explicated in this book is an outgrowth of my previous book, co-authored with Lahra Tatriele, *Wellness Architecture and Urban Design*.[11] Where that book broadened the focused to the seven pillars of wellness, this book focuses on only the spiritual wellness pillar. The following chapters present concepts of wellness as informed by universal spiritual values and qualities that are intended to generate both wellness benefits and concrete approaches to reinvigorating the built environment. They include definitions of wellness and spiritualty and explanations of the wellness pillars, with a focus on the spiritual wellness pillar. They detail the characteristics and benefits, the spatial and built environmental implications of spiritual wellness, and the scalar applications from personal moments to cities. Finally, several narrative vignettes give descriptive examples and first-person experiences with several attribute clusters of the spiritual dimensions of wellness. Part of the book is informed by previous research and scholarly work on both spirituality and wellness, and part is based upon my subjective experiences. Many of the examples cited in this book are based upon qualitative research focused on understanding the experiences, perspectives, and meanings that people attribute to the built environment. The multidimensional set of pursuits, activities, choices and, lifestyles are intended to provide pathways to a greater state of holistic well-being.

> It [a city] is the place where a small boy as he walks through it, may see something that will tell him what to do his whole life.[12]

Phillip James Tabb
Chattahoochee Hills, Georgia

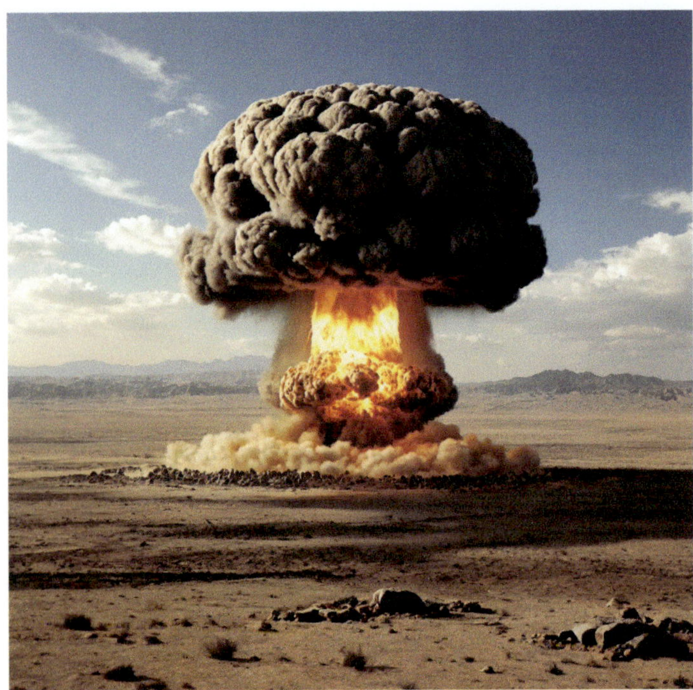

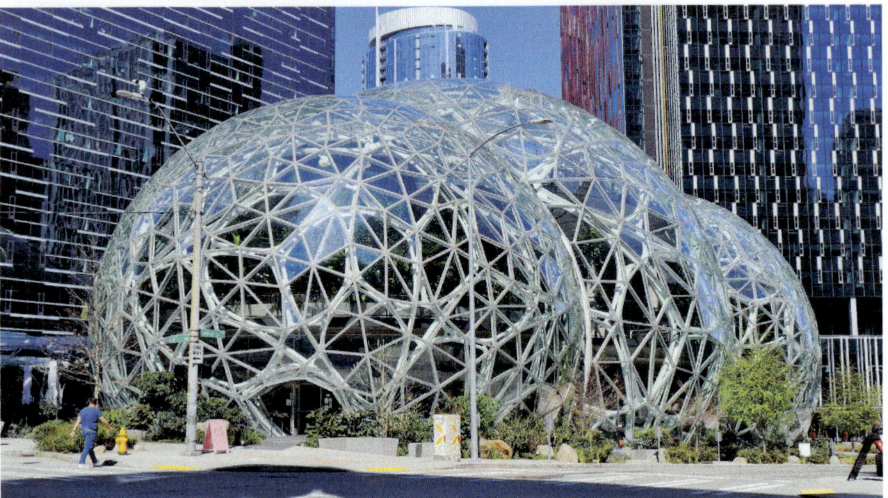

0.8
Two Future Choices: (a) Devastating Nuclear Future or (b) Flourishing Spiritual Wellness

NOTES

1 National Park Service, About Hanford (accessed June 20, 2024), https://www.nps.gov/mapr/about-hanford.htm.
2 Toshi Gomang Stupa (accessed August 20, 2024), https://karmapastupa.org/tashi-gomang-stupa/.
3 Toshi Gomang Stupa (accessed August 20, 2024), https://karmapastupa.org/tashi-gomang-stupa/.
4 This myth was passed on to me by Hanne Strong, who is president of the Manitou Foundation and who, through land grants, has given land in the Crestone, Colorado, area to various spiritual organizations, including the location of the Tashi Gomang Stupa.

5 Attenborough, David, *A Life on Our Planet: My Witness Statement and a Vision for the Future* (New York, NY: Grand Central Publishing, 2020).
6 United Nations, 9.7 Billion on Earth by 2050, but Growth Rate Slowing, Says New UN Population Report (accessed June 20, 2024), https://www.un.org/en/academic-impact/97-billion-earth-2050-growth-rate-slowing-says-new-un-population-report.
7 The Facts (accessed June 20, 2024), https://populationmatters.org/lp-the-facts/?msclkid=a99d444c245614c41e1b223f4db6bbf2&utm_source=bing&utm_medium=cpc&utm_campaign=Population%20Facts&utm_term=facts%20about%20population&utm_content=Population%20Figures%20-%20Exact.
8 Ichioka, Sarah, & Michael Pawlyn, *Flourish: Design Paradigms for Our Planetary Emergency* (Axminster, UK: Triarchy Press, 2021), p. 4.
9 Kristensen, Hans, Matt Korda, Eliana Johns, Mackenzie Knight, & Kate Kohn, Status of World Nuclear Forces (accessed October 12, 2024), https://fas.org/initiative/status-world-nuclear-forces/.
10 Humanitarian Impacts and Risks of Use of Nuclear Weapons (accessed June 20, 2024), https://www.icrc.org/en/document/humanitarian-impacts-and-risks-use-nuclear-weapons#:~:text=A%20nuclear%20weapon%20detonation%20in%20or%20near%20a,the%20environment%2C%20infrastructure%2C%20socioeconomic%20development%20and%20social%20order.
11 Tabb, Phillip & Lahra Tatriele, *Wellness Architecture and Urban Design* (New York, NY: Routledge, 2025).
12 Lobell, Robert, *Between Silence and Light: Spirit in the Architecture of Louis I. Kahn* (Boulder, CO: Shambhala, 1979), p. 44.

Acknowledgements

Thanks goes to Kathryn Schell, Sarah Rae, Senior Editors, and to Selena Hostetler, Editorial Assistant, at Routledge, part of the Taylor & Francis Group, for their guidance and support throughout the completion of this work. They provided great encouragement, enthusiasm and valuable feedback throughout the process. Thanks goes to Dr. Mona Matthews who engaged in many conversations about wellness design and who edited the entire manuscript. Thanks goes to the Global Wellness Institute for initiating the white paper on *Wellness Architecture and Design Pathways*. It was this research effort on my previous book on wellness architecture and design that offered the impetus to further this book into the spiritual realms of wellness. Special thanks to Jennifer Walsh for her foreword and support of my work in the fields of heath, wellness, biophilia and spirituality.

Very special thanks go to my family, especially to my sons Michael and David, and to Shea, Kristin Tabb, to my grandsons Emrys, Caius, James and Jack Tabb, my sister Janice, brother-in-law Richard Nourse, niece Jing Nicholson, and to all my friends. Thanks goes to my Serenbe Community neighbors and colleagues at Texas A&M University who also have supported me in in my scholarly work over the years.

I suppose the book was in part written to all of us now living in the hope the world will evolve so that future generations may enjoy and benefits from fresh, invigorating and more direct experiences of nature and the magic of the sacred world of the architecture and the unknown. I am thankful for all the opportunities to travel abroad as it has given me a greater understanding of the world. The hope is that our planet truly becomes a home.

And very special thoughts go to the memory of my parents, Frank and Tryphosa Tabb, who I am sure would be proud of this book.

1 SPIRITUAL WELLNESS DEFINITIONS AND OVERVIEW

INTRODUCTION

What does it mean to be well? What does it mean to be spiritually well? Health, wellness, and spiritually relevant issues of person and place can indeed give benefits or an advantage that, in part, advances our very survival. Having high levels of wellness with a spiritual focus can enable us to overcome difficulties and flourish, help us to self-actualize, be happy, live longer, and experience life satisfaction. This book does not focus on healthcare architecture or religious buildings per se, but rather it presents preventative principles and premeditated spiritual design concepts aimed at a larger audience of city and building dwellers, visitors, and users of all building types. Hopefully, the principles and design concepts influence wellness in everyday life activities.

In what ways can planning and design solutions contribute to human and environmental health and wellness? Health and wellness benefit both human beings and the environments they inhabit, including natural and built places. Human-centered benefits are directed to the dimensions of wellness that influence our physical bodies, mental health, emotional well-being, social connections, and spiritual growth. Financial health is also seen as a wellness benefit. The environmental-centered benefits are directed to the natural environment around us and the cities and buildings we occupy, as seen in air pollution. The contrast between these two environmental conditions is moving – one is polluted, and the other is endowed with clean air.

Wellness is an everyday process and is inextricably linked to the places where we exist.[1] It is a self-stewardship process with mutually interdependent dimensions focusing on physical, intellectual, emotional, social, financial, environmental, and spiritual dimensions.[2] The places in which we live, work, shop, recreate, dine, and worship and which we otherwise occupy are the contexts within which we interact and function, and, if these places are healthy places, there is a greater chance of achieving wellness. Lifestyles are based on tangible and intangible factors of individuals and groups, and their actions, living behaviors, conditions, habits, and style of living reflect values, attitudes, cultures, and worldviews. For them to become wellness lifestyles means a balanced, holistic, and purposeful choice. The spiritual dimension of wellness offers many tangible and intangible benefits. Spirituality is not a single path or belief system. There are many ways to experience spirituality, and the benefits leading toward well-being are plentiful. To that end, spiritual

DOI: 10.4324/9781003546085-1

wellness is a set of principles, values, beliefs, and morals, with well-being at the center of spiritual practices, behaviors, and lifestyles. The physical environment can positively impact these spiritual wellness qualities.

HEALTH AND WELLNESS

Although health and wellness have been terms used interchangeably, they have different meanings. Health has been referred to as freedom from disease, pain, or defect, with normal physical and mental functions. Health is also considered as a state allowing for coping with all the demands of everyday life. Finally, health is a state of balance within the social and physical environments.[3] The term *haelan* derives from Old English, meaning to make whole, sound, or well.[4] It is a baseline state of well-being. The World Health Organization defines health as "a state of complete physical, mental, and social well-being and not merely the absence of disease."[5] Well-being, as defined by the Stanford Prevention Research Center (SPRC), is "a holistic synthesis of a person's biological, psychological, and spiritual experiences, resulting from interplay between individuals and their social, economic, and physical environments that promotes living a fulfilling life." The SPRC's global longitudinal study, Stanford WELL for Life (WELL), uses new methods to understand, measure, and promote multiple dimensions of well-being across countries and cultures. The study's objective is to understand what it means to be well and how we can increase our well-being, shifting the lens of chronic disease prevention to focus on understanding and enhancing well-being. The built environment in which we live our daily lives can positively impact our well-being.[6]

Wellness is a comprehensive concept encompassing overall well-being. The term *welnes* is derived from the Old English *wel*, meaning abundantly or in good fortune, and *nes*, a word-forming element denoting action. Taken together, wellness suggested behaviors that result in happiness, self-actualization, and optimal health. Wellness was considered the opposite of illness. More recently, Kenneth Cooper further advanced the term with the concept of wellness as a lifestyle.[7] This suggests that human interactions occur in both space and duration of time that frame a wellness experience. Wellness is a process. This includes processes such as holistic living, self-healing, preventative care, and active wellness practices. What we eat, how we move, with whom we interact, and our interactions with nature are contributing factors to wellness. The National Wellness Institute defines wellness as an active process through which we become more aware of, and make choices toward, a more successful existence.[8] The buildings and communities within which we live can also contribute to wellness. Health is considered the goal of well-being, while wellness is the overall journey to that well-being.

When people focus proactively on prevention and improving their vitality, they adopt attitudes and lifestyles that prevent disease, improve health, and enhance their quality of life, sense of happiness and well-being. According to the Berkeley Well-Being Institute, wellness is proactive, preventative, and driven by self-responsibility.[9] The growth of wellness is the extension of this consumer value and worldview. The Global Wellness Institute defines wellness as "the active pursuit

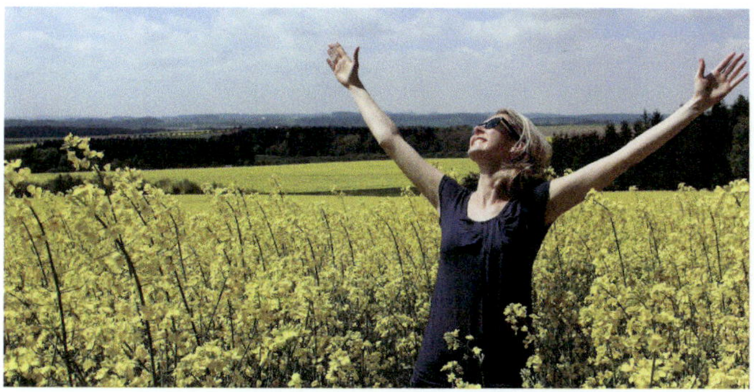
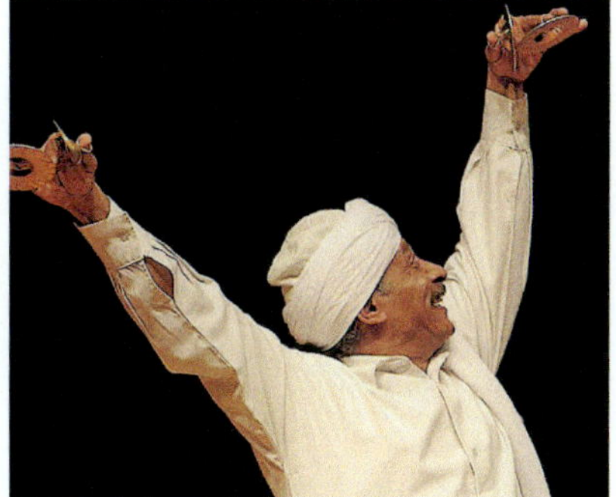

1.1
High-Level Wellness: (a) Spiritual Connections, (b) Wellness Connections

of activities, choices and lifestyles that lead to a state of holistic health."[10] It is an active process of being aware and making choices that lead toward optimal health and well-being outcomes. Closely associated with holistic health, wellness is integrative and multidimensional and includes physical, mental, emotional, social, financial, environmental, and spiritual dimensions. Although considered an individual, proactive pursuit, wellness is influenced significantly by the physical, social, and cultural environments in which we live, including our built environments. Prioritizing wellness as a central concept in the planning and design process can play a significant role in ensuring built environments not only sustain people living in cities, villages, and rural regions but also regenerate and revitalize built areas. This would leave both people and the environment around them better off than before and on a trajectory toward recovery, revival, and flourishment. Following are summary definitions of health and wellness:

- Health refers to the *state* of complete physical, mental, and emotional diseases, and not merely the absence of illness or infirmity. Health includes diagnosis and predisposition of disease and any unexpected injury.
- Wellness refers to a more holistic *process* of balanced, enhanced, and preventative well-being and is more inclusive, adding social, spiritual, financial, and environmental wellness to an active self-directed process and change of lifestyle.

The Garden of Eden is a biblical terrestrial paradise and creation narrative depicted in the Book of Genesis.[11] Its location is reportedly the Hurran Plain in Turkey, and it is ostensibly the home of Abraham.[12] It is described as a fertile crescent and the source of four tributaries. There are three sub-narratives that explain the quality of this paradise, the temptation, and eventual expulsion from the garden. The literal meaning of the word "paradise" is *walled enclosure*. What does this narrative have to do with health and wellness? It suggests an ideal and symbolic connection to wellness, and spiritual wellness in particular. It represents original wholeness, perfect harmony, the natural world as a source of well-being, and the memory of something incredibly valuable lost. So, in some ways, it symbolizes the goal for high-level wellness and happiness as an ideal paradise. In more secular visions, it is the whole Earth as the symbol that possesses the possibility to be a living paradise.

The Eden Project is located in Cornwall, UK, and was designed by Nicholas Grimshaw and completed in 2000. It features two large biomes that cluster with smaller domes. The biomes are enclosed by hexagonal and pentagonal plastic cells that can be inflated or deflated to adjust the insulation levels in response to fluctuating outside temperatures. The biomes enclose multiple complexes covering

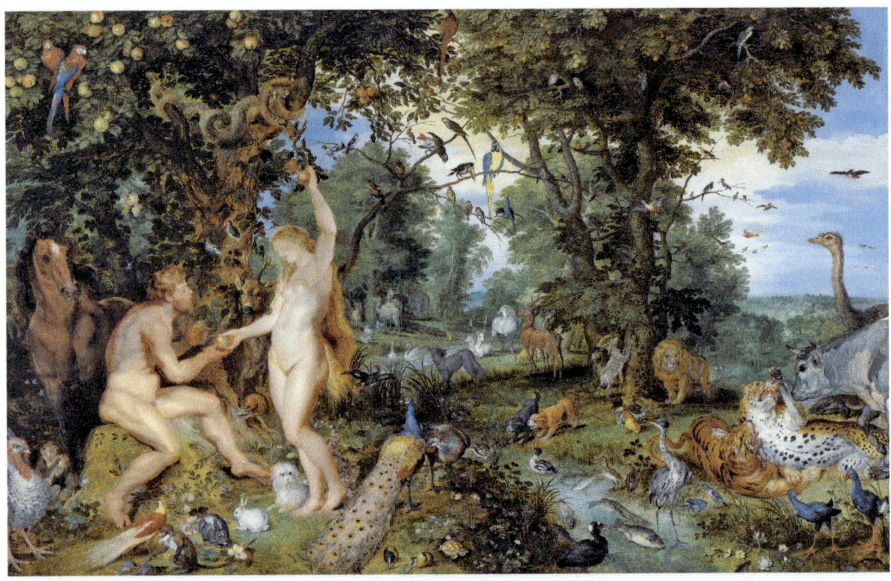

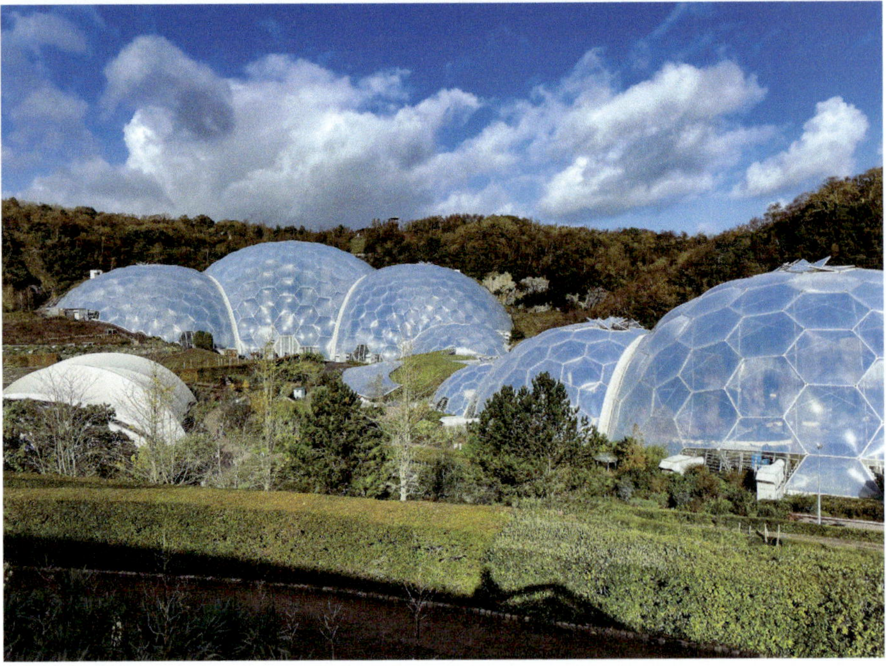

1.2
Two Gardens of Eden: (a) *The Garden of Eden with the Fall of Man* by Jan Brueghel the Elder and Peter Paul Rubens, (b) the Eden Project, Cornwall, United Kingdom

more than 3.9 acres (1.56 hectares) of land and housing over one hundred thousand plants. The tectonic form language is biomorphic and encloses the world's largest manmade rainforest. The biophilic features include access to nature, water, plants, the earth, sensory connections, refuge, living color, natural light, and numinous experiences. The tropical biome was the world's largest enclosed greenhouse, covering more than four acres of land, with over one hundred thousand plants representing five thousand species from many of the climate zones of the world. Refer to Figure 1.2b, which shows the biomes set into the Cornish landscape.

The Garden of Eden narrative and the Eden Project are important in that they suggest an ideal wellness environment from which we evolved and which we lost, and a contemporary Eden Garden functioning as a reminder of the preciousness and beauty of our terrestrial world and the potential, possibility, and harbinger for our future should we agree to move in this direction. The painting by Jan Brueghel the Elder and Peter Paul Rubens is a depiction of the Garden of Eden with the Fall of Man and shows the abundance of the world and the temptation (Figure 1.2a). The challenge, of course, is how to balance the overall population, population growth, and population equilibrium. Also important are the carrying capacities of Earth's valuable natural resources, biodiversity and sustainability, vital human existence, and the vision to create appropriate behaviors and lifestyles that ensure planetary survival and a slowing down of climate change. While the Garden of Eden is based on a religious vision, the Eden Project is the realization of a contemporary secular sacred place, with the intention that, perhaps, the present generations can begin to create a sustainable, balanced, and renewed hope for the future.

SPIRITUALITY

Scholars generally agree that spirituality and religion represent highly overlapping constructs which refer to human beings' relationship to the transcendent, sacred, and ultimate dimensions of existence.[13] Religion refers more to the beliefs, sacred language and rituals, holy texts, traditions, and institutions which are inextricably contextualized by culture.[14] Religious and spiritual experiences, like numinous and awe experiences, comprise two major experiential qualities, those that are ineffable (indescribable) and those that are noetic (possessing hidden or unexplainable knowledge). While the differences between them are sometimes difficult to discern, mystical episodes often accompany these experiences. Spiritual connections to awe experiences include the feeling of being at one with others, the local place, and the larger world; purpose revealing; and containing an element of transcendence and a sense of wonder. And spiritual connections to serenity include feelings of calm and inner peace and slowing of the perception of time. Ways in which religiosity, spirituality, and secularism are differentiated, although blurry, include the following:

1. **Religious experiences** – are devout, more formal, structured, doctrinal, rule-based and community-oriented, have an exclusive worldview, and are about the relationship with and worship and service of a supernatural deity (God, Christ, Allah, Buddha, Moses, Krishna, etc.); at its core, religion is a faith practice. It is

practice founded on belief, faith, and religious apprehension forming an unconditional trust.

2. **Spirituality experiences** – are a life stance of spirituality that does not regard organized religion as the sole or most valuable means of furthering spiritual growth; it is more concerned with inner understandings, purpose in life, and extra-theistic and mystical content, with direct experiences and a universal sense of the "Other" (unknown, sublime, or ineffable) as possessing a greater power or supernatural presence.
3. **Secular spirituality experiences** – are the adherence to spiritual philosophies without adherence to a religion or otherworldly constructs; they are more generalized and cross-cultural, with contemplative practices and a focus on sense of peace, inner life, reflection, interconnectedness, connections to the numinous (the experience itself) and material worlds, and well-being.

According to Gallup, in the United States, approximately 47 percent identify as religious, 33 percent as spiritual, and 18 percent as religiously unaffiliated or neither religious nor spiritual.[15] Worldwide, approximately 84 percent of the population identifies as religious and 16 percent as "*nones*" or non-religious, atheist, agnostic, and spiritual.[16] The term religion comes from the Latin *religionem*, meaning respect for what is sacred. Religion is connecting through an outer experience or source.[17] It focuses on devotion, salvation, self-sacrifice, and an eternal divinity. From a wellness point of view, religion provides a framework for understanding the world and one's place in it, offers social or community support, and provides comfort and hope during difficult times or situations. Even though the world's population favors religion over being spiritually affiliated, this book will focus on a broader use of the term spirituality. The unaffiliated share similar relationships to wellness, especially with respect to the wellness pillars (physical, mental, emotional, social, financial, environmental, and spiritual health). Where religious beliefs tend to be structured, institutionalized, and focused on a higher power, spirituality is more personal, experiential, and inclusive. Secular spirituality is human, nature-centered, and non-religious. According Robert C. Solomon, spirituality is coextensive with religion, and it is not incompatible with or opposed to science or the scientific outlook.[18] Christopher Hitchens, although an atheist, saw the numinous as being valuable while transcendent and not supernatural. The numinous was an appreciation for the amazing insights and workings of the non-material (music, love, landscape) and the natural order as well as an appreciation for the greater aspects of the human experience.[19] Spiritual wellness, then, is a kind of universal spirituality that responds to each of these pillars of wellness in varying degrees and ways. In common, they each seek meaning, purpose, and connections beyond the material world.

The term spirituality derives from the Old French *spirtuel* or *esperituel*, concerning spirit and immateriality, and the Latin *spiritualis*, meaning breath. Spirituality can be understood as a more general, unstructured, and naturally occurring phenomenon, where a person seeks closeness and/or connectedness to a higher power or purpose.[20] This higher power connects through one's own personal experience. Spiritual wellness can connect us to cosmic narratives, original causes (creation myths), spirit of place, source experiences, awe and serene emotions, and purpose in life. Further, it can address existential questions, relieve angst, and effect an experience of a divine presence. Spiritual renewal can occur in a variety of contexts with differing functions or purposes. Exposure to restorative beautiful places can contribute to spiritual renewal. Sometimes referred to as "*thin places*," they can elicit both awe and serene emotions, leading to positive benefits. Serene elicitors develop an inner haven, acceptance, belonging, trust, perspective, contentment, centeredness, and beneficence.[21] Awe elicitors are generally vast triggers within thin places that derive from sources that vary greatly, sparking differing physical, emotional, cognitive, and spiritual responses. These two emotional states create both similar and contrasting wellness benefits.

Spiritual experiences change from secular or profane experiences and places to transcendent ones. Secular space is ordinary space that we experience every day, and this includes unremarkable places. Sacred spaces possess characteristics contributing to charged experiences that include enhanced perception, where the senses are heightened, and where there is a sense of synchronicity and an extrasensory awareness. A spiritual experience goes beyond the ordinary and can be mystical or euphoric, where there is an awareness of the presence of intuitive thoughts, a sense of ultimate peace and well-being, and a degree of surrender. Key to this transcendence is the ability to reduce temporal density and to become more present in experiences of the divine. Transcendent experiences provide shifts with the small self, or individual stress reduction, and prosocial shifts, with alignments greater than the self.[22]

The differences in health and wellness can easily be seen in the architecture that reflects them. Healthcare buildings have long been created to attend to people who are ill, suffering from disease, or recovering from accidents. Early history sees the sick being cared for in their homes and later in churches. Florence Nightingale was influential during the Crimean War of 1853–1856, recognizing the need for clean hospital wards. This included providing patients with access to natural light, air, and landscapes, attention to diet, as well as a clean, sanitary environment. An outgrowth of hospital wards was the creation of the "*pavilion configuration*," which later shifted to a platform typology and, finally, to the layering designs of the larger hospitals of today. In the 1980s, evidence-based research and design, although not a new concept, began to influence the hospital environment.[23] Building types that are associated with health-oriented facilities include hospitals, clinics and medical offices, surgery centers, birthing centers, blood banks, hospices, nursing homes, urgent care facilities, and rehabilitation centers. The images in Figure 1.3 show Florence Nightingale's hospital ward she pioneered during the Crimean War, an interior view of the Maggie's Center in Glasgow, designed by OMA, and the Takaragawa Onsen Osenkaku Hot Springs, in Japan. Each of these demonstrates sensitive healing and wellness qualities and a focus on human experience.

According to a 2021 Forbes article, over 80 percent of people worldwide identify as spiritual or religious, and a 2023 Pew Research Center survey found that

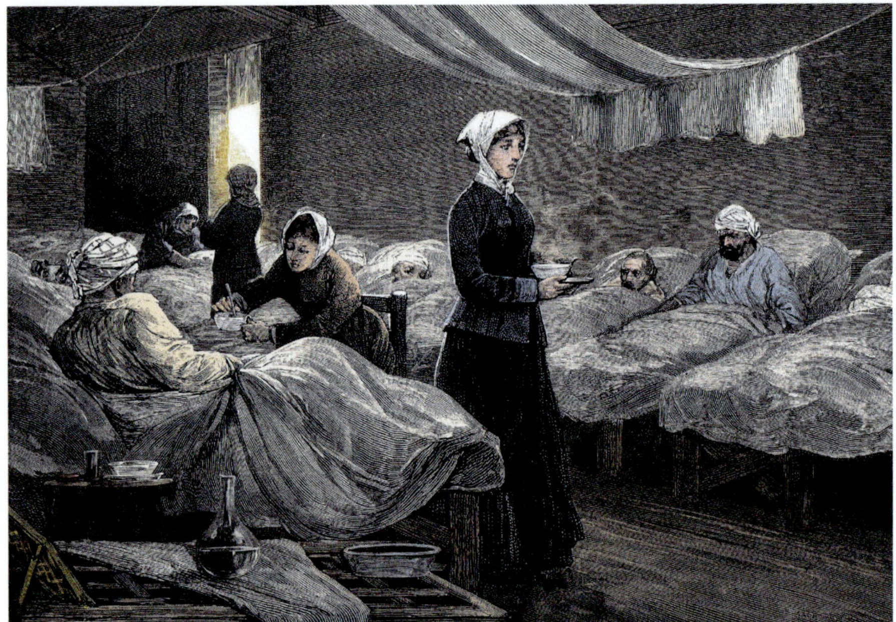

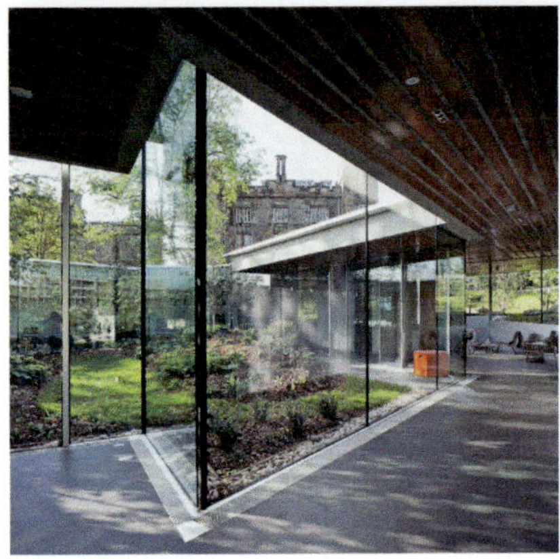

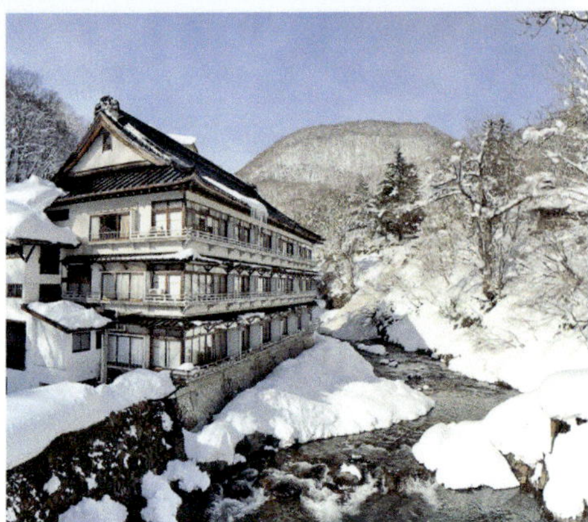

1.3
Wellness Places: (a) Florence Nightingale Hospital Ward, (b) Maggie's Centre, Glasgow, Scotland, (c) Takaragawa Onsen Osenkaku Hot Springs, Japan

70 percent of US adults consider themselves spiritual in some way.[24] There appear to be spiritual values common to various sacred traditions, and it is these sacred traditions that can inform universal spiritual values and spiritual wellness outcomes. Universal dimensions of spirituality seem to share several characteristics that include: an underlying sense of interconnectivity, an energetic experience of unity or oneness, ethical behavior and altruism with care beyond the self, a certain level of mindfulness, and the fabric of relationships as being sacred.[25] The recognized domains of spiritual wellness are connections to self, others, nature (the environment), and the transcendent.[26] Essentially, universal spirituality is a journey of discovery with a shared connection to humanity, nature, and something greater than ourselves. Moreover, it offers a profound connection between our inner worlds and our well-being.

WELLNESS PILLARS

The dimensions or pillars of wellness, developed by Dr. William Hettler in 1976, were originally defined by six approaches constituting a hexagonal model. Hettler's spiritual dimension recognized our search for meaning and purpose in human existence. It included the development of a deep appreciation for the depth and expanse of life and natural forces that exist in the universe.[27] The number of pillars has varied over the years, but they are generally agreed to fall into seven or eight categories. For this work, the seven wellness planning and design benefits are based on the physical, mental, emotional, social, financial, environmental, and spiritual categories.[28] They have been identified through decades of evidence-based health and wellness scholarly and scientific research. A justification for this kind of demarcation is the identification of the varying characteristics of wellness that fit one's present condition and lifestyle. Important is the understanding that all the wellness pillars are interconnected, and together they reinforce one another in contributing to a more inclusive process of well-being. Following are a brief listing and summary of the benefit pillars discussed in further detail in this chapter:[29,30]

1. **Physical wellness** – lower stress and blood pressure, improved respiratory function, increased physical activity and energy, lower obesity levels, weight management, increased healing rates, improved circadian cycles, lower addictions, and improved nutrition.
2. **Mental wellness** – improved cognitive ability and appraisal, increased focus and clarity of mind, increased resilience, reduced anxiety and negative thoughts, awareness of present moment (mindfulness), increased attention restoration and soft fascination, and reduced temporal density.
3. **Emotional wellness** – maintaining healthy relationships, improved mood, lower stress levels, experience of positive emotions (awe, serenity, contentment, wonder, and joy), resilience and positive coping, and experience of inner peace.
4. **Social wellness** – creating community, increased generosity, mutualism, empathy, compassion, helpfulness, enhanced collective concerns, a sense of safety, belonging and security, increased life expectancy, and the experience of prosocial behaviors.
5. **Financial wellness** – increased efficiency and productivity, increased job performance, reduced absenteeism, positive return on investments, increased market distinction and branding, increased facilities owing to economy of scale, and reduced stress over financial matters and security.
6. **Environmental wellness** – lower air pollution and greenhouse gas emissions, cleaner water, greater access to nature, increased biophilic effect, improved biodiversity and regenerative processes, disaster mitigation, and pro-environmental and biospheric behaviors.
7. **Spiritual wellness** – addressing of existential questions, increased self-transcendence, experience of wholeness, positive sense of solving problems, invigorated meaning and purpose in life, spiritual arousal, and increased life satisfaction.

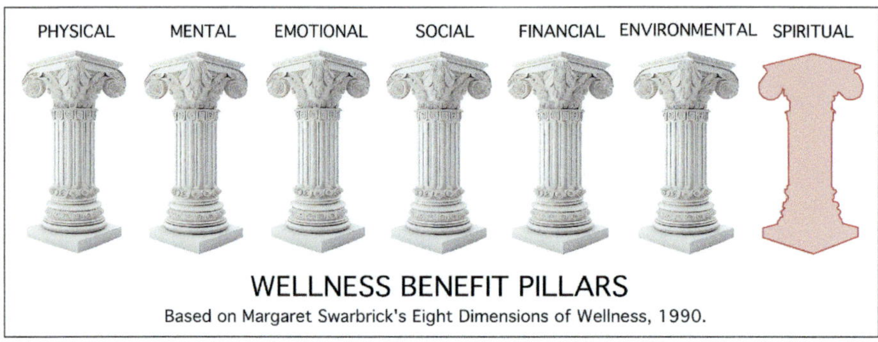

1.4
The Seven Wellness Benefit Pillars

SPIRITUAL WELLNESS PILLAR

Spiritual well-being ultimately represents our connection to ourselves and the greater world around us. It is the ability to experience and integrate meaning and purpose in life through connection with oneself and others, as well as through other contexts such as nature, the arts, religious practices, literature, or something other beyond comprehension.[31] A spiritual experience goes beyond the ordinary and can be mystical or euphoric, where there is an awareness of synchronicity, the presence of intuitive thoughts, a sense of ultimate peace and well-being, and a degree of surrender. Spiritual connections to awe experiences include the feeling of being one with others, immersion within a local place, connecting to the larger world, revealing a life purpose, containing an element of transcendence, and experiencing a sense of wonder. Spiritual connections to serenity include feelings of calm, inner peace, and slowing of the perception of time.

Many are moving away from traditional religious practice but yearn for spiritual connections. Research confirms the link between healthy spiritual connections and mental and emotional health. Spiritual experiences contribute to the reduction of stress and increases in positive mental health, coping strategies, and individual happiness. Religious and spiritual experiences, like numinous and awe emotions, comprise two major experiential qualities, those that are ineffable (indescribable) and those that are noetic (possessing hidden or unexplainable knowledge).[32] Focusing on spirituality in healthcare means caring for the whole person, not just their disease. Spiritual wellness combines with other benefit pillars to produce new insights and perspectives, peace of mind, increased kindness and generosity, more social connections with improved relationships, and greater physical health.

Spiritual dimensions of wellness are about active pursuits, lifestyle choices, and preventative care measures incorporating spiritual experiences leading to processes of holistic well-being. What is important is the frequency (*how often*), duration (*how long*), accessibility (*how easy*), and quality (*how much* or *how intense*) of these wellness experiences.[33] Spiritual well-being ultimately represents our connection to ourselves and the greater world around us. It is the ability to experience and integrate meaning and purpose in life through connection with oneself and others, as well as through other contexts such as nature, the arts, religious practices, literature, or something other beyond comprehension.[34] A spiritual

1.5
Spiritual Pillar Architectural Examples: (a) Ribbon Wedding Chapel, Japan, (b) Brion Cemetery, Italy, (c) New Gourna Village Mosque, Egypt

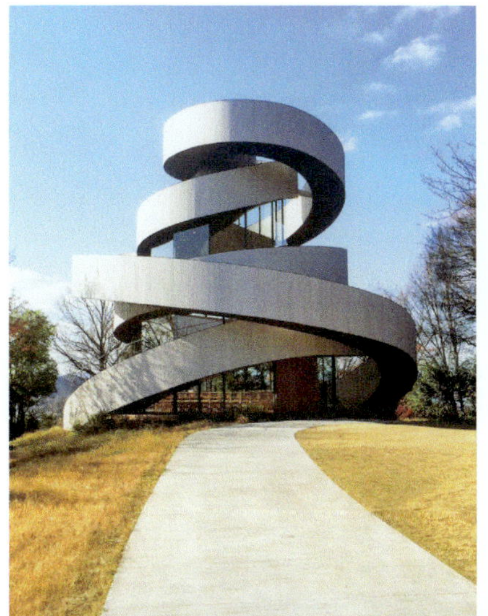

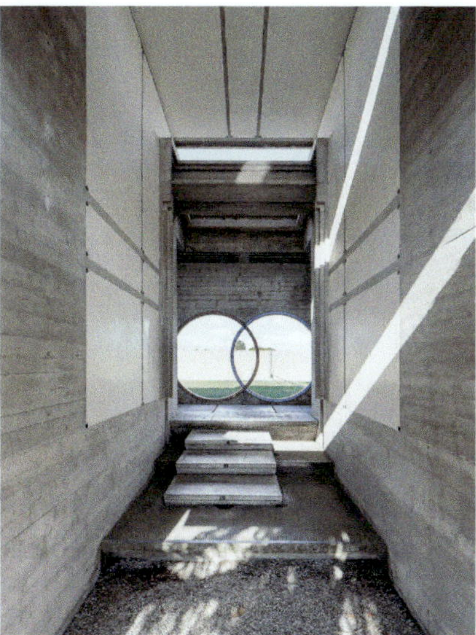

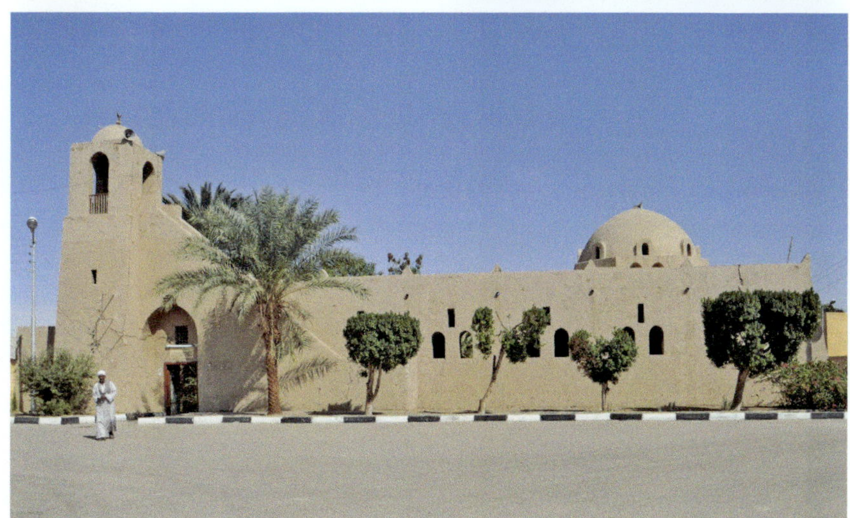

experience goes beyond the ordinary and can be mystical or euphoric, with an awareness of synchronicity, the presence of intuitive thoughts, a sense of ultimate peace and well-being, and a degree of surrender. Spiritual connections to awe experiences include the feeling of being one with others, the local place and the larger world, revealing purpose, containing an element of transcendence, and a sense of wonder. Spiritual connections to serenity include feelings of calm, inner peace, and slowing of the perception of time. Figure 1.5a shows the Ribbon Chapel located in Hiroshima, Japan, which was designed by Hiroshi Nakamura & NAP Architects and built in 2013. The building is an architectural metaphor referred to as the "Ribbon Chapel" because of its dual spiraling staircases embodying the act of marriage. Figure 1.5b shows the vesica passageway in the Brion Family Cemetery in Italy, deigned by Carlo Scarpa and built between 1968 and 1979. And Figure 1.5c is the New Gourna Village Mosque by Hassan Fathy, built in 1945, which illustrates the beautiful sculpted earthen forms, designed with the adobe earth as secular sacredness and a mosque form and geometry as spiritual sacredness. The intentional use of geometry, spatial generosity, natural light, and integrity of materials contribute to the sacred qualities of these places.

THE SPIRITUAL DIMENSION

The spiritual wellness pillar is made of defining dimensions and attribute categories. Spiritual wellness dimensions are three characteristic categories. Attributes are particular qualities of a particular dimension of spiritual wellness and help define and provide actionable direction. The dimensions explored in the next chapter include (1) place-based attributes, (2) experience-based attributes, and (3) process-based attributes. These dimensions of place, experience/behavior, and process capture the range of benefits associated with spiritual wellness, which range from biophilic principles and awe experiences to practicing altruism, patience, and mindfulness.

Design responses to these characteristics involve a variety of strategies. Spiritually oriented wellness strategies are a mutually supporting set of design approaches that serve as prime actionable elicitors. Importantly, these strategies need to be considered interdependently across the various scales of the built environment. The three dimension concepts – place, experience/behavior, and process – are all interconnected and can influence each other. *Places* can shape our *experiences*. For example, visiting a historical landmark or sacred well can be a powerful educational or spiritual experience. *Experiences* can influence our *behavior*. For instance, a positive experience at a "third place" neighborhood café with friends might make you more likely to return. *Behaviors* can be shaped by *processes*. For example, the meditating process can influence our behavior by relaxing us and making us more present. And *processes* can occur within *places*. For example, the process of photosynthesis occurs in plants, and, correspondingly, the process of finding the unity and harmony, numinous, purpose in life, and life satisfaction can influence our process of living in high-level wellness places. The spiritual wellness dimensions and attributes discussed in the following chapters include the following:

1. **Place-based attributes** – locations and settings that represent distinctive, therapeutic, and cherished qualities of a place that elicit experiences and behaviors toward individual and collective goodness, wellness, and spirituality.
2. **Experience-based attributes** – spiritual wellness benefits gained through interactions and engagements through unique, inspiring, and beautiful direct experiences.
3. **Practice and process attributes** – actions and practices including mindfulness, selflessness, benevolence, compassion, and participation, practices that are intentional and inclusive, flourishing with deeper connections and enhanced well-being.

The dimensions of places, experiences, and processes form specific characteristics that solicit desired spiritual wellness outcomes. They elicit connections to ourselves and the greater world around us. They increase awareness of synchronicity and the presence of intuitive thoughts, purpose, and an element of transcendence. They help us address and process existential issues in life. Further, they produce inner peace, a sense of wonder, and a slowing of the perception of time. The attributes are specific characteristics and carriers of spiritual wellness places, experiences, and processes. They are defining qualities and active pursuits, lifestyle choices, and preventative care measures incorporating qualitative experiences and leading to holistic well-being.

SUMMARY

The spiritual dimensions involve guiding beliefs, principles, and values that help give direction in life and, in the context of this work, help in maintaining wellness lifestyles and achieving high-level wellness. They include beneficial experiences, behaviors, life processes, and lifestyle choices. The spiritual process is a connection to one's higher power and/or purpose, through a belief system, set of principles, or other activities that align with one's personal values. The wellness dimensions in part inform spiritual and wellness design approaches to the built environment. Spiritual wellness is inclusive as it incorporates each of the other six pillars. It includes lifestyles full of a self-defined balance of spiritual wellness habits that include good sleep and rest, a healthy diet, productive and active lives, contact and participation with others, and spiritual connections to nature and, in the context of this work, the built environment around us.[35]

Wellness as a concept is relatively new, and its applications to the spiritual pillar of wellness and the design fields are rare, especially at the urban design and planning scales. However, the breadth of concerns around wellness and the history of the wellness movement over the past 50 years is an indication of how important the issue is. Physical designs embodying spiritual wellness strategies are arousing and full of wonder, express awe, are vital and alive, and transcend the ordinary experiences in life. They employ significant numbers and geometry and/or are serene, soulful, authentic, biophilic, and beautiful and are charged with a certain (divine) energy. This underlies the importance of planning and design strategies to support an integrated model for preventable measures for health and wellness, and positive lifestyle choices that are in part defined by this spiritual pillar of wellness. Access to these measures should occur daily in order to realize the greatest potential of their benefits. The built environment does not occur outside of the larger context. The NASA photograph taken from the space station shows the Earth and Sun as a reminder of this larger context (Figure 1.6). The following chapters discuss the various spiritual wellness pillar attributes according to the place-based, experience-based, and process-based dimensions.

The spiritual realm informs (1) our values, which in turn affects (2) our behaviors and lifestyles, which directs (3) planning and design objectives within the built environment, which (4) generates positive wellness benefits, and, finally, (5) which elicits spiritual wellness outcomes. It is important to see this continuum from intentions through outcomes. It is the purpose of the following chapters to address this process, from values, built environment, behaviors and lifestyles, and wellness

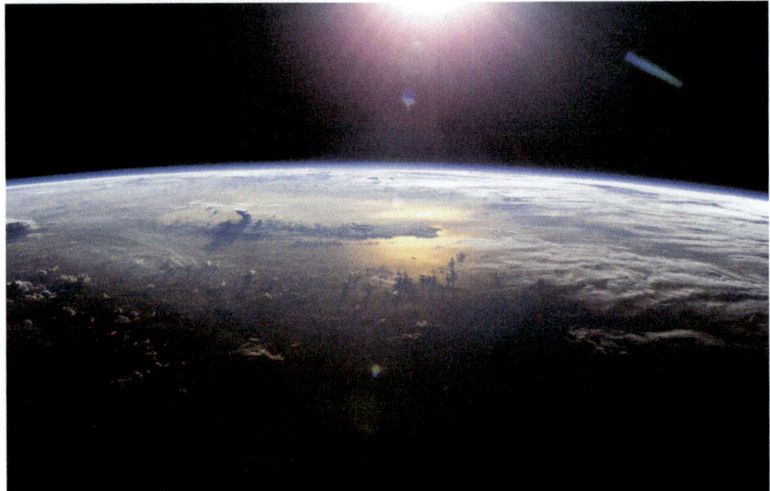

1.6
The Spiritual Dimension of Wellness

benefits to spiritual wellness. First is an investigation of the dimensions of spiritual wellness, then followed by planning and design strategies at varying scales. It is the purpose of the following three chapters to further explain and expand upon the concepts of place-based, experience-based, and process-based spiritual wellness attributes. These dimensions and attributes cultivate spiritual wellness by shaping our behaviors and grounding our actions in meaningful ways, fostering deep personal connections and responsible engagements with life's journey.

NOTES

1 Gesler, Wilber M., *Healing Places* (Lanham, MD: Rowman & Littlefield, 2003).

2 National Library of Medicine, Dimensions of Wellness: Change Your Habits, Change Your Life (accessed August 21, 2024), https://www.ncbi.nlm.nih.gov/pmc/articles/PMC5508938/.

3 Sartorius, Norman, Meaning of Health and Its Promotion (accessed November 20, 2023), https://www.ncbi.nlm.nih.gov/pmc/articles/PMC2080455/.

4 Guidotti Tee L., The Literal Meaning of Health (accessed July 10, 2012) https://www.tandfonline.com/doi/abs/10.1080/19338244.2011.585096?journalCode=vaeh20#:~:text=The%20English%20word%20"health"%20derives,%2DIndo%2DEuropean%20root%20"*.

5 World Health Organization, Health and Well-Being (accessed April 14, 2025), https://www.who.int/data/gho/data/major-themes/health-and-well-being#:~:text=The%20WHO%20constitution%20states%3A%20%22Health,of%20mental%20disorders%20or%20disabilities.

6 Standford WELL for Life (accessed July 21, 2023), https://med.stanford.edu/wellforlife.html.

7 Cooper, Kenneth H., *Overcoming Hypertension: Dr. Kenneth H. Cooper's Preventative Medicine* (New York, NY: Bantam Books, 1990).

8 National Wellness Institute, About Wellness (accessed July 10, 2013), http://www.nationalwellness.org/?page=AboutWellness.

9 Berkeley Well-Being Institute, Definition of Wellness: Meaning, Dimensions, and Examples (accessed July 21, 2023), https://www.berkeleywellbeing.com/wellness-definition.html.

10 Global Wellness Institute, What Is Wellness? (accessed June 1, 2013), https://globalwellnessinstitute.org/what-is-wellness/.
11 The Holy Bible (London, UK: Oxford University Press).
12 Schuster, Ruth, On Harran Plain Where Adam and Eve Fell to Earth, Legend Reigns (accessed July 21, 2024), https://www.haaretz.com/archaeology/2022-05-23/ty-article-magazine/on-harran-plain-where-adam-and-eve-fell-to-earth-legend-reigns/00000180-f6cf-d469-a5b4-f6ff6aec0000.
13 McClintock, Clayton, Elsa Lau, & Lisa Miller, Phenotypic Dimensions of Spirituality: Implications for Mental Health in China, India, and the United States (accessed June 23, 2024), https://www.frontiersin.org/journals/psychology/articles/10.3389/fpsyg.2016.01600/full#:~:text=Analyses%20of%2040%20spirituality%20measures,oneness%20with%20other%20beings%20in.
14 Geertz, Clifford, *The Interpretation of Cultures: Selected Essays*, Vol. 5019 (New York, NY: Basic Books, 1973).
15 Jones, Jeffrey, In U.S. 47% Identify as Religious, 33% as Spiritual (accessed July 5, 2024), https://news.gallup.com/poll/511133/identify-religious-spiritual.aspx#:~:text=Which%20of%20the%20following%20statements,religious%20and%2018%25%20as%20neither.
16 Wasserman, Pam, World Population by Religion: A Global Tapestry of Faith (accessed July 5, 2024), https://populationeducation.org/world-population-by-religion-a-global-tapestry-of-faith/#:~:text=Today%2C%20some%2085%20percent%20of%20people%20around%20the,%2831%25%29%2C%20Islam%20%2824%25%29%2C%20Hinduism%20%2815%25%29%2C%20and%20Buddhism%20%287%25%29.
17 Aletheia, Spirituality vs Religion: 11 Differences (with Pros + CONS LIST) (accessed July 5, 2024), https://lonerwolf.com/spirituality-vs-religion/#h-what-is-spirituality.
18 Soloman, Robert C., Secular Spirituality (accessed March 20, 2025), https://forum.philosophynow.org/viewtopic.php?t=23392
19 Hitchens, Christopher, The HITCH Series: The Numinous (accessed July 23, 2024), https://www.youtube.com/watch?v=PMId7vH_Mik.
20 Joseph, R.P., B.E. Ainsworth, L. Mathis, S.P. Hooker, & C. Keller, Incorporating Religion and Spirituality into the Design of Community-Based Physical Activity Programs for African American Women: A Qualitative Inquiry. *BMC. Res. Notes*, 10(506), 2017. 10.1186/s13104-017-2830-3 [PMC free article] [PubMed] [CrossRef] [Google Scholar].
21 Tabb, Phillip James, *Thin Place Design: Architecture of the Numinous* (New York, NY: Routledge, 2024).
22 Transcendence and Wellbeing (accessed September 24, 2023), https://www.mybestself101.org/transcendence-well-being.
23 Burpee, Heather, History of Healthcare Architecture (accessed August 15, 2023), http://www.mahlum.com/pdf/HistoryofHealthcareArchBurpee.pdf.
24 Google, AI Overview (accessed July 23, 2024), https://www.google.com/search?q=what+percentage+of+the+world+is+spiritual&sca_esv=6dff3b47ea39d1e5&sxsrf=ADLYWIINN1Dc9PGBx0V3EYjC1IZiIESj4g%3A1721747975546&ei=B8qfZonwIJPdwN4P_puBmAY&oq=how+many+people+identify+as+being+spiritual&gs_lp=Egxnd3Mtd2l6LXNlcnAiK2hvdyBtYW55IHBlb3BsZSBpZGVudGlmeSBhcyBiZWluZyBzcGlyaXR1YWwqAggBMgoQABiwAxjWBBhHMgoQABiwAxjWBBhHMgoQABiwAxjWBBhHMgoQABiwAxjWBBhHMgoQABiwAxjWBBhHMgoQABiwAxjWBBhHMgoQABiwAxjWBBhHSI1MUOIEWLAtcAF4AJABAJgBS6ABuAKqAQE1uAEByAEA-AEBmAICoAJGmAMA4gMFEgExIECIBgGQBgeSBwEyoAfoDQ&sclient=gws-wiz-serp.
25 McClintock, Clayton, Elsa Lau, & Lisa Miller, Phenotypic Dimensions of Spirituality: Implications for Mental Health in China, India, and the United States (accessed June 23, 2024), https://www.frontiersin.org/journals/psychology/articles/10.3389/fpsyg.2016.01600/full#:~:text=Analyses%20of%2040%20spirituality%20measures,oneness%20with%20other%20beings%20in.

26 Fisher, John, The Four Domains Model: Connecting Spirituality, Health and Well-Being (accessed September 2, 2024), https://www.mdpi.com/2077-1444/2/1/17.

27 Hettler, William, The Six Dimensions of Wellness Model (accessed July 21, 2024), https://static1.squarespace.com/static/5aced79796e76f98f1bcb075/t/5b64cd0d575d1fb39f6ac159/1533332749875/SixDimensionsFactSheet.pdf.

28 Swarbrick, Margaret, Mapping Mental Health: Dr. Swarbrick & The Eight Wellness Dimensions (accessed August 15, 2023), https://alcoholstudies.rutgers.edu/mapping-mental-health-dr-swarbrick-the-eight-wellness-dimensions/.

29 Moorthy, Kailas, & Valentina Cereda, Wellness Benefits, Chapter 2, Wellness Architecture and Design Pathways, Global Wellness Institute, 2023.

30 Tabb, Phillip James, & Lahra Tatrirle, *Wellness Architecture and Urban Design* (New York, NY: Routledge, 2025).

31 Predojevic, Anja, Spiritual Wellbeing (accessed June 1, 2023), https://www.stress.org.uk/spiritual-wellbeing/#:~:text=Spiritual%20wellbeing%20ultimately%20represents%20our%20connection%20to%20ourselves,art%2C%20literature%2C%20nature%20or%20something%20greater%20than%20oneself.

32 VanderWeele, Tyler, Spirituality Linked with Better Health Outcomes, Patient Care (accessed June 8, 2023), https://www.hsph.harvard.edu/news/press-releases/spirituality-better-health-outcomes-patient-care/.

33 Tabb, Phillip James, *Thin Place Design: Architecture of the Numinous* (New York, NY: Routledge, 2024), p. 193.

34 Predojevic, Anja, Spiritual Wellbeing (accessed June 1, 2023), https://www.stress.org.uk/spiritual-wellbeing/#:~:text=Spiritual%20wellbeing%20ultimately%20represents%20our%20connection%20to%20ourselves,art%2C%20literature%2C%20nature%20or%20something%20greater%20than%20oneself.

35 Swarbrick, Margaret, Wellness in Eight Dimensions (accessed October 2, 2024), https://www.center4healthandsdc.org/uploads/7/1/1/4/71142589/wellness_in_8_dimensions_booklet_with_daily_plan.pdf.

2 PLACE-BASED ATTRIBUTES OF SPIRITUAL WELLNESS

INTRODUCTION

Lifestyles are based on tangible and intangible factors of individuals and groups. Their actions, living behaviors, conditions, habits, and style of living reflect their values, attitudes, cultures, and worldviews. The three attribute dimensions – place-based, experience-based, and process-based – identify concepts that help define and explain the characteristics and qualities of spiritual wellness. The place, experience, and process are each interconnected and can influence each other. *Places* can shape our *experiences*. *Experiences* can influence and be shaped by *processes*. And, circling back, *processes* occur within *places*. This chapter focuses on the place-based attributes as they feature and are specific to a particular location, natural or built. According to Wilbert Gesler, "healing and place are inseparable."[1] Healing, therefore, includes physical, cultural, social, environmental, and energetic qualities. The attributes, in turn, become important determinants for the design of spiritually oriented wellness places.

One of the oldest tenets of geography is the concept of place, with three defining characteristics, namely location, locale, and sense of place. Location is the specific position of a particular point on Earth. Locale is the physical setting that supports relationships between people and spatial settings. And sense of place is the identity, perception, spirit, or emotion attached to a particular place. Places obviously vary from the most mundane and secular places to highly charged or sacred places. A charged place is one that contains an energy or presence, whether it is a natural, social, cultural, historic, symbolic, or physical energy. Experiences of charged places can alter perception, create a loss of self-awareness, and generate feelings of connectedness with physiological sensations. Health and wellness factors are also connected to place and further discussed in this chapter.

Yi-Fu Tuan makes a distinction between space and place, as they co-exist within the world in which we live. "What begins as undifferentiated space becomes place as we get to know it better and endow it with value."[2] Space is abstract, and place is endowed with definition and meaning. In this regard, space is amorphous, intangible, or pragmatic, where place embodies location, diverse meaning, personal involvement, and reflection. According to John Donat, "places occur at all levels of identity, my place, your place, street, community, town, city, regions, country and continent, but places never conform to tidy hierarchies of classification."[3] Yet,

DOI: 10.4324/9781003546085-2

according to Gary Snyder, of all the memberships with which we identify, it is place that has the greatest potential for healing.[4]

According to theologian Belden Lane, there are a set of principles that are phenomenological categories of what he called "mythogenesis."[5] These characteristics of experience or axioms of sacred places pre-exist our encounter with thin places. They underly the way in which these places ignite the imagination and they provide an interesting way to understand the nature of sacred places. The axioms do not represent a human-centric view, but rather a view beyond our control.

The first axiom is that a sacred place is not chosen, it chooses. This suggests a place-centered origin and source. Sacred places are not determined by human-centered perspectives or in deterministic ways but are chosen by the land, *genius loci*, or a higher presence. While design intentions are important, they do not guarantee connections to this higher presence. It is the energy and presence of an otherworldly, unknown, or divine source that seek us out. The second axiom is that these places can be ordinary places, ritually made extraordinary, where ritual acts are performed that set them apart from secular space. This suggests a different state of mind and participatory respect for the places, and that sacred places are abundantly located everywhere. The third axiom is that these places can be trod upon without being entered, where recognition is existentially discerned, meaning that sacred places are related to increased levels of openness and elevated consciousness. The last axiom is that the impulses within these places are both centripetal (local) and centrifugal (universal), and that the sacred nature of the spaces is not confined to a single locale. This axiom allows for serene moments at the intimate scale and cosmic experiences at the larger scale. It also suggests that a divine source both can be expressed locally, such as a beautiful flower or flickering candle, and, according to Lane, can be simultaneously larger and smaller, never confined to a single locale, such as a colorful sunset, rainbow, or starlit night sky. These axioms underlie the place-based dimension of spiritual wellness.

DIMENSIONS OF SPIRITUAL WELLNESS

Dimensions are broad categories of aspects of well-being and benefit outcomes. The spiritual wellness dimension leads to sustainable behaviors and lifestyles, increased stewardship, physical changes to the built environment, and increased care for the natural environment. These behaviors are in part informed by certain attributes, which can produce positive spiritual wellness design strategies. Where dimensions are broad groupings of spiritual wellness experiences, the attributes represent specific characteristics and qualities defining the connections between spirituality and well-being.

Attributes are varied. Some attributes also include specific places that are either extraordinary, beautiful, spiritually charged, or thin, or have healing or restorative qualities. Other attributes are experiences and emotional responses to specific elicitors, such as the unknown, the numinous, and serenity, or the awe emotions from experiences of vastness – threat, beauty, ability, virtue, and supernatural causality.[6] Attributes also derive from daily routines and practices such as forest bathing, meditation, mindfulness, presence, and gratitude. And finally, some attributes derive from processes and standards of behavior or codes of conduct that are ethical, moral, principled, noetic, or altruistic. Each of these dimensions is affected by the environment and the qualities of experience they provide. Dimensions represent concepts, categories, and perspectives and contain specific attributes, qualitative descriptions, and desirable outcomes.

The dimensions or pillars of wellness, developed by Dr. William Hettler in 1976, were defined originally by six approaches constituting a hexagonal model.[7] This wellness model is one of the most widely recognized and applied models, with six interdependent dimensions: physical (the combination of exercise and eating habits), intellectual (emotional intelligence and mental health), emotional (awareness and acceptance of feelings), social (contribution to environment and community), occupational (job satisfaction and productivity), and spiritual (the search for meaning and purpose in life). These dimensions function as distinct, yet interdependent, areas of health and wellness indicators. This work focuses on the spiritual dimension of wellness, which is defined by three attribute categories: place-based, experienced-based, and process-based outcomes. The spiritual wellness dimension does not necessarily involve religious activities as, according to Tony Robbins, it is considered the highest level of life's mastery.[8]

Attributes are defining qualities of experience and can be specific physical characteristics of the spiritual wellness dimension. Since the spiritual dimension of wellness is about active pursuits, lifestyle choices, and preventative care measures incorporating experiences leading to processes of holistic well-being, the attributes represent the places, experiences, and processes by which this is achieved. Furthermore, the attributes are not necessarily singular patterns, but rather they are interdependent qualitative experiences. And finally, an attribute is a quality, property, or set of values or principles regarded as a characteristic or inherent part of the spiritual wellness dimension. The dimension categories and their specific attributes of spiritual wellness are discussed in detail in this and the next two chapters.

PLACE-BASED ATTRIBUTES OF SPIRITUAL WELLNESS

One of the oldest tenets of geography is the concept of place, with several defining characteristics, mainly location, locale, function, and sense of place. Yi-Fu Tuan sees place occurring in widely divergent contexts that are centers of felt value and meaning.[9] This people–place connection includes attributes relating to the spirit of a place or the energetic qualities of a particular locale. It includes the connection to biophilia and the human love of nature and affiliation with natural processes. It includes the attraction to thin places, which are locations or settings where a thin veil or experiential threshold exists between the earthly world in which we live and the heavenly spiritual world and possess an energy that is qualitatively different. Moreover, place-based attributes include third places, locations away from home and work that serve as places for frequent encounters, social interactions, and prosocial behaviors. Other attributes are included within this dimension, including sanctuary places, healing landscapes, religious and spiritual spaces, and ritual or ceremonial places. Finally and importantly, place-based attributes are human interactions with specific cultural and geographic settings, sites, and environments that elicit spiritual wellness benefits.

Spiritual wellness is an ongoing process of self-discovery and active participation shaping the deepest part of us, including our beliefs, values, feelings, behaviors, and lifestyle practices. The spiritual realm possesses its own characteristics contributing to charged experiences that include enhanced perception, where the senses are heightened or enlarged, and there can be an extrasensory awareness. The wellness benefits in part are achieved through design as the dimensions inform the design opportunities in the built environment. Many of the attributes have a more direct impact upon design opportunities in the built environment, whereas others have secondary effects on attitudes, convictions, and sensibilities thereby influencing the placed-based dimensions including *spirit of place*, *biophilia*, *third places*, and *thin places*.

The placed-based attributes are essentially places that serve as inherent elicitors by their location, geographic features, purpose, function and use, historic or cultural significance, or spatial quality. As elicitors, they contain an energy or presence, whether it is a natural, social, cultural, historic, symbolic, or physical energy. This energy can be sensed and felt, and some places are more charged than others. This may occur because of the profound historic or cultural meaning tied to the place, the dramatic features of a natural site, or the quality of the architecture. Michael Brill explains that, when immensely charged places are experienced, they trigger very powerful feelings, and that, when other total strangers are in these places, their responses are much the same, creating a sudden and strong bond between them.[10] A summary of spiritual wellness place-based attributes follows:

1. **Spirit of place and original cause** – represent distinctive and cherished qualities of places that sometimes are thought to possess guardians, spirits, or creation myths.
2. **Biophilic places** – have an innate tendency for connections to nature and life processes.
3. **Thin places** – locations where a thin veil exists between the earthly world in which we live and the heavenly spiritual world that is qualitatively different.
4. **Third places** – locations away from home and work that serve as places for frequent encounters and social interactions.
5. **Sanctuary places** – physical locations that provide a sense of peace, security, refuge from the stresses of daily life, and rejuvenation; also refer to passive survival spaces advantageous for survival, offering basic necessities and access to natural resources in emergency situations.
6. **Healing environments** – used to produce medicinal plants and considered therapeutic landscapes serving as places of recovery, restoration, and forest bathing, facilitating spiritual renewal.
7. **Religious spaces** – places that focus on spiritual and wellness practices such as monasteries, ashrams, churches, chapels, temples, cathedrals, mosques, spiritual retreats, cemeteries, and pilgrimage sites.

8. **Ritual and ceremonial spaces** – places that foster active participation, transformative routines, numinous, awe, and serene experiences, meditation practices, forgiveness, and gratitude.

Attribute of Spirit of Place

Spirit of place gives meaning, value, emotion, identity, and mystery to place and, in the context of this chapter, it gives spiritually oriented health and wellness benefits. They are most often found in natural environments, but also can be found in urban places as well. The ancient world viewed certain places as being occupied by gods, spirits, or guardian deities who require propitiation. Often, they embody the presence of animals, special beings, and narrative layers of history. The natural world is most often the source of the spirit of place, either through its energetic qualities or geography. The beauty and energetic qualities of a special place can amplify, vitalize, charge, and inspire spiritual or transcendent experiences. Often, these experiences are characterized by emotional connections, altered perceptions, feelings of connectedness, embodied narratives, ethereal experiences, and an ancient stirring of the archetypal first place.

Spirit of place and sense of place are often interchangeable and have received considerable attention from social scientists in recent years. Research has indicated that a person's sense of place is influenced by several factors, including the built environment, socio-economic status (SES), well-being, and health.[11] Spirit of place is associated with the concept of *genius loci*, known as the protective spirit of place. It is defined by both tangible (physical, natural, and built features) and intangible (mythic, historic, cultural associations) elements. Spiritual benefits include connections to the sacred character of a place, including the unique, distinctive, and cherished qualities. The design implications suggest understanding the specific location, geography, history, and cultural significance and the presence of local features and local cues from the site.

The spirit of place, the unique character and atmosphere of a location, can significantly impact our well-being. Places that evoke feelings of peace and tranquility, such as serene gardens or calming natural settings, can promote relaxation and lower stress hormones. Awe-inspiring environments such as mountains or beaches can uplift your mood and spark feelings of joy and optimism. Locations rich in history or cultural significance can connect you to something larger than yourself and foster a sense of belonging and purpose. Spending time in nature or engaging in spiritual practices in designated spaces can promote mindfulness and self-awareness.

Today, the spirit of place is a concept used by a variety of disciplines, including architecture, urban planning, and environmental psychology. It is seen as an important factor in creating healthy, livable communities. The spirit of place fosters a sense of identity and belonging for those who inhabit or visit it. Modern conceptions of spirit of place delve deeper than simply aesthetics or ambiance. It is a multifaceted concept that acknowledges the interplay between tangible and intangible elements. Preserving cultural heritage and historical sites is seen as a way to safeguard the spirit of place and to recognize that a growing focus on the connection between spirit of place and mental and emotional well-being is possible.

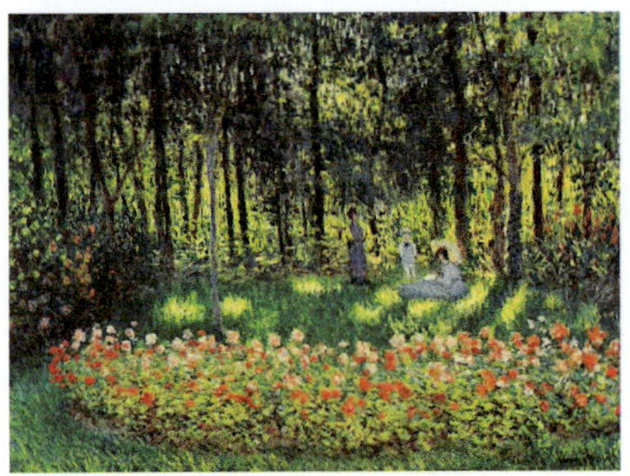
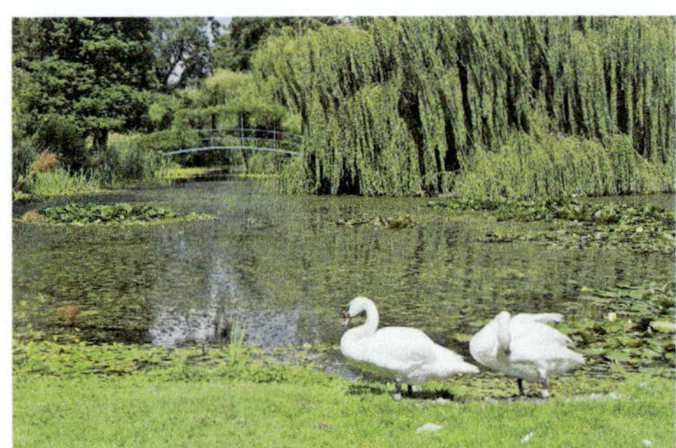

2.1
Spirit of Place: (a) Monet Garden at Highnam Court, United Kingdom, (b) Monet's *Au Jardin*, France

The wellness implications of spirit of place suggest a resonance, a sense of belonging, and evoke positive emotions. The spiritual implications are an unforeseen influence with a profound presence which amplifies sensory experiences and feelings of synchronicity. The paintings and gardens of Claude Monet exemplify the inspiring tranquility of place. In 1890, Monet started renovating his garden, inspired by serene scenes from the Japanese prints he collected. He diverted a stream to form a pond, planted willows and bamboo on the shores, filled the pond with water lilies, then crossed the pond with a wooden footbridge (Figure 2.1a). Inspired by his own garden and painted in 1875, Monet's *Au Jardin* is an intimate space defined by trees, flowers, grass turf, and beams of soft sunlight (Figure 2.1b).

Attribute of Biophilic Places

Biophilia's epistemology derives from the two Greek terms, *bio*, meaning "life," and *philia*, meaning "affection or friendly feeling toward." The attraction we have to nature is toward its beauty, wonder, rich diversity of life, and vitality. It also is ascribed to abstract manifestations – the diversity of shapes, forms, patterns, and colors found in the living natural world, all of which can inform designs within the built environment. The biophilic principles have evolved from a re-evaluation of the Western worldview and its interplay with nature, human beings, and the built environment. Our role is to respect nature and build accordingly. The design implications suggest consideration of the numerous biophilic attributes, especially the place-based, natural form-based, and light- and space-based attributes.[12]

Stephen Kellert, in 2008, developed a restorative design approach and paradigm in which there were 72 comprehensive attributes of biophilic design.[13] These attributes are intended to influence various outcomes, including wellness and spiritual outcomes. The first outcome is to respect, restore, and respond to the larger natural context within which we live. This includes the ecological regions and climatic contexts. The second outcome is to respond repeatedly and sustainably to interactions with nature and the renewable technologies they support. The third outcome is to support placemaking and the positive urban forms and social interactions that can result from it. The fourth outcome is to promote health and wellness behaviors and lifestyles through positive experiences with both the natural and built environments. And the fifth outcome is to create the opportunities for spiritual connections to nature and the experiences of sacred places, true sustainability, and high-level wellness.

Spirituality is intertwined with biophilia in several profound ways. Biophilia taps into this deep respect and reverence for the natural world. This includes a sense of awe and wonder at nature's vastness, intricate ecosystems, and constant change. Such respect and reverence can evoke a sense of awe and wonder that transcends the everyday. This feeling of connection to something larger than ourselves is a cornerstone of many spiritual traditions. Biophilia reflects interconnectedness that reminds us that we are part of a web of life. Spiritual practices often emphasize this interconnectedness, fostering a sense of belonging and responsibility toward the natural world. Renewal and healing include spending time in nature, which is known to foster a calming and restorative effect. Similarly, spiritual practices often aim to cultivate inner peace and well-being. Nature can provide a space for reflection, meditation, and a return to a more grounded state. Nature's beauty and resilience can inspire a sense of purpose and meaning in life. Spiritual practices often explore our place in the universe and how to live a meaningful life. By fostering biophilia, we can cultivate a deeper appreciation for the natural world, which enriches our spiritual lives and fosters a sense of connection to something greater than ourselves.

Our ancient ancestors were hunter-gatherers whose lives were intertwined with the wilderness, endless grasslands, dense forests, and vast stretches of green landscapes. Hence, deep inside us is an instinctual connection and understanding that much health and wellness can derive from nature. Forests and trees in particular are particularly appealing as they provide oxygen, shelter, food, building materials, safety, windbreaks, and, in some cases, water. On a spiritual level, trees reflect connections with things greater than ourselves and they ground to the earth with their roots and to heaven with their branches and leaves. Forests were the source of myths and mystery and were often seen as enchanting. Also, they were home to certain gods and spirits, and, often, certain trees were seen as holy and considered worthy of spiritual respect. Although not a new concept, forest bathing was promoted in Japan in the early 1980s by the Japanese Ministry of Agriculture, Forestry and Fisheries as *shinrin-yoku*, literally meaning "taking in nature," where taking in the qualities of the forest, its atmosphere, or, in a broader sense, experiencing all of nature is a wellness emersion process. Forest bathing significantly improves physical and psychological health. Benefits include stress reduction, encouragement of physical activity, creation of positive moods, improvement in sleep patterns, strengthened immune system, lowered blood pressure, reduced concentrations of cortisol, and lower pulse rate.

The wellness implications of biophilia are improved physical, mental, and emotional health. Typical among these benefits is increased physical activity, stress reduction, a feeling of calmness, improved heart health and cognitive function, and improved sleep. The spiritual implications lie in the deep connection or bond between nature and humans, resulting in emotional peace, spiritual renewal, and connections to the unknown. The photographs in Figure 2.2 show a man forest bathing by walking across fallen logs over a stream and a woman enjoying the softness of the leaves on the forest floor and the filtered sunlight. It is biophilia's love of nature and life processes that can bring wellness to both people and place.

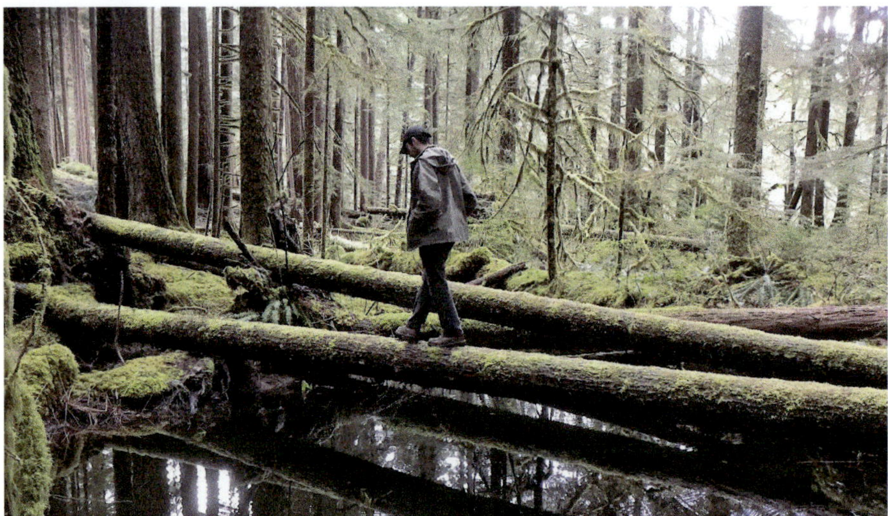

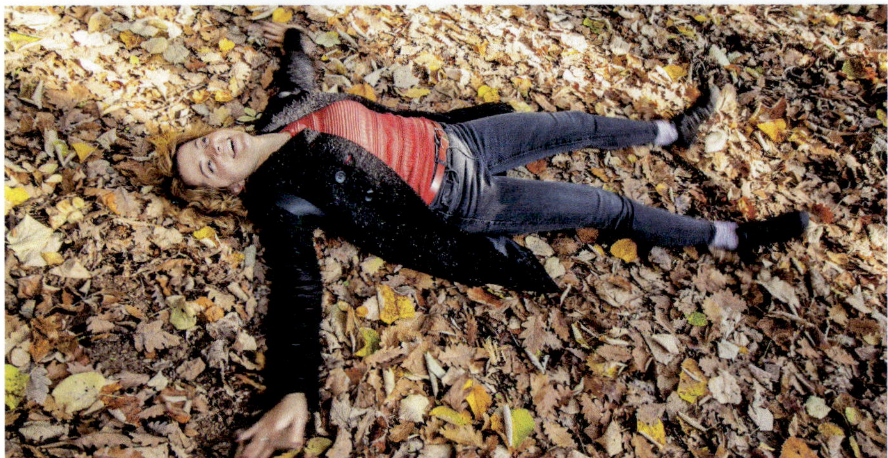

2.2
Biophilic Places: (a) Nature Walk, (b) Forest Bathing

Attribute of Thin Places

Exposure to restorative beautiful places can contribute to spiritual renewal. Sometimes referred to as "*thin places*," they can elicit both awe and serene emotions leading to positive benefits. Spiritual experiences can be fostered in places of refuge and sanctuary. Refuge is withdrawal into a safe, sheltered, and protected asylum from danger. Spaces like these can occur either indoors or outdoors and create opportunities for quiet solitude, peacefulness and relaxation, spiritual renewal, change in moods, reduced stress, and isolation from/with communicable diseases such as COVID-19. Third places, such as coffee shops, hair salons, and malls, are places where people meet to socialize, express themselves, and support one another. These sanctuary spaces enrich social interaction and elicit a sense of community and belonging outside of the home and workplace.[14] Therefore, spiritual renewal can occur in a variety of contexts with differing functions and purposes.

Religious and spiritual sites and sacred architecture have consistently had the intention to create a more fluid threshold and transcendent connection between heaven and earth, deity and human, and parish or community and religious institutions and belief systems. Non-theistic believers might see these places and the wellness benefits as opportunities to experience awe, wonder, nature, and the present. Especially charged spaces in many ways are similar to any other building, requiring foundations, structure, heating and ventilating systems, and responses to fire regulations. Yet, an additional responsibility exists to create spaces that can become charged, possibly elicit transcendent experiences, and support health and wellness behaviors.

With the experience of such places there often is a "*cross state retention*" or a renewal that is remembered. Religious and spiritual benefits comprise two major experiential qualities, those that are ineffable (indescribable) and those that are noetic (possessing hidden or unexplainable knowledge). The design implications suggest the need to provide thin places, charged places, or transcendent places with certain functions or purposes. These include graves, cemeteries, burial grounds, purification and healing sites, sacred plant and animal sites, quarries, astronomical observatories, shrines, temples and effigies, fertility sites, mythic and legendary sites, historic sites, and places of spiritual renewal, healing, and wellness.

What makes thin places important is complex and involves understandings of both the nature of place and emotion theory. They are accessible to everyone and make us feel we are part of something greater than ourselves. Thin places provide us opportunities to step outside of ourselves and our everyday lives and give us new perspectives and experiences that are self-transcendent and outside our normal range of experience. They give us experiences, even if momentary, that are extraordinarily beautiful, incredibly tranquil or contemplative, and insightful. According to Mindie Burgoyne, *thin places* are places in which a svelte veil exists between our secular world and the sacred, where an energetic connection and nexus can more easily be made.[15] The exact nature of this veil is not really known, but certainly is sensed.

Veils, beyond their literal associations as garments with ceremonial significance, are defined as things that cover, conceal, or disguise. They are permeable membranes of perception. Thin places are also considered veils. As veils, they initially maintain a certain sense of separation as well as a concealment and closeness to something magical, unknown, sacred, or divine; later, they become thinner, more transparent, and accessible to a source and source experience. The veil in this sense can be experienced as part or whole of the thin place. As a space, the veil has a special function. It serves to make both a spatial and temporal pause and transition.

Thin places are mesmerizing places that form a transitional experience and often alter our perception of time. Thin places seem to possess a charge. A charged place contains an energy or presence, whether it is a natural, social, cultural, historical, symbolic, or physical energy. This energy can be sensed and felt, and some places are more charged than others. This may occur because of the profound

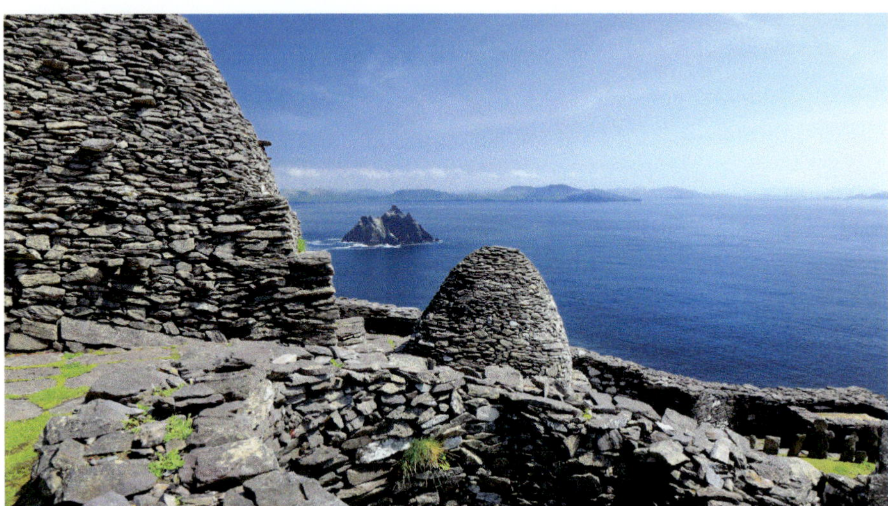

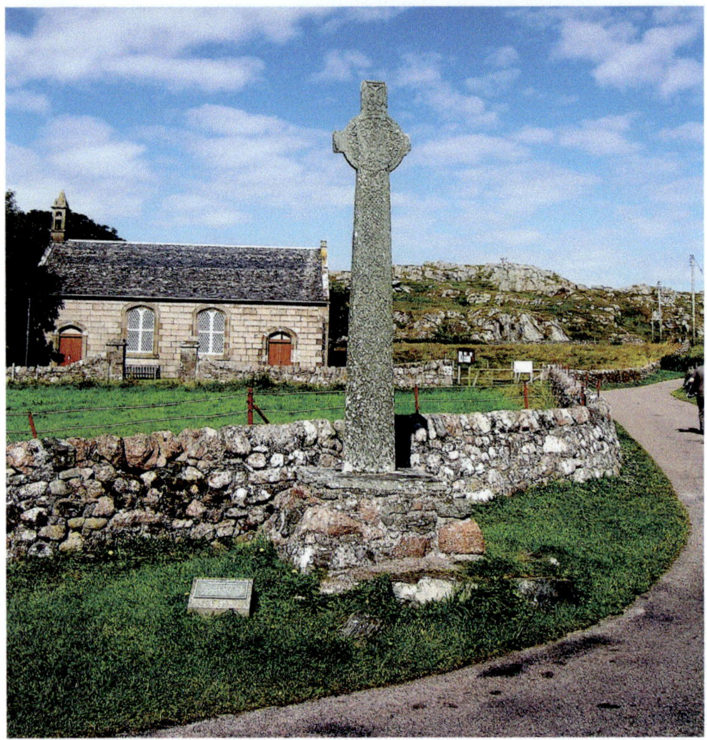

2.3 Thin Places: (a) Skellig Island, Ireland, (b) Iona, Scotland

historical or cultural meaning tied to the place, the dramatic features of a natural site, or the quality of the architecture. Charged places carry, reveal, and have a narrative capacity. According to Michael Brill, the experiences of charged places derive from universal and transcultural commonalities about place.[16] The charge comes from either a species-wide, cultural, or personal resonance from the place and from within. In the context of this work, charged places transform us through both wellness and spiritual benefits.

Benefits occur in personal growth; health and wellness; prosocial outcomes, with increases in generosity, helpfulness, and compassion; and sensitivity of an environmental awareness supporting preservation, stewardship, and spiritual sensibilities. Thin place experiences help us to be more tolerant and less afraid of uncertainty, assist in rescaling ourselves and our circumstances, and contribute to both health and wellness. At the heart of thin places are the emotional responses and spiritual wellness experiences they create and support. Moreover, the outcomes from these emotional responses also vary from inner personal insights to accelerating transformative moments. Figure 2.3 illustrates two recognized thin places, located in Ireland and Scotland.

Attribute of Third Places

Ray Oldenburg developed the concept of third places. He posits that certain settings, separate from the most familiar (home, work), support social engagement by fostering encounters with familiar people and new acquaintances within a safe place. They may include coffee shops, theaters, gyms, cafés, bars (pubs), parks, libraries, places of worship, or friends' houses, where everyone spends the most time outside of home and work. Third places can help alleviate feelings of boredom and loneliness, create a playful atmosphere, and maintain a healthy work–life balance and are key to fostering a sense of community. Other wellness benefits include boosting mood, reducing stress, and increasing our self-esteem. Third places can be exclusionary, disallowing certain populations, political orientations, behaviors, and already-marginalized populations. The design implications include provisions of walkable commercial centers with a mix of services, public spaces, and locally owned businesses serving as third places.

Spiritual third places are those special spaces outside of home and work that nurture the soul and cultivate a connection to something greater than oneself. These havens can be physical locations or even activities that provide a sense of peace, meaning, and belonging. Places of worship, such as churches, temples, mosques, and other religious institutions, can offer a sense of community, shared values, and spiritual connection. Nature sanctuaries – serene natural settings such as forests, mountains, or beaches – can provide a sense of awe, peace, and connection to a higher power. Creative spaces, including art studios, music schools, or even your own home, can become a spiritual third place if they allow you to express yourself and connect with your creativity, a source of inspiration for many. The key characteristic of a spiritual third place is that it allows you to step outside the busyness of daily life and separate from home and workplace to connect with your inner self and something more significant.

Third places are a concept addressed by Robert Putnam that are social spaces separate from home and work, offering crucial civic engagement and community building.[17] Third places, such as pubs, coffee shops, hair salons, farmers' markets, malls, places of worship, and community gardens, are places where people meet to socialize, express themselves, and support one another. These third spaces enrich social interaction, a sense of community, and belonging outside of the home and workplace.[18] Third places provide opportunities for re-engaging lost social capital, which is a spiritual wellness benefit. This sense of belonging can nourish the spiritual need for connection and purpose. Engaging in activities in third places can provide a sense of meaning and purpose beyond work and family obligations. And exposure to third places can broaden our understanding of the world and challenge our own assumptions, fostering spiritual growth and empathy. Third places are also a context for expressing generosity.

The wellness benefits of third places include a surprising range of healing benefits. They can promote well-being by reducing stress and loneliness. Third places provide a supportive social environment where you can connect with others, reducing feelings of isolation and fostering a sense of belonging. They can improve mental well-being through engagement in casual conversations and shared

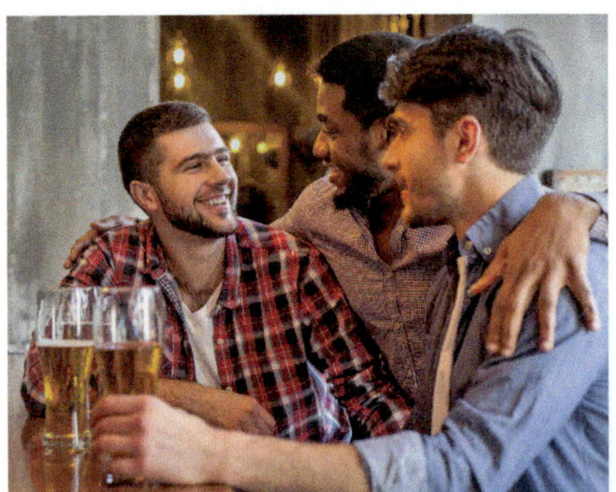

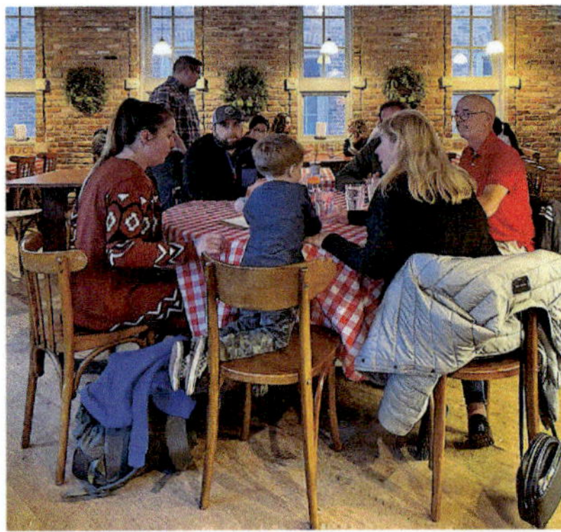

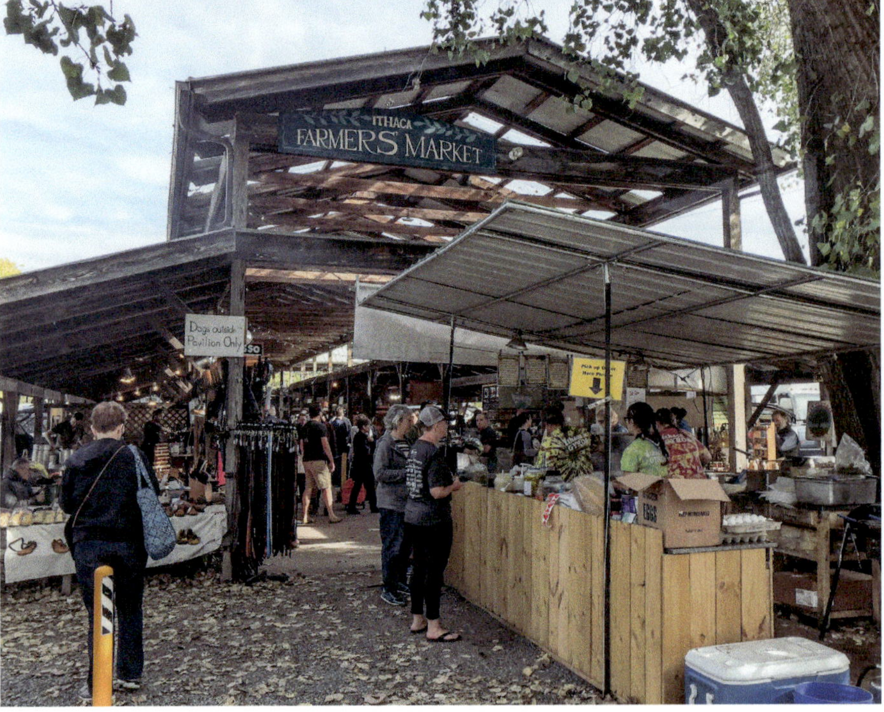

2.4
Third Places: (a) Pub in Cork, Ireland, (b) Family at the Blue Eyed Daisy Café, Serenbe, Georgia, (c) Ithaca, New York Farmer's Market

activities in a welcoming atmosphere, which can boost mood and combat feelings of anxiety and depression. They can enhance cognitive function when socially oriented third places connect you to your community and provide opportunities to contribute your skills and interests, fostering a sense of purpose and fulfillment. The wellness implications of third places are that they can help build relationships with people who share your interests or values and can provide a strong social support network, crucial for overall well-being. The spiritual implications of third places are that they foster space to find renewal, purpose, and a sense of peace but also, most importantly, to connect to others – family, friends, and even strangers. The images in Figure 2.4 show a few third place social settings.

Attribute of Sanctuary Spaces

Sanctuary spaces can occur in varying forms, sizes, and locations, from special alcoves in a bedroom or a home office space to a favorite hiding place in the woods or vacation spot. They can occur throughout everyday experiences or on special occasions. They are nurturing and personal. Children's treehouses or forts are a favorite sanctuary space allowing for intimacy, comradeship, creativity, and solitude. Google is known for its unique and varying workspaces that serve to provide privacy, focus, and opportunities to recharge. Sanctuary spaces are also found in natural beauty spots, spiritual and thin places, therapeutic environments, and wellness retreats. During COVID-19, such spaces allowed isolation and limited physical contact with fellow employees. The wellness benefits of such interesting environments include sources for renewal, relaxation, and quiet. Experiences within them can reduce stress and overstimulation, can strengthen the immune system, and can improve mood and positive feelings.

Silence facilitates deeper, more self-reflective, and peaceful moments in the context of a noisy world.[19] Moments of silence can be transitions to transcendent experiences of awe and serenity. The health benefits are mental clarity, decreased stress, lower blood pressure and heart rate, reduced cortisol, improved sleep, and increased focus and positive moods. Sanctuary spaces are nurturing, comforting, and therapeutic and provide protection and a safe haven. They support social healing, can be sacred, and can include workshops, storm shelters, bedroom alcoves, treehouses, children's forts, bathtubs, and even baby cribs.

The term *passive survivability* was coined by Alex Wilson in 2005 in the wake of Hurricane Katrina. According to Wilson,

> Passive survivability can be achieved by incorporating the sustainable design features that have been so actively promoted by the green building community: such design features include cooling-load avoidance strategies, capabilities for natural ventilation, a highly efficient thermal envelope, passive solar gain, and natural daylighting.[20]

Passive survivability refers to the ability to maintain critical life-support conditions if those conditions have been shut off for an extended time. Passive survivability is intended for houses, apartment buildings, and emergency shelters in the event of extended systems failures, especially for electricity, water, and heating fuel. The wellness design strategies provide a range of healthy, safe, and productive buildings during normal and catastrophic events.

Passive survival places share key characteristics that make them naturally advantageous for survival in an emergency situation. These locations provide protection from the elements (sun, wind, rain, extreme temperatures) and potential hazards such as wildlife. Examples include caves, rock overhangs, dense forests with good overhead cover, fallout shelters, and other structures designed for resiliency and sustainability. Ideally, these places offer access to basic necessities for survival with minimal effort. This could include a freshwater source (streams, springs), natural sources of food (edible plants, fruits), materials for building a fire (dry tinder, firewood), or renewable energy sources and technologies. Passive survival places often have features that contribute to a comfortable or tolerable environment, such as areas with natural wind barriers, sufficient sunlight for warmth (or shade in hot climates), and good drainage to avoid flooding. While these characteristics enhance chances of survival, they are not a guarantee.

Another area of sanctuary places is the prepping movement (disaster preparedness), which no longer is a fringe obsession. Now it has roots in individualism and self-reliance. Recent elicitors for this movement include the 9/11 attacks; increasing natural disasters; social unrest, particularly in the context of a bifurcated political climate; and the COVID-19 pandemic. The wellness benefits of this movement include reduced anxiety, increased self-reliance, mindfulness around sustainability and resource utilization, and an increase in community bonds. On the downside, there also can be excessive worry and increased financial costs. The spiritual benefits include building inner strength, increasing a sense of connectedness to nature, a focus on life purpose and meaning, and renewed gratitude.

Immigrant camps are sanctuary places that can be very challenging environments for spiritual well-being. Approximately 22 percent of the world's refugee population lives in refugee camps – an estimated 6.6 million people.[21] The stress of displacement, separation from loved ones, and uncertainty about the future can take a toll on mental and spiritual health. Many immigrants experience trauma during their journeys, which makes it difficult to connect with their spirituality. However, creating designated spaces for prayer, meditation, cultural gatherings, or religious services can offer a sense of normalcy and belonging. The spiritual wellness benefits in these environments are limited but can include coping with shared values and circumstances and developing spiritual bonds and communities from within.

An unprecedented 68.5 million people live as refugees, asylum-seekers, stateless people, and internally displaced people in precarious situations around the world.[22] Sanctuary cities combat closed borders, detention, and deportation; communities across the country are proclaiming sanctuary city status. Cities throughout the world find solutions and ways to protect refugees. Unfortunately, the tendency toward rising nationalism is confronting sanctuary asylums worldwide.

Climate change, which affects sea levels, will inevitably cause further migrations inland. It is causing the global mean sea level to rise in two ways. First, glaciers and ice sheets worldwide are melting and adding water to the ocean. Second, the volume of the ocean is expanding as the water warms.[23] Coastlines are shrinking owing to the sea level rise and land erosion. According to the World Economic Forum, 410 million people could be at risk from rising sea levels by 2100.[24] Sea levels along the coastline are estimated to rise 10–12 inches by 2050, with specific amounts varying regionally, mainly owing to land height changes. Sea level also matters in a horizontal direction. A rule of thumb is that 1 inch of vertical change in sea level translates into 100 inches of horizontal loss on a flat beach or marsh.[25] With 12 inches of sea level rise, it translates to 1200 inches, or 100 feet, horizontally. An estimated 267 million people live in coastal areas worldwide. For future growth and development, should we not be thinking of safer locations?

Relocation can cause stress, disruption of social networks, loss of cultural heritage, and uncertainty and can exert a toll on mental health. Wellness is enhanced by removing direct threats, which should improve physical health, enhance mental well-being, and create more certainty. Even though the spiritual benefits of moving

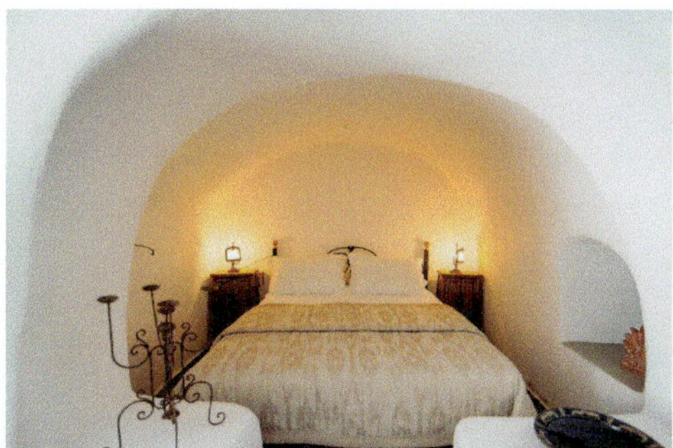

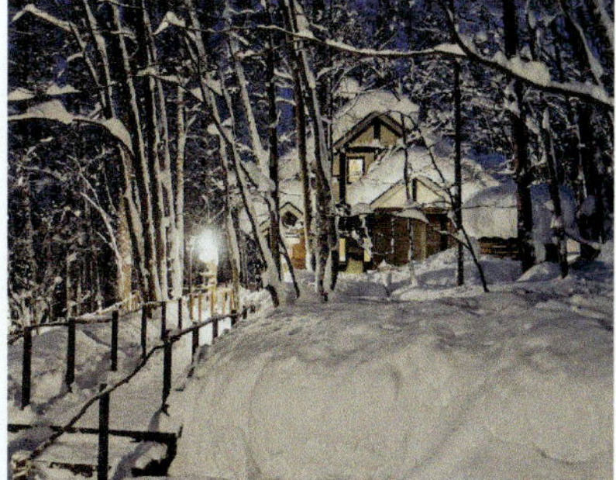

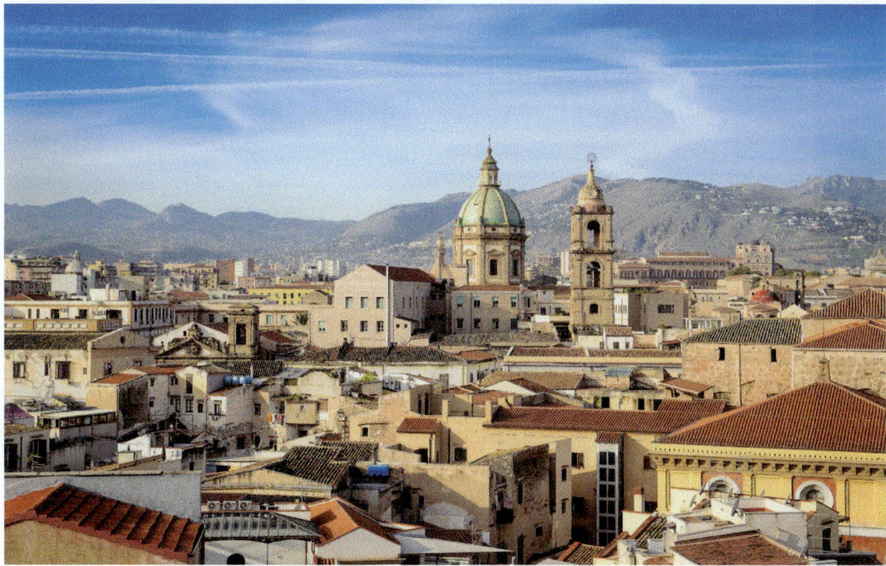

2.5
Sanctuary Places: (a) Oia, Santorini, Bedroom Alcove, (b) Warm Cabin in Snowstorm, (c) Palermo, Italy, Sanctuary City

to higher inland ground come with challenges, they could be uplifting and create opportunities to redefine home and its relation to nature, community, resilience, and the new physical location. The dimension of sanctuary places offers a multitude of spiritual wellness strategies. The images in Figure 2.5 show the sanctuary of a cozy bedroom, a woodland cottage, and an aerial view of Palermo Sanctuary City.

Attribute of Healing Environments

Healing environments range from gardens to entire communities. For Wilbert Gesler, "healing and place are inseparable."[26] While most landscapes possess an intrinsic appeal and offer benefits to humans, healing gardens suggest improved health and wellness outcomes and are, therefore, considered therapeutic landscapes. Therapeutic environments or sanctuaries are considered safe spaces specifically designed for physical, social, psychological, and spiritual healing. They are generally plant-dominated environments purposefully designed to facilitate interaction with the healing elements of nature. They serve as places of recovery, and restoration of the mind, body, and soul. Healing gardens have a long history, most likely beginning with ancient Egyptian, Persian, and Greek cultures with landscapes of medicinal plants. In the Middle Ages, monastic compounds provided enclosed and protected gardens for herbal remedies and dietary prescriptions.

Healing gardens are used to produce medicinal plants, while others may be developed for ornamental plants and their serenity healing. They often are a part of hospitals, healthcare, and aging-in-place settings. Healing gardens have appeared worldwide and, according to Roger Ulrich, they help reduce pain, improve sleep, reduce stress and anxiety for patients and their families, lower infection occurrence, and improve patient satisfaction.[27] Therapeutic gardens often engage with the active and deliberate needs of particular populations, whereas healing gardens, on the other hand, generally aim for a more passive involvement and are designed to provide benefits to a diverse population with many differing needs.

While many homeowners spend weekends maintaining traditional lawns and landscapes, there is an opportunity to have life-giving and food-producing landscapes with positive benefits. Edible gardens can take several forms, from gardens to orchards, streetscapes, and micro-farms. Edible gardens provide healthy food and great accessibility. Typically found in these gardens are fruit trees, culinary herbs, and vegetables. In addition to producing food, there is a positive social aspect to creating edible landscapes. Edible landscapes double as food-producing gardens and *foodscapes*, as well as ornamentals full of color and seasonal change. Edible ornamentals can provide beauty, shade, and food, in addition to helping conserve water, reduce pollution, and provide habitat for wildlife.

In addition to *shinrin-yoku*, forest bathing is a central example of biophilia, with the love of and affiliation with nature. Long-term benefits derive from the combination of the physical activity of slowly walking and being present in the surrounding nature, breathing in oxygen-rich air, and exposure to the presence of the phytoncides or natural oils of the forest. Forest bathing significantly improves physical and psychological health. Other benefits are stress reduction, encouragement of physical activity, creation of positive mood, improving sleep patterns, strengthening the immune system, lowering blood pressure, decreasing concentrations of cortisol, reducing pulse rate, enhancing the biophilic effect, reversing the "nature deficit disorder,"[28] and encouraging pro-environmental behaviors. Forest bathing exposes us to lower levels of salivary cortisol concentrations and higher levels of tree-produced phytoncides, which in turn improve human immune systems with increased levels of white blood cells with natural killer (NK) cell activity.

Forest bathing is recommended for a minimum of 20 minutes a day, although a two-hour period is recommended for the full benefits. Walking quietly, opening the senses, periodic pauses, and finding a thin place or special spot to stop and attune to the place can elicit the best results. Two experiences often occur. The first is a serene, calming, or relaxing experience, safe from the negative aspects of nature and filled with sensual experiences. The second is an inspiring or insightful experience evoking states of mind and mindfulness. Forest bathing can be awakening and instinctual and evoke a sense of aliveness and awe. It can also be amplified with therapeutic guided tours and retreats. With forest bathing, caution should be exercised in certain situations. According to Agnieszka Olszewska-Guizzo, darker, denser elements of nature could be non-beneficial to health and even dangerous.[29] However, the experience of what is called an "awe walk" and "wild awe" is both safe and exhilarating and can be positive for health and wellness.

Benefits also include stress and tension reduction; improved respiratory system; lowered blood pressure; increased mental activity and powers of concentration; improved mental health, memory, and mood, endocrine, and immune system activity; encouragement of social interaction; contribution to a spirit of place; and support for prosocial and pro-environmental behaviors. Health and wellness benefits can also be derived from desert, meadow, and glacial bathing. The two outdoor healing environments illustrated in Figure 2.6 are the Saturnia Thermal Baths in Tuscany and the Badi Bani Khalid Oasis in Oman. Throughout history, thermal baths have been used for relaxation and healing. They offer mineral-rich water from natural springs with numerous health benefits.

Figure 2.6c is a Native American sweat lodge located in Crestone, Colorado.[30] The sweat lodge is an extraordinary expression of the combinatory use of the elements and their effects on healing and wellness. Similar to the Scandinavian sauna, it utilizes fire, earth, and water to create steam or hot air, which in turn purifies the body by dehydrating various toxins in the body. Traditionally, it is a small dome-like structure made with willows and an animal skin or blanket covering. A hole is dug out in the center, where fire-heated dry river rocks are placed. A small bucket and ladle are ceremoniously used to periodically pour water on the hot rocks. The healing effects are said to be extraordinary; however, care must be observed because the effects can be fatal.

Healing environments, both natural and human-made, are becoming more popular as evidenced by the growing wellness tourism, spa, personal care, nutrition, and real estate trends.[31] Not only are healing environments increasingly becoming destinations, they are also being integrated into home designs. Going far beyond the small medicine cabinet in the family bathroom of the 1950s, today, wellness considerations include safe site locations, favorable climate regions, incorporation

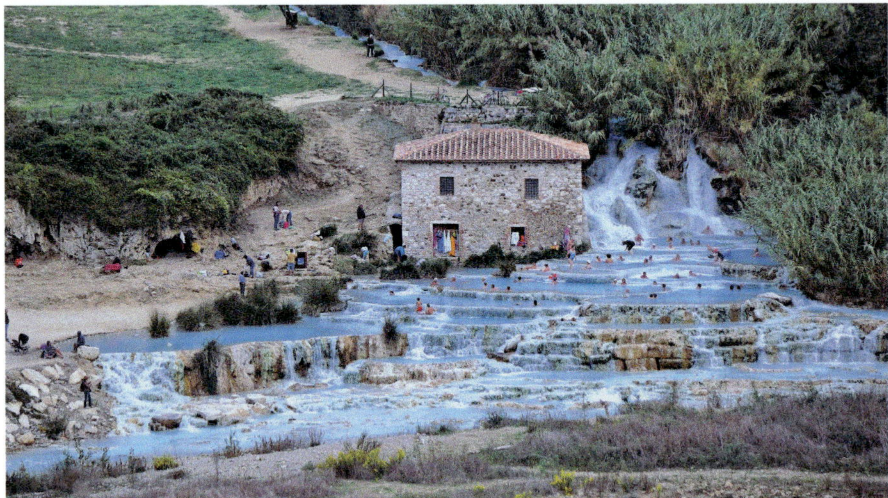

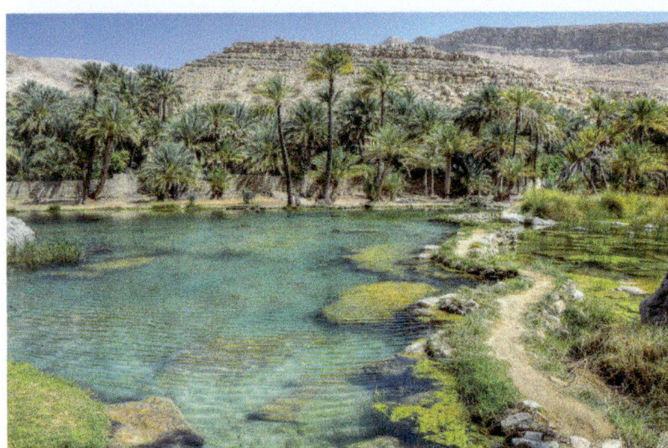

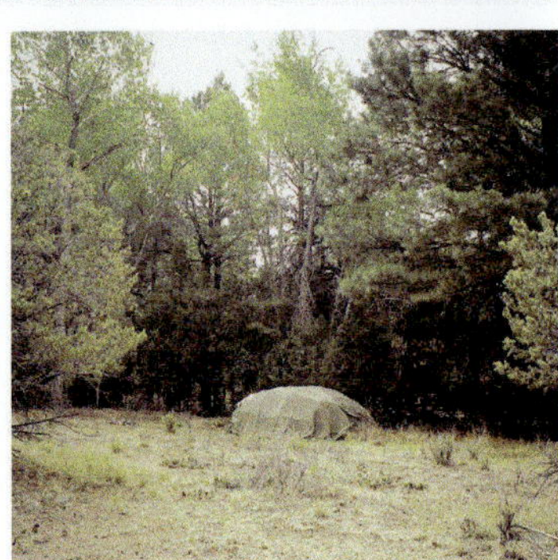

2.6 Healing Environments: (a) Saturnia Thermal Baths, Tuscany, (b) Badi Bani Khalid Oasis, Oman, (c) Sweat Lodge, Crestone, Colorado

of healing gardens, views of nature, use of non-toxic building materials, increased natural light, and inclusion of sanctuary spaces. And many homes are now accommodating spiritual spaces designed for contemplation, meditation, ceremonies, and inspiration.

Attribute of Religious Places

Religious and spiritual experiences go beyond the ordinary and can be mystical or euphoric, where there is an awareness of synchronicity, presence of intuitive thoughts, a sense of ultimate peace and well-being, and a degree of surrender. Religious and spiritual places share similar characteristics, yet they have some differences. The function of religion has been to provide social cohesion and solidarity, to enforce religious-based morals and norms, and to offer answers to existential questions.[32] Religions have typically evolved through the lives, teachings, and beliefs of historical or archetypal figures. Religions are regarded as holy, sacred, absolute, spiritual, divine, and worthy of unconditional reverence. According to Albert Einstein, the religion of the future will be a cosmic religion transcending a personal god and avoiding dogma and theology.[33] According to Kamitsis and Francis, spirituality can be defined as an individual's inner experience and/or belief system that gives meaning to existence and subsequently allows them to transcend the present context.[34] And, to Christina Puchalski, MD, spirituality is the aspect of humanity referring to the way in which individuals experience their connectedness to the moment, to self, to others, to nature, and to the significant or sacred.[35]

Similarities of religious and spiritual sites and sacred architecture have consistently had the intention to create a more fluid threshold and transcendent connection between heaven and earth, deity and human, and parish or community and religious institutions and belief systems. Spiritual and religious spaces vary in spatial organization, programmatic function, internal–external focus, and open universal uses versus more specific, directed liturgical programs.

Contemplative environments support a more conscious way of living when spiritual and/or contemplative practices are brought into everyday life. Living is concentrated and focused within a single place where the discipline of everyday survival functions is woven into a contained, seamless, ritualistic, and repetitious sequence of contemplative and spiritual activities. Contemplative environments generally have a strong sense of identity, serene atmosphere, and a comprehensible form.

Wellness is impacted by religious space through solace, meaning, and purpose, a sense of belonging, and community support. Owing to the vast diversity of religious life worldwide, religious spaces and buildings vary as well. While the specific functions, traditions, sizes, and locations vary greatly, there are certain spiritual wellness characteristics they seem to share. These include locations in special sites (geological and historical), the use of natural light, spatial generosity, and denominational symbolism contributing to the salient meaning of the religious experience.

Religious space can vary greatly, as seen with the examples in Figure 2.7. The MIT Chapel is intimate, and the skylight and light column are inspiring. The Hagia Sophia is large in scale, uplifting, and monumental. And, finally, the Western Wall in Jerusalem has a commanding presence with its historic significance, physical size, and connection to the Temple Mount and other adjacent structures. The wellness implications of religious space in the context of spiritual wellness include spatial generosity, formal geometry, dramatic use of light, a sense of uplifting and verticality, and a strong sense of place. The benefits are the experience of awe, presence, feelings of something larger than ourselves, and a sense of connectedness (to a higher power).

Attribute of Ritual and Ceremonial Spaces

Rituals are structured, often symbolic, actions performed individually or collectively. The core characteristics are behaviors that are patterned and repetitive, symbolic, most often social, and sometimes rule-based. With many rituals, invariance and consistency occur over time. Often, rituals incorporate sacred objects and ritualized spaces. Rituals can be religious ceremonies, cultural celebrations, or personal routines. Examples include baptisms, communion, weddings, funerals, meditation, exercise regimens, and third place visits. Rites of passage, calendrical events, and communion gatherings are also considered rituals. These include celebrations of crepuscular light and skies.

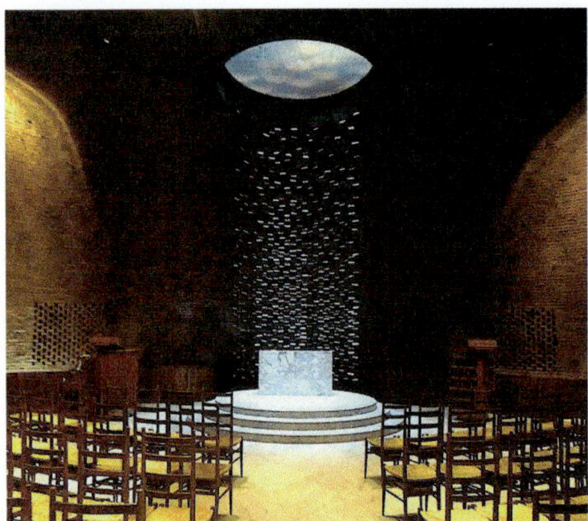

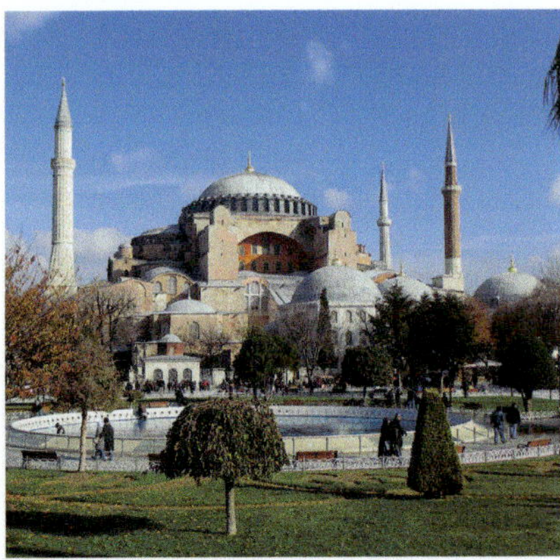

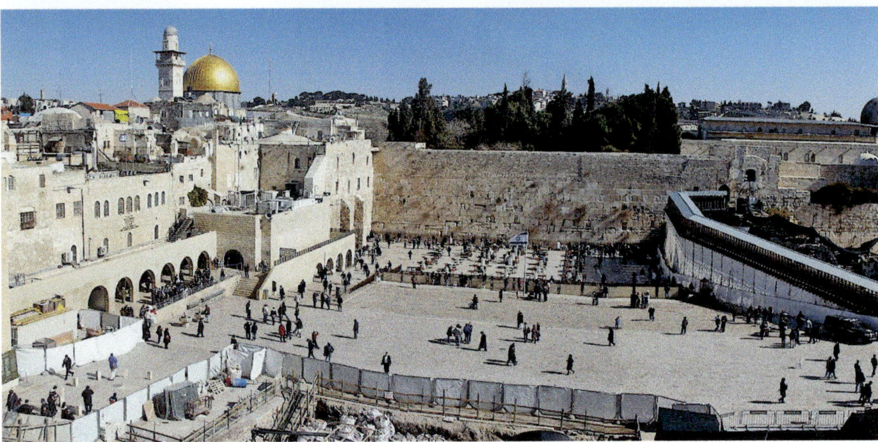

2.7 Religious Places: (a) MIT Chapel, Cambridge, Massachusetts, (b) Hagia Sophia Mosque, Istanbul, Turkey, (c) Western Wall, Jerusalem, Israel

Ceremonial spaces are designated as settings for performances, celebrations, rituals, and a wide range of ceremonies. They are found worldwide for cultural, educational, political, spiritual, and religious purposes. Spatially, they typically have a strong focal point, distinct boundary, and organized seating arrangements. Types of ceremonies vary greatly from rites of passage and religious practices to holiday and seasonal ceremonies. Ceremonial participation within places we occupy can occur in groups as well as individually.

Wellness behaviors and lifestyle practices need to occur on a daily basis. Ritual occurs when ordinary behavior is repeated until it forms recognizable patterns. Rituals become imbued with emotion. They can be calming in the context of uncertainty. Rituals can help transform difficult emotions into cathartic experiences, promoting emotional well-being.[36]

Ceremonial participation provides a sense of grounding in the present moment, helping individuals connect with their surroundings and themselves. For individuals, rituals and the most ordinary of actions become transformed into symbolic expressions, their meaning reinforced each time they are performed. The architectural implications for ceremonial design suggest focus on circulation and passage,

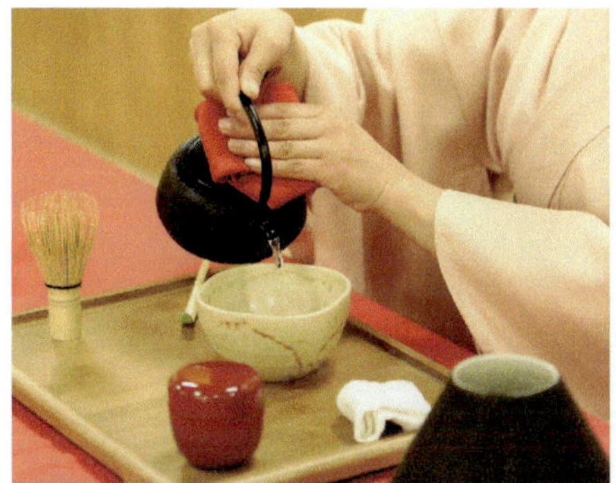

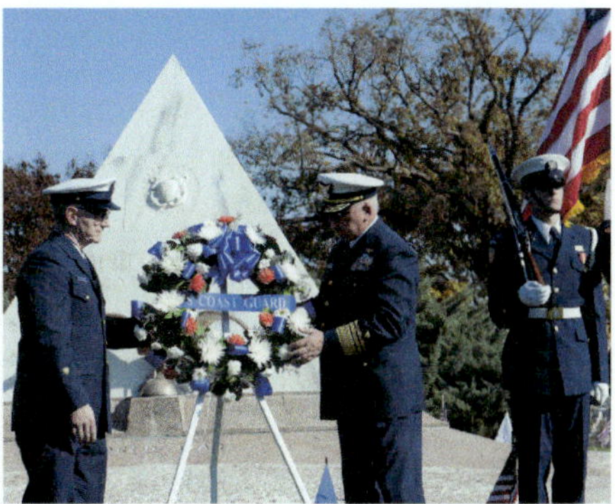

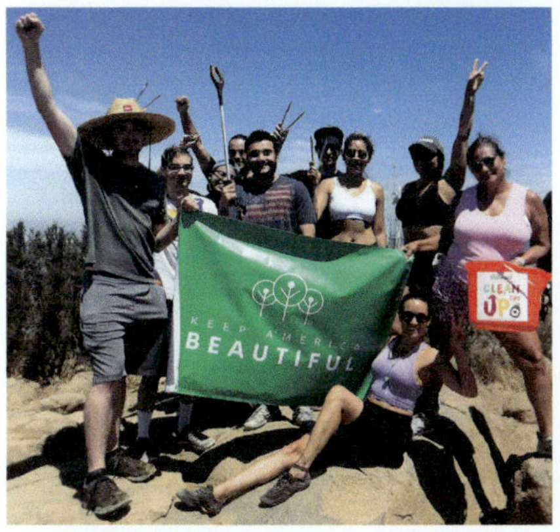

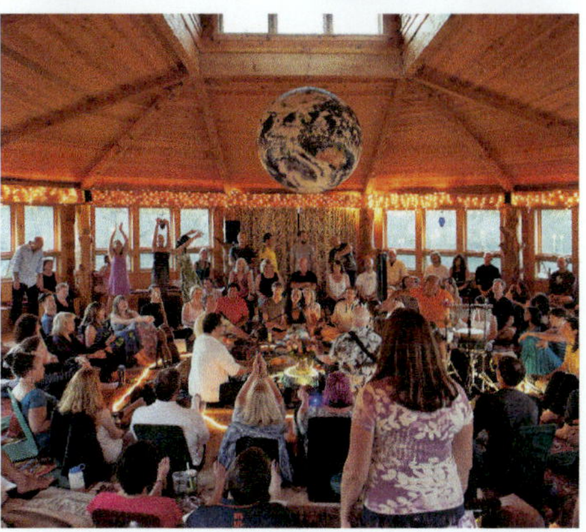

2.8 Ritual and Ceremonial Places: (a) Japanese Tea Ceremony, (b) Arlington Cemetery Veteran's Day Ceremony, (c) Earth Day Celebration, (d) StarHouse Sacred Seasons' Ceremony, Boulder, Colorado

sense of bounding, use of centralized geometry, use of light and symbolic elements, and emphasis on flexibility and adaptability. In planning, it might suggest provision of accessible public space.

There are many types and occasions for ritual and ceremonial space that are celebrated individually or collectively, from birthdays to religious holidays. For example, all chairs are not ceremonial places, as they normally function to accommodate seating for a myriad of purposes – to rest, to eat, to drink, to work, to watch, and even to drive. However, in some instances, they can serve to create special ceremonial experiences. Something as little as lighting a candle can be mesmeric and transformative, especially for young children. Throughout the day, going outdoors, relaxing, gardening, or preparing a special meal can also be an opportunity for a ceremonial experience. Yearly cycles present opportunities for ceremonies with special events, anniversaries, birthdays, and religious holidays. Figure 2.7 illustrates a few ceremonial spaces, including the intimate tea ceremony, a Veteran's Day Memorial ceremony at Arlington Cemetery, and seasonal ceremonies at the All Seasons Chalice in Boulder, Colorado.

The placed-based attributes are places that serve as elicitors by their location, geographic features, purpose, function and use, historic or cultural significance, or spatial quality.

SUMMARY

As discussed in this chapter, health and wellness are inextricably linked to place. The importance of place cannot be overstated, as both wellness and spiritual experiences are rooted in the places we occupy. The spiritual dimensions of wellness help inform place design through the wellness pillar – physical, cognitive, emotional, social, financial, environmental, and spiritual benefits. They produce pro-individual, prosocial, and pro-environmental behaviors. In spiritual wellness, there are specific attributes and desired outcomes, some of which produce benefits that overlap with the other dimensions. The place-based dimensions focus on the ways in which places shape our connections, experiences, behaviors, and lifestyles, especially toward health, well-being, and spirituality experiential outcomes. These places can be natural wonders, religious sites, healing gardens, personal sanctuaries, or even a favorite chair. The place-oriented attributes have direct application to design at all scales. For the attributes that follow in the next chapters, experience-based attributes describe multiple connections to transcendent experiences and well-being, and process attributes occur over time and address more holistic and deeper personal issues. These attributes have derived directly from definitions and research and reflect a broad view of spiritual wellness.

NOTES

1 Gesler, Wilbert M., *Healing Places* (Lanham, MD: Roman & Littlefield, 2003), p. 1.
2 Tuan, Yi-Fu, *Space and Place: The Perspective of Experience* (University of Minnesota, 1977).
3 Donat, John, *World Architecture 4* (London, 1967), p. 9.
4 Snyder, Gary, *Sacred Place: The Presence of Archetypal Patterns in Place Creation* (Self-published by Phillip Tabb, 1996).
5 Lane, Belden, *Landscapes of the Sacred: Geography and Narrative in American Spirituality* (Baltimore, MD: Johns Hopkins University Press, 1988), p. 19.
6 Allen, Summer, The Science of Awe (accessed October 20, 2021), https://ggsc.berkeley.edu/images/uploads/GGSC-JTF_White_Paper-Awe_FINAL.pdf.
7 Hettler, William, The Six Dimensions of Wellness Model (accessed August 20, 2024), https://www.researchgate.net/figure/Circular-model-of-wellness-by-Ardell-1977_fig1_335339647.
8 Robbins, Tony, The Keys to Spiritual Wellness (accessed September 1, 2024), https://www.tonyrobbins.com/blog/the-keys-to-spiritual-wellness.
9 Tuan, Yi-Fu, *Space and Place: The Perspective of Experience* (Minneapolis, MN: University of Minnesota Press, 1977), p. 179.
10 Brill, Michael, *The Origin of Charged and Mythic Landscapes: A Speculation* (Self-published May 16, 1991).
11 National Institutes of Health, Sense of Place and Health in Hamilton, Ontario: A Case Study (accessed September 24, 2023), https://www.ncbi.nlm.nih.gov/pmc/articles/PMC3400750/.
12 Kellert, Stephen R., Judith H. Heerwagen, & Martin Mador, *Biophilic Design: The Theory, Science, and Practice of Bringing Building to Life* (New York, NY: John Wiley, 2008).
13 Kellert, Stephen R., Judith H. Heerwagen, & Martin Mador, *Biophilic Design: The Theory, Science, and Practice of Bringing Building to Life* (New York, NY: John Wiley, 2008).

14 National Institutes of Health, Closure of "Third Places"? Exploring Potential Consequences for Collective Health and Wellbeing (accessed September 24, 2023), https://www.ncbi.nlm.nih.gov/pmc/articles/PMC6934089/.

15 Burgoyne, Mindie, About Mindie Burgoyne (accessed November 24, 2024), http://thinplacestour.com/about-mindie-burgoyne/.

16 Brill, Michael, *The Origin of Charged and Mythic Landscapes: A Speculation* (Self-published May 16, 1991).

17 Putnam, Robert, *Bowling Alone: The Collapse and Revival of American Community* (New York, NY: Simon & Schuster, 2001).

18 National Institutes of Health, Closure of "Third Places"? Exploring Potential Consequences for Collective Health and Wellbeing (accessed September 24, 2023), https://www.ncbi.nlm.nih.gov/pmc/articles/PMC6934089/.

19 Tabb, Phillip James, *Biophilic Urbanism: Designing Resilient Communities for the Future* (New York, NY: Routledge, 2019).

20 Wilson, Alex, Passive Survivability: A New Design Criterion for Buildings (accessed January 12, 2020) https://www.buildinggreen.com/feature/passive-survivability-new-design-criterion-buildings.

21 UN Refugee Agency, Refugee Camps Explained (accessed July 1, 2024), https://www.unrefugees.org/news/refugee-camps-explained/ .

22 Argerious, Natalie Bicknell, What Does a Sanctuary City Look Like? (Accessed July 10, 2024), https://www.theurbanist.org/2018/09/24/what-does-a-sanctuary-city-look-and-feel-like/.

23 Lindsey, Rebecca, Climate Change: Global Sea Level (accessed July 12, 2024), https://www.climate.gov/news-features/understanding-climate/climate-change-global-sea-level.

24 Masterson, Victoria, Stephen Hall, & Madeleine, North, Sea Level Rise: Everything You Need to Know (accessed July 12, 2024), https://www.weforum.org/agenda/2024/07/rising-sea-levels-global-threat/.

25 NASA, The Waters are Rising on NASA's Shores (accessed July 12, 2024), https://earthobservatory.nasa.gov/images/86655/the-waters-are-rising-on-nasas-shores.

26 Gesler, Wilbert M., *Healing Places* (Lanham, MD: Roman & Littlefield, 2003), p. 1.

27 Natural Design for Better Health: An Interview with Dr. Roger Ulrich (accessed October 12, 2023),
https://naturesacred.org/natural-design-for-better-health-an-interview-with-dr-roger-ulrich/.

28 Louv, Richard, *Last Child in the Woods: Saving our Children from Nature-Deficit Disorder* (Chapel Hill, NC: Algonquin Books, 2008).

29 Olszewska-Guizzo, Agnieszka, *Neuroscience For Designing Green Spaces* (London, UK: Routledge, 2023), p. 133.

30 This sweat lodge was built by a Native American Elder from Alberta, Canada, my oldest son, Michael, and me in the summer of 1988 in Crestone, Colorado. It was constructed with 16 overlapping willow branches and covered with a large tarp. In the center was a small pit for the heated rocks. Directly to the east of the entry was a small dirt ceremonial mound and a fire pit to heat the rocks. The lodge was used for various rites of passage and healing ceremonies.

31 Global Wellness Institute, Wellness Industry Trend Reports (accessed November 9, 2024), https://globalwellnessinstitute.org/industry-research/industry-trends/.

32 Saroglou, Vassilis, Awe Activates Religious and Spiritual Feelings and Behavioral Intentions (accessed December 8, 2021), https://psycnet.apa.org/record/2011-24221-001.

33 Eistein, Albert, 100+ Famous Quotes about Religion (accessed November 9, 2024), https://thequotesarchive.com/quotes-about-religion/.

34 Kamitsis I., & A. Francis, Spirituality Mediates the Relationships between Engagement with Nature and Psychological Wellbeing. *J. Environ. Psychol.* 36 136–143, 2013. Schneider,

K. J., The Phenomenology of Awe (accessed November 10, 2021), https://www.psychologytoday.com/us/ blog/awakening-awe/201806/the-phenomenology-awe.

35 Pulchalski, Christina, Religion vs. Spirituality: And the Difference between Them (accessed January 9, 2022) https://chopra.com/articles/religion-vs-spirituality-the-difference-between-them.

36 Karlovits, Stephanie, The Why: Understanding the Power of Ceremony for Mental Health (accessed June 30, 2024), https://merkababedesigns.com/blogs/merkablog/ceremony-and-mental-health-rituals-for-healing-and-resilience.

3 EXPERIENCE-BASED ATTRIBUTES OF SPIRITUAL WELLNESS

INTRODUCTION

In what ways can planning and design solutions contribute to human and environmental health and wellness? Health and wellness benefit both human beings and the environments they inhabit, including both natural and built places. Human-centered benefits are directed to the dimensions of wellness, including our physical bodies, mental health, emotional well-being, social connections, and spiritual growth, as seen with illness and joy. Financial health is also seen as a wellness benefit. The environmental-centered benefits are directed to the natural environment around us and the cities and buildings we occupy. Wellness is an everyday process and is inextricably linked to the places where we exist.[1] The places in which we live, work, shop, recreate, dine, and worship and otherwise occupy are the contexts within which we interact and function, and, if these places are healthy places, there is a greater chance of achieving wellness, especially spiritual wellness.

The experienced-based attributes serve the self-stewardship process of focusing on the physical, intellectual, emotional, social, financial, environmental, and spiritual dimensions of wellness. They are encounters and lived experiences occurring over time. Many of the attributes act as triggers or elicitors of spiritual wellness outcomes, such as the numinous, awe, serenity, and transcendent experiences. Others are results or consequences, such as the noetic processing, the feelings of synchronicity, and the uncertainty or exhilaration of the unknown. The experience-based attributes also include the unity experience with its connection to a world larger than ourselves.

The numinous has been broadly used to describe sacred experiences. In his chapter in the book *The Idea of the Numinous*, psychiatrist Lionel Corbett suggests that it is the quality of the numinous experience that is important and not its specific content.[2] These experiences occur through a variety of channels, including dreams, visionary experiences, and experiences of nature, and through the body. In the context of this work, they also occur through experiences of certain natural, architectural, and urban settings. Corbett further identified characteristics of a numinous or mythic state experience as the ineffable, having noetic and cognitive content; they are transient and produce positive effects.

The experience-based spiritual wellness dimension is made with numerous attributes that are holistic experiences that foster deeper connections with oneself, others, and higher powers. They are transformational in that they require us

DOI: 10.4324/9781003546085-3

to think beyond the commonplace and consequently require accommodation. The need for accommodation is common to each of the emotional responses associated with spiritual wellness – numinous, awe, serene, synchronicity, noetic, and unity experiences. Hence, the accommodation process is the adjustment or attempt to make sense of new or transformational experiences within pre-existing mental structures that often are initially difficult to assimilate. The new experiences challenge our existing concept of ourselves and the world around us through numinous, awe-inspiring emotions and spiritual experiences that require us to adjust our cognitive schema to accommodate them.

EXPERIENCE-BASED ATTRIBUTES

Lifestyles are based on tangible and intangible factors of individuals and groups and their actions, living behaviors, conditions, and habits. Furthermore, styles of living reflect values, attitudes, cultures, and worldviews. For them to be wellness lifestyles means they reflect a balanced, holistic, and purposeful choice. In other words, the experiences we have can contribute to outcomes of both wellness and spiritual wellness. These are highly personal and can vary from person to person. The experience-based attributes help define spiritual wellness design strategies and elicit spiritual wellness outcomes. The following eight experiences outline and describe experienced-based attributes. They trigger strong physiological responses and spiritual emotions, support personal values, emotional balance, and mindfulness, and help connect us to the larger world around us.

1. **Numinous experiences** – have an engaging power and are typically momentary and associated with fascination, wonder, mystery, tranquility, and even terror.
2. **Awe experiences** – are human emotions associated with vastness, diminished focus on self, changing time perception, and the need for accommodation, and can be overwhelming.
3. **Serenity experiences** – are sustained inner peace, tranquility, calm, and trust; they are sedating and free from anxiety and need accommodation in terms of cognitive and emotional readjustments.
4. **Synchronicity and coincidences** – are where circumstances and personal experiences have simultaneous meaning connections.
5. **Noetic experiences** – are the notion that spiritual experiences reveal an otherwise hidden or inaccessible knowledge and feelings of connection to something beyond ourselves.
6. **Transcendence and spiritual renewal** – are experiences of moving beyond ordinary limitations, including connections to spiritual wellness.
7. **Experiences of the unknown** – are things that cannot be described through other experiences, with a special character we can feel without being able to give it clear conceptual expression.
8. **Unity experience, sense of oneness** – is a profound experience encompassing a deep sense of interconnectedness, harmony, and oneness, becoming a single whole with the world around us. It dissolves the illusion of division and separateness.

Attribute of the Numinous

The numinous is defined as arousing spiritual or religious emotion. The term derives from the Latin *numen*, meaning "a nod of the head," implying divine approval and now associated with arousing spiritual, transcendent, or mysterious emotion.[3] It was brought into contemporary theory by Rudolf Otto in 1917 when he characterized these emotional responses as elicited by fascination (potent charm), mystery (astonishing wonder), and/or terror (overwhelming power). According to Robert Spitzer, the numinous creates opposites. *Mysterium tremendum* is a sense of something mysterious, amazing, generating boundless mystical wonder, entrancing, and often eliciting an overwhelming sense of diminution, humility, and awe emotional responses, especially in the presence of a spiritual power and utter vastness. *Mysterium fascinans* is a sense of something fascinating, desirable, good, caring, enchanting, and comforting. It attracts, lures, captivates, contains reassurance, joy, and grace, and elicits serene emotional responses, especially with intimate, beautiful scenes of nature or of home.[4] The design implications suggest creating spaces that are fascinating and mysterious.

The wellness benefits of the subjective experience of the numinous include enhanced resilience, increased mindfulness and serenity, hope and optimism, improved social connections, and, finally, spiritual connections. There are also physical benefits of the numinous, such as stress and anxiety reduction through peace and tranquility, lower blood pressure, and better sleep. The spiritual benefits of the numinous include the experience beyond the ordinary, the mysterious, something greater than oneself, and finding deeper meaning in life. This includes connections to a higher source and the experience of the emotion awe. It is the ability to experience and integrate meaning and purpose in life through connection with oneself and others, as well as through other contexts such as nature, the arts, religious practices, literature, or something other and beyond comprehension.[5] William James, in his seminal work *The Varieties of Religious Experience: A Study of Human Nature* (originally published in 1902), identified four characteristics that are important in understanding the nature of a numinous experience:[6]

1. **Numinous experiences are ineffable** – defying the normal expression of ordinary conceptual language.
2. **Numinous experiences are noetic** – they have cognitive content and produce an overwhelming sense of clarity.
3. **Numinous experiences are transient** – usually less than a half hour, but rarely more than a few hours.
4. **Numinous experiences are passive** – they produce positive affects in the grip of superior power and can produce healing.

Figure 3.1a is an image of an enchanting forest with indistinct and mysterious light beyond it in the background. The numinous in this regard activates an instinctual, even survival-based, emotion in which all the senses are activated, generating a keen sense of presence. Enchantment, wonder, mystery, and even those emotional experiences elicited by terror, as defined by Otto, can activate a fight-or-flight response. Figure 3.1b is a view from the inside of a dark cave looking

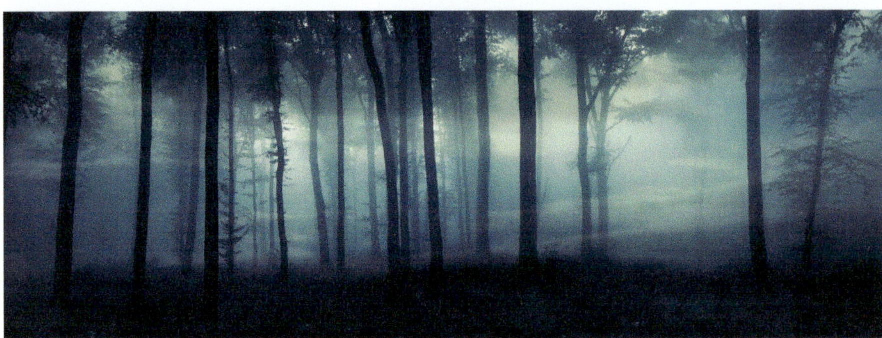

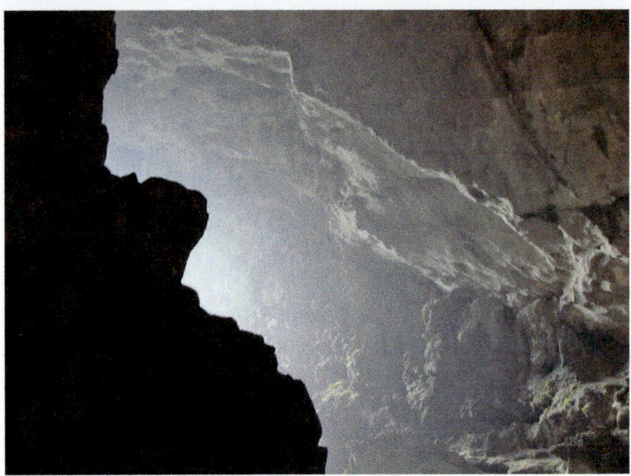

3.1 Numinous Attribute: (a) Enchanted Forest, (b) Mysterious Cave

outward to a brilliant light. It is reminiscent of Plato's allegory of the cave in the seventh book of his *Republic*, in a dialogue between Plato's brother, Glaucon, and his mentor, Socrates.[7] In this allegory, humanity is seen as chained while dwelling deep in a cave where shadows were projected onto the back wall of the cave showing objects placed in front of a fire behind them. This was the cave's inhabitants' apparent reality. One of the inhabitants, the philosopher, was able to break away, climb out of the cave, and experience the world in full light, moving metaphorically into the world of real truth and beauty. No longer was his reality shadows and reflections on the wall but rather the experience of a real presence – the sky, sun, moon, mountains, and natural life. The philosopher's experience was certainly a numinous one.

The wellness and spiritual aspects of the numinous are mostly expressed through profound, meaningful and purposeful, otherworldly, unusual, and ineffable architectural space that can elicit numinous experiences through awe, wonder, and fascination. To illustrate, there are relatively contemporary building designs that appear intentionally awkward and unstable and can evoke the numinous sense of terror. As defined, the wellness benefits are mental and emotional and can contribute to a sense of well-being and life satisfaction and elicit connections that are larger than ourselves.

Attribute of Awe

Awe is defined as an emotional response to perceptually vast stimuli that transcend current frames of reference. These include dramatic natural environments, extraordinary architecture, beautiful cities, charismatic figures, extraordinary concepts or ideas, and music and art. Awe experiences are vast and elicit ineffable wonder and fascination, and positive emotional valences and transformations. These experiences challenge our concept of self and the world around us and bring awareness to the process of adjusting or making sense of pre-existing mental structures and emotional states that were unable to be assimilated during the experience. Awe, in its more contemporary conception of a sacred experience, de-emphasizes the importance of fear in favor of ineffable wonder, fascination and mystery, and positive emotional valences and transformations.

In a 2018 publication, research showed a 6-factor scale for measuring awe emotion.[8] The 6-factor scale included time, self-loss, connectedness, vastness, physiological (physical) sensations, and accommodation. Awe elicitors are generally vast triggers in thin places that derive from sources that vary greatly, sparking differing physical, emotional, cognitive, and spiritual responses. These two differing emotional states create both similar and contrasting wellness benefits, where time perception in awe experiences slows down for some, and, for others, time is expanded. Self-diminishment is the reduction of the salient aspect of self, such as one's own body or its size relative to a natural sacred place or extraordinary building. Perceptual vastness is beyond measure and is much larger than the self and things that one does not fully understand.

In 2018, Summer Allen published an article titled "The Science of Awe,"[9] where she presented the idea of *flavors of awe*. They were threat, beauty, ability, virtue, and supernatural causality. The design implications of these flavors suggest designs with vastness and high emotional arousal, uniqueness of form and material, spatial generosity, abundant natural light favoring ineffable wonder and fascination, and connections to the unknown. They do provide a broad view of the elicitors of an awe experience beyond those associated with the physical environment, including the effects of changes in time perception, loss of self-awareness, sense of connectedness, experience of vastness, and physiological and cognitive responses.

Refer to Figure 3.2a, which shows the scalar difference of a person viewing the vast Grand Canyon, and Figure 3.2b, showing the extraordinary beauty and wonder of Machu Picchu in Peru, in contrast with the unusual buildings in Figures 3.2c and 3.2d. The Riverside Museum, in Scotland, and Dancing Building in Prague, in the Czech Republic, are unique, dramatic, and in some ways unsettling and can elicit awe emotions. Keltner and Haidt proposed an explanation of the awe flavors that do provide a broad view of the elicitors of an awe experience beyond those associated with the physical environment, as follows:[10]

1. **Threat-based awe** – is the awe likely accompanied by fear; stimuli that elicit threat-based awe may include a charismatic leader such as Adolf Hitler or an extreme weather event such as an electrical storm.

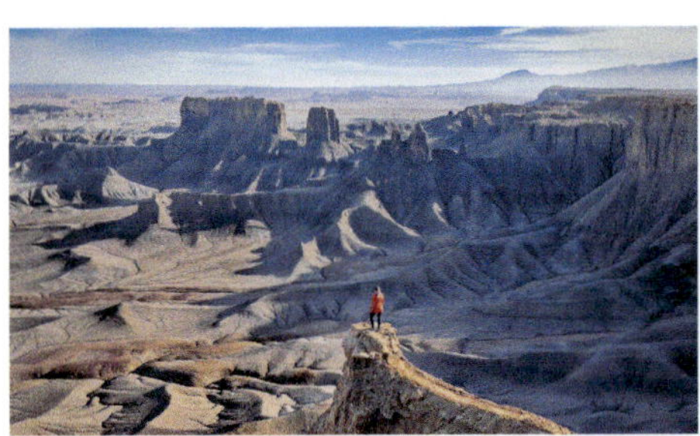

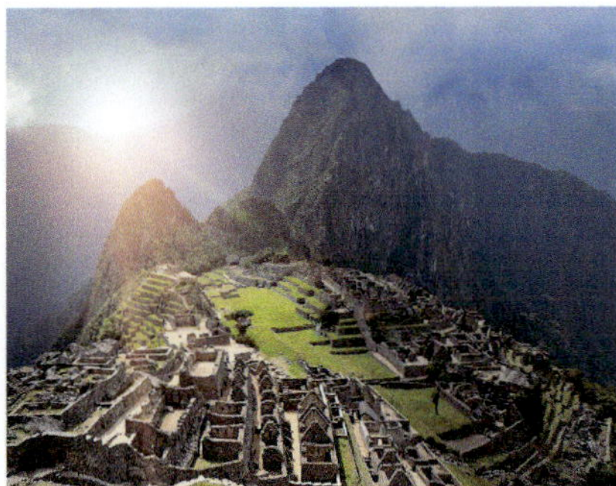

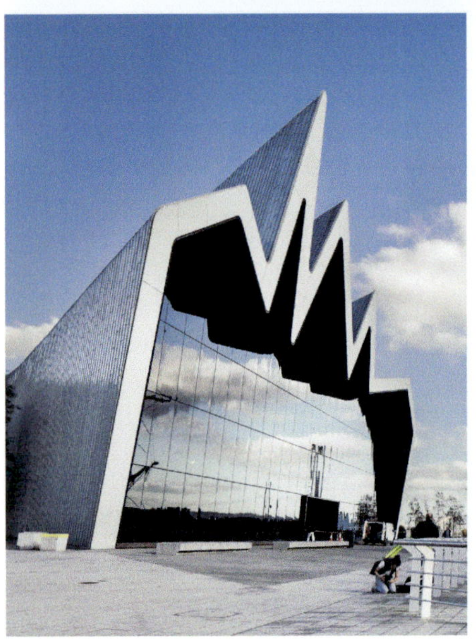

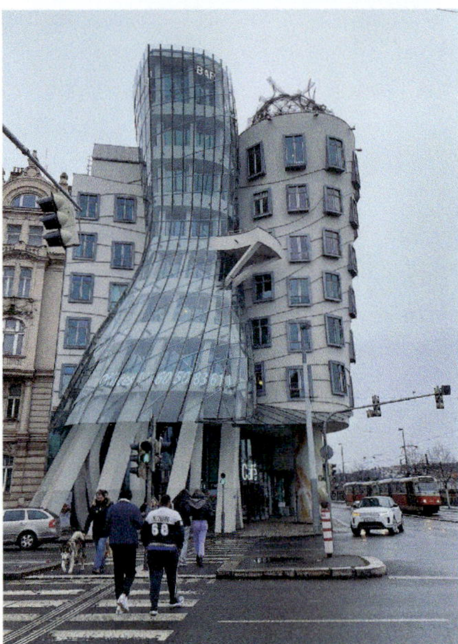

3.2
Awe
Attribute: (a) Grand Canyon, Arizona, (b) Machu Picchu, Peru, (c) Riverside Museum, Scotland, (d) Dancing Building, Prague, Czech Republic

2. **Beauty-based awe** – is the awe flavored with "aesthetic pleasure" and may be elicited by a person, a natural scene (e.g., the Grand Canyon), or a work of art (e.g., Monet's *Water Lilies*).
3. **Ability-based awe** – is the awe thought to co-occur with admiration of a person's "exceptional ability, talent, and skill." Examples include seeing an especially talented musician or stellar athlete.
4. **Virtue-based awe** – is the awe one feels when in the presence of someone displaying virtue and strength of character and would likely be accompanied by feelings of elevation. An example of virtue-based awe might be the result of reading about the lives of saints or generous philanthropy.
5. **Supernatural causality-based awe** – is the awe one might experience if one saw an angel, a ghost, or a floating object; it will be tinted with an "element of the uncanny," which can be terrifying or glorious, depending on the source.

The wellness and spiritual aspects of awe experiences are profound and may be in need of accommodation. Awe design characteristics are vast, monumental, impactful, and consequential. The triggers most related to spiritual wellness places include natural scenery and extraordinary buildings and monuments with evidence of great skill, particularly related to building craftsmanship and the inclusion of beautiful examples of art. These include national parks; the Northern Lights; extraordinary buildings such as the Taj Mahal, the Great Pyramids, the Acropolis, or Chartres Cathedral; places of memory such as cemeteries and memorials; battle sites; places that are compellingly serene such as parks, gardens, or holy wells; sites that are highly religious or mystical; and sites for night sky watching. The wellness benefits are mental and emotional and can contribute to and certainly can elicit connections to aspects larger than ourselves.

Attribute of Serenity

Serenity and its relationship to emotion theory, health and wellness, and spirituality first appeared in the nursing literature in the mid-1960s when it was identified as important to terminally ill patients. It focused on persons facing emotional stress, physical illness, and even death. Based on the nursing profession's evidence-based serenity research, nurses were able to develop health intervention strategies. Serenity is defined as sustained inner peace.[11] Serenity experiences are peaceful, tranquil, calm, even sedating, as well as free from anxiety. Its accommodation comes in the form of emotional readjustment. Serene elicitors develop an inner haven, acceptance, belonging, trust, perspective, contentment, centeredness, and beneficence.[12]

Another scale was initially developed in the 1960s that defined serenity, with nine factors, as a sustained state of inner peace and spiritual well-being and universal appeals to a large population of diverse persons.[13] These experiences challenge our concept of self and the world around us and are the accommodation process of adjusting or making sense out of pre-existing mental structures and emotional states that were unable to be assimilated during the experience. The design implications suggest a high degree of interacting with nature, serene gardens, water features, tranquil forms, and soulful materials. The positive benefits of serenity include appreciation of the moment, formulation of a more refined sense of self, a strong sense of groundedness, and the sense of congruence and gratitude.

The serenity scale is an analysis of the measure of spirituality and well-being relative to acceptance, inner haven, and trust.[14] It is predicated on the idea that serenity is related to peace of mind and an inner peace unaffected by external events or factors. This scale was initially developed by Kay Roberts and Cheryl Aspy to provide a number of wellness factors and characteristics published in the *Journal of Nursing Measurement* in February 1993, that will help inform design strategies. The scale is based on a conceptual framework of critical attributes for patients to better cope with harsh circumstances. Their development of a serenity scale involved nine factors:

1. **Inner haven** – inner source awareness and strength, peace of mind, experience of inner quiet and calmness that is not dependent upon external events, and feeling security and serenity, self-view, and long-range perspective.

2. **Acceptance** – perspective of self and life events, being present-centered, having benevolence, forgiving oneself, accepting situations that cannot change, being able to let go, and feeling serenity.
3. **Belonging** – a close and intimate affiliation or relationship, feeling connected and not feeling isolation or loneliness.
4. **Trust** – life events happen within a larger spiritual context, trust; in the life plan, seeing good in painful events and trusting that everything happens as it should.
5. **Perspective** – taking action to create change; hindsight into the past, foresight into the future, and insight into the present.
6. **Contentment** – free of excessive stress and worry about the future and what one cannot have, satisfaction with present material goods, and contentment with what is.
7. **Present-centered** – time orientation shifts from mainly past to the present, letting go of regret and anger.
8. **Beneficence** – the disposition for doing good, acts of kindness and good will, helping, sharing, forgiveness, and a positive and mindful regard for others.
9. **Cognitive restructuring and emotional restoration** – as in awe emotions, there is the need for cognitive appraisal and restructuring.

Serenity emotions are foundational for spiritual wellness in that they provide calm and peacefulness which support mindfulness, presence, meaningfulness, and reflection. Serene emotions elicit physiological relaxation responses of lower heart rate and slower and deeper breathing in sync with one another, relaxation of muscles, and a state of deep rest. Serene design characteristics are intimate and introspective and can be profound. They occur in places of memory such as cemeteries and memorials; battle sites; or places that are compellingly serene such as parks, gardens, or holy wells, sites that are highly religious or mystical, and sites for night sky watching. The wellness benefits are mental and emotional and can contribute to and certainly can elicit connections that are larger than ourselves. Also, they support a sense of self, a strong sense of groundedness, and a sense of congruence and gratitude. The wellness and spiritual aspects of serenity experiences are calming and stress relieving, and are in need of time for emotional readjustment or accommodation. Figure 3.3 shows a pastoral scene along a calm winter stream.

Attribute of Synchronicity

Synchronicity is a phenomenon in which people interpret two separate – and seemingly unrelated – experiences as being meaningfully intertwined, even though no evidence exists that one led to the other or that the two events are linked in any other causal way. Often, they appear to be serendipitous juxtapositions, as in the photography of Denis Cherim.[15] While it is difficult to depict synchronicity with specific images, their occurrences are something that most people experience that result in awe and wonder, shifts in perspective, enhanced sense of connection, and something larger than ourselves. Carl Jung saw synchronicity as "meaningful coincidences."[16] Furthermore, synchronicity can be interpreted as guides or signs from higher powers offering a sense of purpose or direction in life. They strengthen

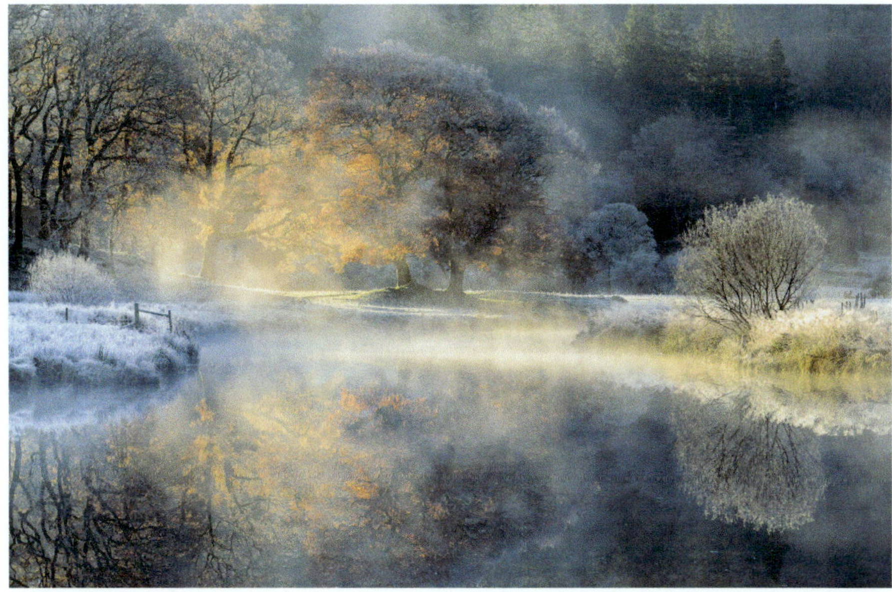

3.3
Serenity Attribute with Serene Autumn Mist and Gentle Stream

connections to a larger whole and appear to be connected to events that feel significant. There can also be experiences leading to something greater than ourselves. They can lead to heightened perception. The design implications suggest open-ended, shared, and multifunctional spaces that are easily circulated or intuitively navigated and allow for the unexpected. To Jung, synchronicity was the simultaneous occurrence of a certain psychic state with one or more external events which appear as meaningful parallels to the momentary subjective state.[17] How does this relate to spiritual wellness?

Spiritual wellness is personal and, therefore, can reinforce the sense of life purpose and direction through affirming recurring patterns. It encourages mindfulness and being present in the moment and it reveals connections to things beyond ourselves. In fact, purpose and meaning can be enhanced, amplified, and affirming. Further, synchronicity wellness is being open to and noticing meaningful coincidences related to one's current situation, especially during periods of change and uncertainty. Synchronicity reinforces connections to the unknown, the universe, and things greater than ourselves. According to Dana Klisanin, engaging with synchronicity aids in "rewilding the psychic." This means re-establishing connections to deep-seated awareness of interconnectedness and meaningful coincidences, and a process of returning to a more intuitive and nature-connected state of mind.[18] When we experience synchronicity, it serves as a reminder that we are part of a larger tapestry woven with intention and energy beyond ourselves, and something of significance. Several benefits of experiencing synchronicity include:

1. **Sense of connectedness** – the awareness of the interdependence of all living things and that we are part of an interdependent web of life.
2. **Meaningful patterns** – where two or more independent events, having no apparent causal connection, form meaning patterns.

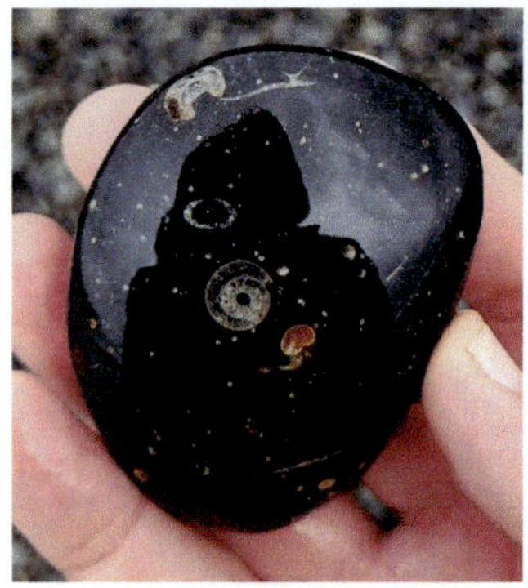
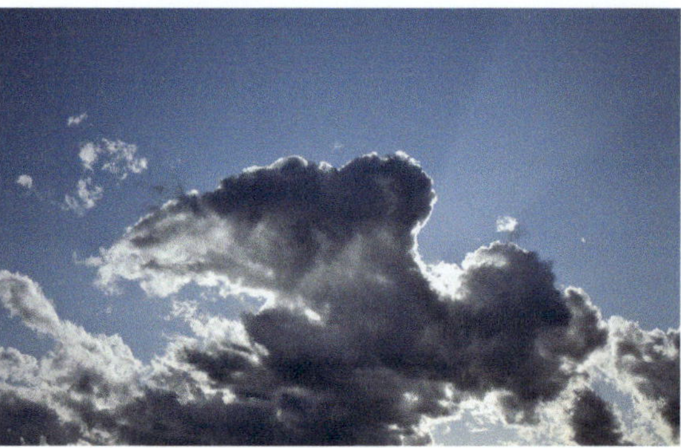

3.4
Synchronicity Attribute: (a) Rock and Embedded Universe, (b) Angel Cloud in the Sky

3. **Enhancement of self-awareness** – reflecting on synchronicities can reveal deeper thoughts and emotions where internal and external realities intertwine in remarkable ways.
4. **Rewilding the psyche** – reviving this deep-seated awareness, and re-establishing our connections with aspects of our humanity that have been suppressed or forgotten in the fast-paced modern world.[19]

According to Rodrick Main, synchronicity experiences can casually occur, connected to a common source.[20] The coincidence can mirror external events or experiences with internal ones. The wellness and spiritual aspects of synchronicity experiences are a process of returning to a more intuitive and nature-connected state of mind. These experiences can inform purpose in life and intentionality. They foster connections and interconnectedness which generate prosocial behaviors, gratitude, unity experiences, and deeper feelings that appear greater than ourselves. While it is difficult to visually represent synchronicity, Figure 3.4 suggests the dual qualities of random backgrounds (rocks and clouds) superimposed with suggestions of other images (cosmos and angels). Synchronicity, here, refers to meaningful coincidences that seem to have no causal relationship, yet it is a subjective experience where two or more phenomena connect in a way that feels significant to the observer.

Attribute of Noetic Experiences

The term "noetic" derives from the Greek *nous*, meaning implicit understanding or way of direct knowing, and the Greek *noetikos*, meaning intellectual. Noetic experiences can be noetic by carrying information or knowledge that later can be assessed and assimilated. They are illuminations and revelations possessing hidden or unexplainable knowledge. According to William James, noetic experiences include inner wisdom, direct knowing, depth of insights, and subjective understanding.[21] Noetic knowing is a state of knowledge separate from our intellect and it comes with a sense of authority. It, too, is an intuition, insight, gut feeling, or hunch about something. Noetic experiences are instinctual, intuitive, and full of importance. The implications of the unknown do not have direct implications for design; however, noetics in design can emphasize intuition and connections to users' inner worlds. Noetic transformation begins with a subjective experience of inner knowing and then follows a continuing process of exploration and practice, leading to the enrichment of both the individual and the collective.[22]

Some positive qualities of noetic experiences are interconnectedness, entrancement, allure, and impelling motive power.[23] Furthermore, noetic experiences often transcend the perception of our five senses. This transcendence is what Helané Wahbeh refers to as a "noetic signature" and is one's unique process for receiving and expressing non-traditional kinds of communications. In a study on noetic signatures, there were 12 characteristics that were common to noetic experiences. Some of these characteristics included inner knowing through emotions, embodied sensations, cognitive knowing, visualization or mental imagery, and self-knowing and inner voice.[24] Sensations such as goosebumps, chills, tingles, dizziness, temperature differences, and visions were present with noetic information. The notion that noetic experiences are ineffable, transient, contain feelings of unity, and reveal an otherwise hidden or inaccessible knowledge can elicit both spiritual and wellness benefits. Among the characteristics of a noetic experience are the following:

1. **Emotional knowing** – when one feels or experiences others' emotions and goes beyond ordinary empathy, where you relate to someone else's emotions.
2. **Embodied sensations** – experience of sensations such as goosebumps, smells, visions, tastes, sounds, dizziness, tingles, or vibrations in your body when you are accessing noetic information.
3. **Cognitive knowing** – knowing when something is true about people, places, or situations that could not be known or inferred by rational thought.
4. **Visualization** – use of visualization or mental imagery to manifest things in your life or in the world as intention has an influence.
5. **Inner voice** – noetic information comes to you through an inner voice.

Noetic attributes are non-physical as they describe certain ineffable experiences. However, certain physical design strategies may contribute to a de-materialization of physical spaces thereby helping to enable transformative experiences to occur. There are designs that help in grounding, centering, and experiencing the moment. The image in Figure 3.5 suggests the cognitive process of reading and expanding the imagination with thoughts of possible spiritual wellness experiences that are larger than ourselves. Wellness benefits include the physical outcomes of reduced risk of heart and respiratory diseases, increased self-esteem, and reduced stress and anxiety.[25] The spiritual aspects of the noetic are mostly expressed through experiences that are profound, meaningful, and purposeful. There are no specific physical design characteristics of the noetic; however, otherworldly, ineffable architectural space can elicit noetic experiences. The wellness benefits are mental and emotional, can contribute to a sense of well-being and life satisfaction, and can elicit connections that are larger than ourselves.

Attribute of Transcendence

Spiritual experiences change from secular or profane experiences and places to transcendent ones. Secular space is the ordinary space that we experience every day, and this includes unremarkable places, whereas sacred space possesses its

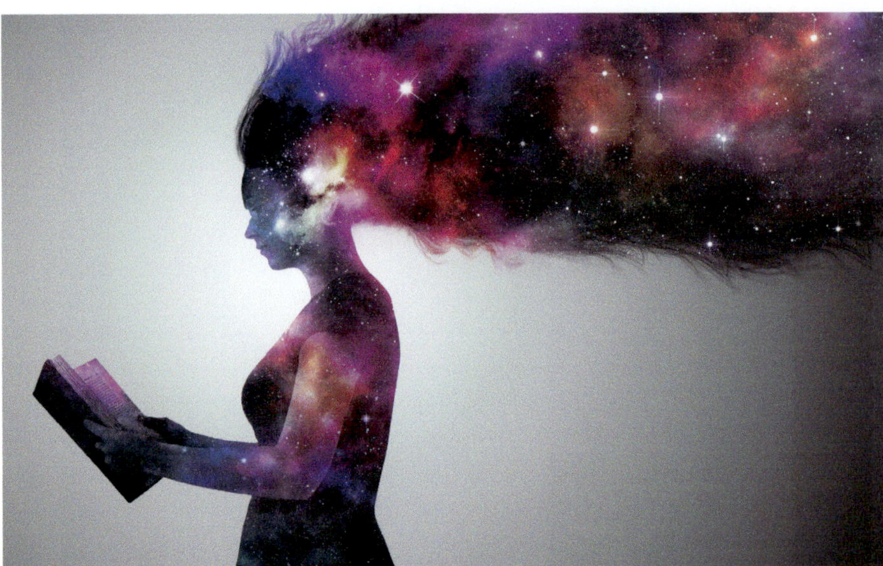

3.5
Noetic Attribute of Woman Reading Book with Cosmic Imagination

characteristics contributing to charged experiences that include enhanced perception when the senses are heightened. There is a sense of synchronicity and an extrasensory awareness. Transformation is a paradigm shift in one's worldview, behaviors, and attitudes.[26] A spiritual experience goes beyond the ordinary and can be mystical or euphoric, accompanied by an awareness of the presence of intuitive thoughts, a sense of ultimate peace and well-being, and a degree of surrender. Key to this transcendence is the ability to reduce temporal density and to become more present in experiences of the divine or the unknown. Transcendent experiences provide shifts with the small self or individual stress reduction and prosocial shifts with alignments greater than the self.[27] Spiritual experiences include the feeling of being one with others, a local place, and the larger world and are purpose-revealing, containing an element of transcendence and a sense of wonder. The design implications suggest going beyond the ordinary with designs that evoke meaning or tell a story and use space generosity and ineffable light.

Transcendent spaces embody certain qualities that help render them ineffable. The Oculus building, designed by Santiago Calatrava and opened in 2016, is a wonderful example of a public-spirited transcendent space with its soaring skyward, positive form and breathtaking, luminous interior (Figure 3.6). While it is such a dramatic space, it has a surprising feeling and sense of quiet and serenity. It embodies the concept for hope. Contributing to the transcendent experience is the flight-like exterior and lightness of form, the vertical emphasis of the naturally lit space, the luminous quality of light, the rhythmic ribbed structure, and, as illustrated in Figure 6.3b, the upward movement of the stair. The symbolism of the building as a dove taking flight suggests hope, peace, and transcendence. It functions as a transit hub, for it connects to 12 subway lines, and, further, can be symbolic as a portal, connections, and for movement. This is a remarkable expression of transcendence for a non-religious building type. Both images are luminous and

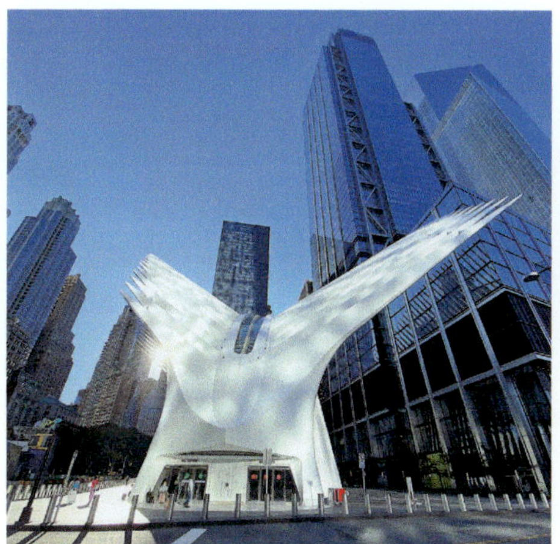
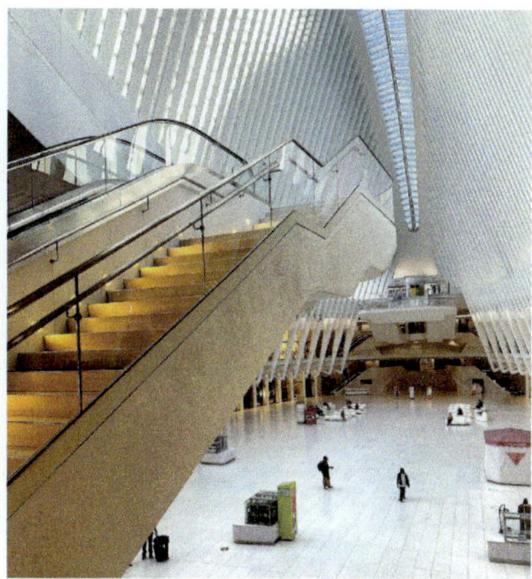

3.6
Transcendence Attribute: (a) Oculus Exterior, New York, (b) Oculus Interior, New York

inspiring, simultaneously representing a crossroads from across the world to a secular cathedral. And, to Carrie Meyer, it is a phoenix rising from the ashes of a post-9/11 world.[28]

Transcendent experiences often induce a sense of peace and calm, which can help alleviate stress and anxiety. Feelings of awe, wonder, and connection associated with transcendence can uplift moods and outlook on life. Transcendent experiences can foster a sense of connection with a higher power. This connection can provide comfort, guidance, and a sense of belonging in the universe. Experiencing transcendence can provide a sense of meaning and purpose in life, contributing to overall emotional well-being.[29] Further, it can provide experiences that are larger than ourselves. Transcendence can also cultivate prosocial and pro-environmental behaviors.

Attribute of the Unknown

The word "unknown" is derived from the Old English word "unġecnāwen," meaning not known or discovered. In early Greek philosophy, "the Wholly Other" was considered that which was immeasurable, and the use of sacred geometry helped transcend corporeal materiality.[30] Experiences of the "Wholly Other" evoke an alluring sense of the unknown, utter presence, pinnacle of self-inclusiveness, and completing with consecrative grace. Eric Weiner describes the Wholly Other as a dwelling place of the gods, and the realm of angels, ghosts, fairies, mythic creatures, and nature spirits.[31] The unknown can also be described as being mysterious, wonderous, uncertain, and paradoxical.

The unknown seems to possess a spiritual affinity, and its energy and presence are of an otherworldly, unknown, or divine source. The implications of the unknown generally do not have direct implications for design, yet they do emphasize open-endedness and future-oriented forms and materials. The unknown reflects design experiences that are ineffable or are full of light. Benefits might relieve the anxiety around the unknown or, in some cases, inspire positive experiences of the unknown. An image of the unknown is quite difficult

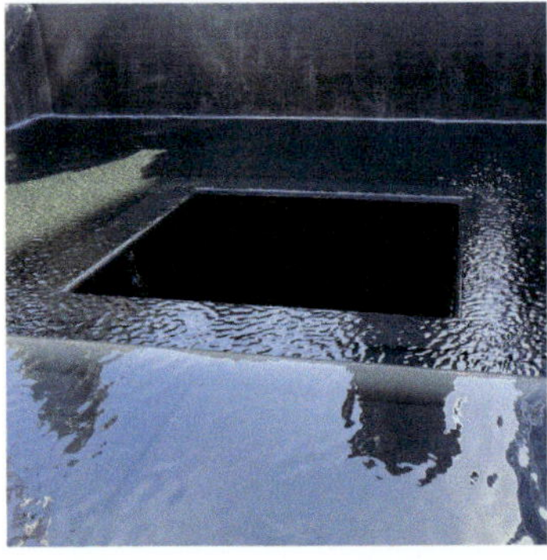

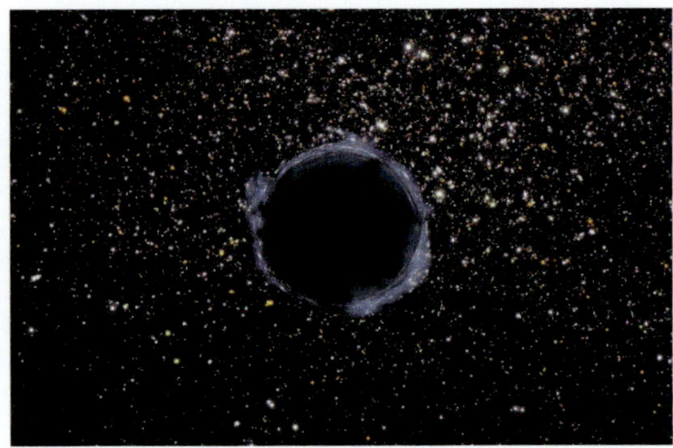

3.7 Unknown Attribute: (a) 9/11 Memorial Pool, New York, (b) Dying Star

to find; however, it can be depicted as something that is mysterious, unfathomable, ethereal, and vast, as in the 9/11 memorial pools "reflecting absence" (Figure 3.7a) or the image of a dying star and black hole taken by the James Webb Space Telescope (Figure 3.7b). Both images express an unfathomable unknown that creates an emotional stirring and spiritual provocation from within. Three characteristics describe the unknown:

1. **The divine or supernatural is unknowable** – we are incapable of fully knowing the mysteries of life or having explicit answers to our existential questions.
2. **Something beyond ourselves** – allows for focus on positive emotions, gratitude, acceptance, and peace. Rather than "larger than ourselves," as in purpose, mission, a commitment that goes beyond our human contrivances, the unknown is "beyond ourselves."
3. **Mysterious and uncertain** – there is an element of intrigue and mystery with a wide range of emotions.

The wellness and spiritual aspects of the unknown are mostly expressed through experiences that are profound, meaningful, and purposeful. There are no specific physical design characteristics of the unknown; however, otherworldly, ineffable architectural space can elicit spiritual wellness experiences. The wellness benefits are mental and emotional, can contribute to a sense of well-being and life satisfaction, and can elicit connections that are larger than ourselves. Stepping outside comfort zones and embracing uncertainty open us to new possibilities and perspectives. Additionally, experiences of the unknown lead to deeper understandings of ourselves and the larger world and can elicit profound spiritual growth.

Attribute of Unity Experience

Unity suggests we are not separate entities but rather interconnected threads in the grand tapestry of existence. Simply put, all diverse elements dissolve into a single unity. Oneness, wholeness, inclusiveness, completeness, and totality describe a state of interconnectedness and a sensation of abundance that transcend our individual selves. On a global sale, it is recognizing that we are all inhabitants of this planet, and that our actions have far-reaching consequences. As an experience, it becomes the simultaneity of cognitive unity, temporal unity, and spatial unity. Unity experience is an elegant way that reflects the universe and our concept(s) of a higher power. The unity experience seems to express in two ways, sometimes separately and sometimes simultaneously:[32]

1. **The division of unity** – where something whole divides and separates into harmonious and proportionally integrated parts.
2. **The creation of unity** – where parts relate and come together into a compressible whole, becoming increasingly more inclusive.

The design implications suggest the use of balance, harmony, cohesion, and comprehensiveness. As a design approach to building and urban planning, holistic design encompasses all aspects of the project and its impacts on the site and users, the embodied energy needed to create it, and the larger built and natural environments. Designs employ visual harmony, repetition, rhythms, proximity, and balance. Unity designs connect to the immediate surroundings as well as the larger cosmic context. Figure 3.8a shows migrating herd of zebra in the African savannah of the Serengeti, with the uniformity of their stripes. The stripes are intended to create an indivisibility and homogeneity, confusing predators and preventing them from identifying individual zebras. Not only is this an example of unity but also it is one showing an evolutionary process of de-materializing. The unity of purpose of more than 1.5 million animals migrating annually through Tanzania and Kenya, following seasonal rains, is recognized as one of the "Seven Wonders of the Natural World."[33] Unity expresses in many different ways in nature. This includes a clear night sky full of millions of stars, on a ship on open seas, or within a whiteout snowstorm. Figures 3.8b and 3.8c show animals believed to express the universe or cosmos – the turtle's back and the curvature of the elephant's trunk, back, and tail. The colorful thistle and the incredible 1970 Apollo 17 photograph of Planet Earth taken from our moon is the first image of our whole Earth and a symbol of a living unity. To Lionel Corbett, the unity or union experience occurs with the divine, in which there is no sense of a separate self, no distinction between oneself and others or between oneself and the world.[34]

Unity is also expressed within the urban environment where individual elements dissolve into a single cityscape, giving the place identity and a sense of unity. With each of these expressions of wholeness there is a sense of disillusioning of the parts into a singularity of experience. Figure 3.9 illustrates two urban examples where color is a unifying urban design element. Bodrum, in Turkey, has predominantly white buildings that wash the landscape uniformly, while Burano, in Italy, is uniform with its varied colored buildings. Unity in wellness design fosters a sense of harmony and cohesion, ultimately enhancing well-being by creating balanced, supportive, and intuitive environments.

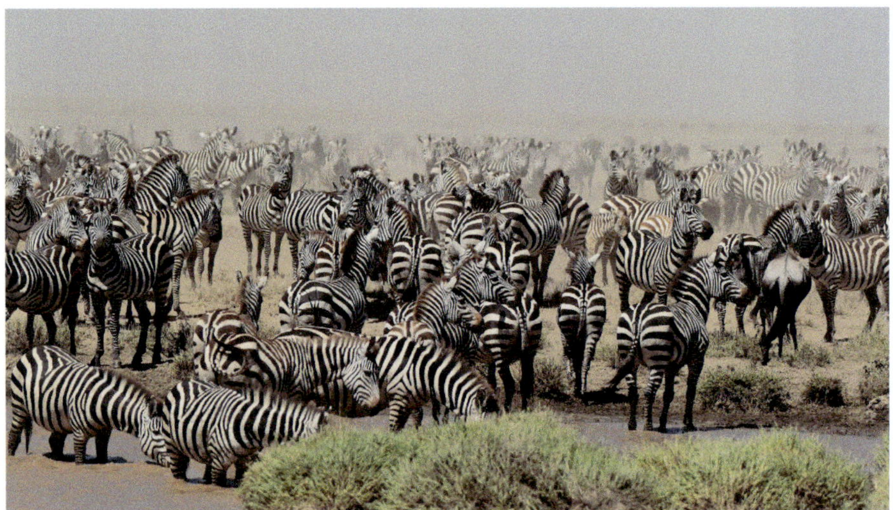

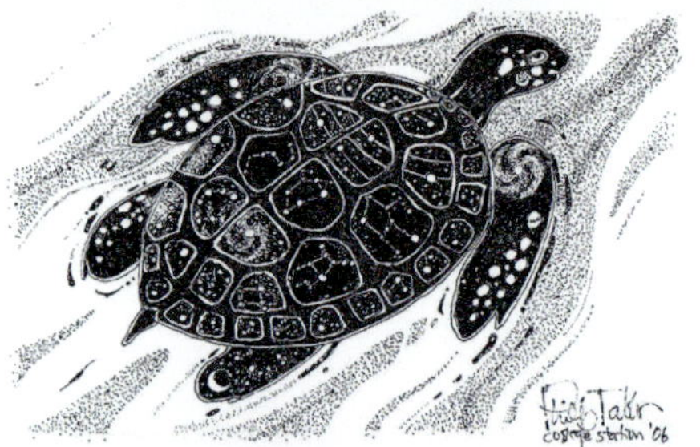

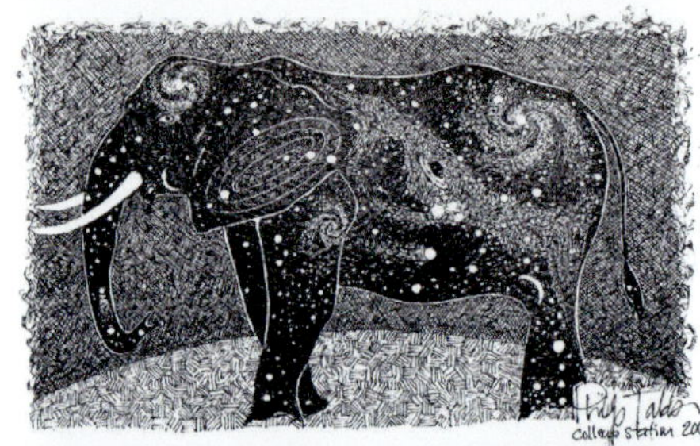

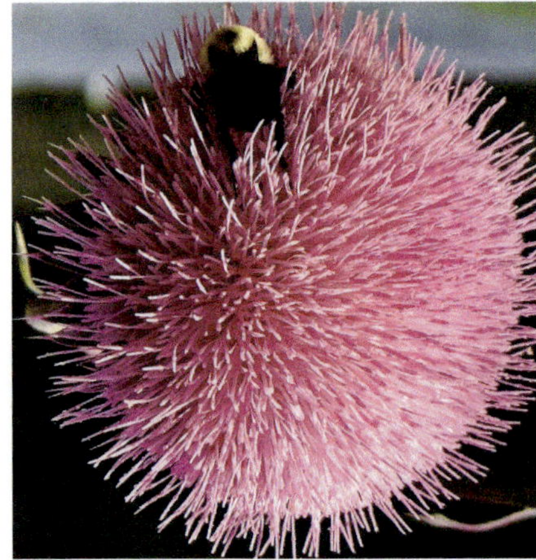

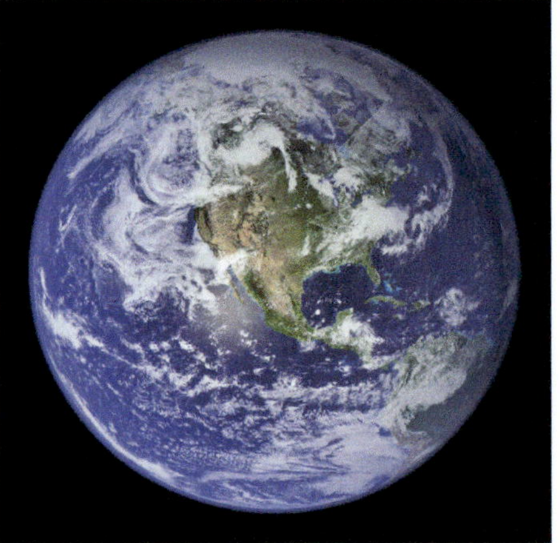

3.8
Unity Experience Attribute: (a) African ZebraintheSerengeti, (b) CosmicTurtle, (c) Cosmic Elephant, (d) SphericalThistle, (e) Planet Earth

SUMMARY

Spiritual wellness is an ongoing process of self-discovery and active participation shaping the deepest part of us, including our beliefs, values, feelings, behaviors, and lifestyle practices. The wellness benefits are in part achieved through design as the dimensions inform the design opportunities in the built environment. Many

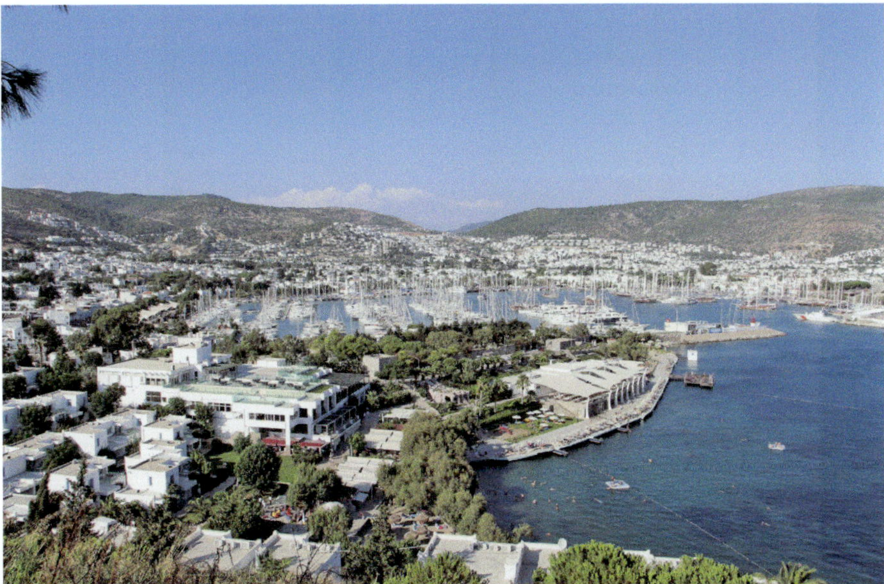

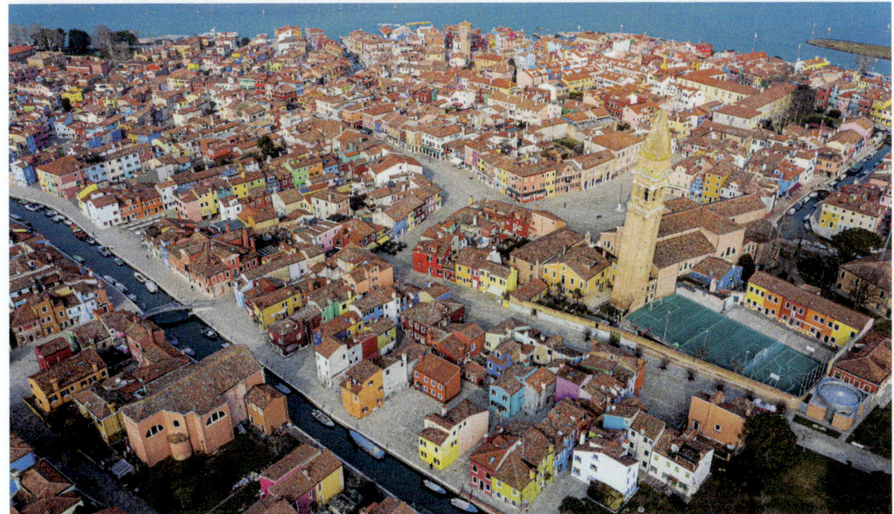

3.9
Urban Unity Experience: (a) Uniform White Buildings in Bodrum, Turkey, (b) Varied Colors with Complexity of Urban Space in Burano, Italy

of the attributes have a more direct impact upon design opportunities in the built environment. Some attributes have secondary effects on the environment, with attitudes, convictions, and sensibilities that may influence planning and design decisions. The place-oriented attributes have direct application to design at all scales. The experience-based attributes describe multiple connections to transcendent experiences and well-being. And the next chapter focuses on process attributes that occur over time and address more wholistic and deeper personal issues. These attributes derive directly from definitions and research and reflect a broad view of spiritual wellness.

NOTES

1 Gesler, Wilber M., *Healing Places* (Lanham, MD: Rowman & Littlefield, 2003).
2 Casement, Ann, & David Tacey, Eds., *The Idea of the Numinous: Contemporary Jungian and Psychoanalytic Perspectives* (London, UK: Routledge, 2006), pp. 53–54. James, William, *The Varieties of Religious Experience* (Whitefish, MT: Kessinger, 1902), pp. 288–290.
3 Wikipedia, Numinous (accessed July 10, 2022), https://en.wikipedia.org/wiki/Numinous.
4 Spitzer, Robert, Rudolf Otto's 'Mysterium Tremendum et Fascinans' of the Numinous Experience (accessed September 12, 2022), https://blog.magiscenter.com/blog/rudolf-ottos-mysterium-tremendum-et-fascinans-in-our-experience-of-the-numen.
5 National Institutes of Health, Suffering a Healthy Life – On the Existential Dimension of Health (accessed September 24, 2023), https://www.ncbi.nlm.nih.gov/pmc/articles/PMC8830493/.
6 James, William, *The Varieties of Religious Experience: A Study of Human Nature* (Cambridge, MA: Harvard University Press, 1985).
7 Plato (Translator Benjamin Jowell), *The Republic*, Book VII (Heritage Press, 1944).
8 Yaden, D.B., S.B. Kaufman, E. Hyde, A. Chirico, A. Gaggioli, J.W. Zhang, & D. Keltner, The Development of the Awe Experience Scale (AWE-S): A Multifactorial Measure for a Complex Emotion (accessed October 4, 2021), https://psycnet.apa.org/record/2018-35661-001.
9 Allen, Summer, The Science of Awe (accessed August, 20, 2024), https://ggsc.berkeley.edu/images/uploads/GGSC-JTF_White_Paper-Awe_FINAL.pdf.
10 Keltner, Dasher, & Jonathan Haidt, Approaching Awe, a Moral, Spiritual, and Aesthetic Emotion (accessed October 10, 2022), https://www.tandfonline.com/doi/abs/10.1080/02699930302297.
11 Roberts, K., and T. Messenger, Helping Older Adults Find Serenity, *Geriatric Nursing*, 14(6), 1993, p. 14. Roberts, Kay, & Cheryl Aspy, Development of the Serenity Scale. *Journal of Nursing Measurement*, 1(2), 1993, pp. 155–156.
12 Tabb, Phillip James, *Thin Place Design: Architecture of the Numinous* (New York, NY: Routledge, 2024).
13 Roberts, Kay, & Cheryl Aspy, Development of a Serenity Scale. *Journal of Nursing Measurement*, 1(2), 1993 (accessed August 20, 2022), https://www.researchgate.net/publication/15347724_Development_of_the_Serenity_Scale.
14 Roberts, Kay, & Cheryl Aspy, Development of a Serenity Scale. *Journal of Nursing Measurement*, 1(2), 1993 (accessed August 20, 2022), https://www.researchgate.net/publication/15347724_Development_of_the_Serenity_Scale.
15 Cherim, Denis, Coincident Project (accessed July 20, 2024), https://denischerim.com/coincidenceproject.
16 Main, Rodrick, Ed., Synchronicity, in *Jung on Synchronicity and the Paranormal* (London, UK: Taylor & Francis, 1951), pp. 91–98.
17 Main, Roderick, *The Rupture of Time* (New York, NY: Routledge, 2004), p. 39.
18 Klisanin, Dana, Synchronicity: Enhance Well-Being via Meaningful Coincidences (accessed July 12, 2024), https://www.psychologytoday.com/us/blog/digital-altruism/202306/synchronicity-enhance-well-being-via-meaningful-coincidences.
19 Klisanin, Dana, Synchronicity: Enhance Well-Being via Meaningful Coincidences (accessed September 9, 2024), https://www.psychologytoday.com/us/blog/digital-altruism/202306/synchronicity-enhance-well-being-via-meaningful-coincidences.
20 Main, Rodrick, Ed., Synchronicity, in *Jung on Synchronicity and the Paranormal* (London, UK: Taylor & Francis, 1951), p. 30.
21 James, William, *The Varieties of Religious Experience* (Whitefish, MT: Kessinger, 1902).
22 Helané Wahbeh, C. Vieten, G. Young, A. Cartry-Jacobsen, D. Radin, & A. Delorme, Transformative, Noetic, and Transpersonal Experiences during Personal Development Workshops (accessed July 3, 2024), https://digitalcommons.ciis.edu/cgi/viewcontent.cgi?article=1046&context=advance-archive.

23 Otto, Rudolf, *The Idea of the Holy* (Oxford, UK: Oxford University Press, 1958), p. 67.
24 Helané Wahbeh, C. Vieten, G. Young, A. Cartry-Jacobsen, D. Radin, and A. Delorme, Transformative, Noetic, and Transpersonal Experiences during Personal Development Workshops (accessed July 3, 2024), https://digitalcommons.ciis.edu/cgi/viewcontent.cgi?article=1046&context=advance-archive.
25 AI, Noetics and Wellness (accessed October 20, 2024), https://gemini.google.com/app?utm_source=google&utm_medium=cpc&utm_campaign=2024enUS_gemfeb&gad_source=1&gbraid=0AAAAApk5BhkQNuoamgSl4z7edozMTntMM&gclid=Cj0KCQjwj4K5BhDYARIsAD1Ly2q10hVNv0dtquwleekhJXcQ0B4TmZVYKYA5TxcPIRFp9kZ7mBXF3eMaAgIIEALw_wcB&gclsrc=aw.ds.
26 Neal, J.A., B.M. Bergmann Lichtenstein, & D. Banner, Spiritual Perspectives on Individual, Organizational and Societal Transformation. *Journal of Organizational Change Management,* 1999, pp. 175–186. *OECD Guidelines on Measuring Subjective Well-being* (Paris: OECD, 2013).
27 Transcendence and Wellbeing (accessed September 24, 2023), https://www.mybestself101.org/transcendence-well-being.
28 Meyer, Carrie, A Phoenix Rising from the Ashes: The Oculus and the 911 Memorial (accessed July 20, 2024), https://www.carriemyers.blog/2017/07/05/a-pheonix-rising-from-the-ashes-the-oculus-and-the-911-memorial/.
29 AI, Transcendence and Wellness (accessed October 20, 2024), https://gemini.google.com/app?utm_source=google&utm_medium=cpc&utm_campaign=2024enUS_gemfeb&gad_source=1&gbraid=0AAAAApk5BhkQNuoamgSl4z7edozMTntMM&gclid=Cj0KCQjwj4K5BhDYARIsAD1Ly2q10hVNv0dtquwleekhJXcQ0B4TmZVYKYA5TxcPIRFp9kZ7mBXF3eMaAgIIEALw_wcB&gclsrc=aw.ds.
30 LYNN, The Vast Immeasurable Dimensions of God's Love (accessed November 10, 2022), https://www.tickledpinklife.com/2014/01/the-vast-immeasurable-dimensions-of-gods-love/.
31 Weiner, Eric, Where Heaven and Earth Come Closer (accessed June 30, 2024), https://www.nytimes.com/2012/03/11/travel/thin-places-where-we-are-jolted-out-of-old-ways-of-seeing-the-world.html.
32 Tabb, Phillip James, *Thin Place Design: Architecture of the Numinous* (New York, NY: Routledge, 2024). p. 62.
33 Seven Wonders, Serengeti Migration (accessed July 20, 2024), https://sevenwonders.org/serengeti-migration/.
34 Corbett, Lionel, *The Sacred Cauldron: Psychotherapy as a Spiritual Practice* (Ashville, NC: Chiron, 2015), p. 59.

4 PRACTICE- AND PROCESS-BASED ATTRIBUTES OF SPIRITUAL WELLNESS

INTRODUCTION

In what ways can planning and design solutions contribute to human and environmental health and wellness? Health and wellness benefit both human beings and the environments they inhabit and include both natural and built places. Human-centered benefits are directed to the dimensions of wellness, including our physical bodies, mental health, emotional well-being, social connections, and spiritual growth, as seen with illness and joy. Financial health is also seen as a wellness benefit. The environmental-centered benefits are directed to the natural environment around us and the cities and buildings we occupy, as experienced with clean air and water. The contrast between these two environmental conditions is obvious – one is polluted, and the other is endowed with clean resources. Wellness is an everyday process and is inextricably linked to the places where we exist.[1] The places in which we live, work, shop, recreate, dine, worship, and otherwise occupy are the contexts within which we interact and function, and, if these places are healthy places, there is a greater chance of achieving wellness.

PROCESS-BASED ATTRIBUTES AND OUTCOMES

Lifestyles are based on tangible and intangible factors of individuals and groups. These factors are process-oriented and are evidenced in actions, living behaviors, habits, and styles of living. They reflect values, attitudes, cultures, and worldviews. Importantly, for them to become wellness lifestyles means one makes balanced, holistic, and purposeful choices. There is a difference between experience-based and process-based attributes of wellness. Experiences tend to be personal and subjective, while processes are more objective, measurable, and sequential. However, in the context of spiritual wellness, processes are experiences that evolve over time. Processes attend to healthy places and experiences over time and include intentional well-being and spiritual practices. According to Halbert Dunn, there is not necessarily an optimum level of wellness that can be attained, but rather wellness is a direction in progress.[2] Another important concept related to wellness processes is that of integration, meaning for whole health, and it requires a balance of all the attributes and prevention processes.[3] This is to suggest that high-level wellness is not a static state, but rather it is a process, a direction, and progress toward whole spiritual wellness. A summary list of practice- and process-based attributes follows:

DOI: 10.4324/9781003546085-4

1. **Presence and mindfulness** – the state of being physically connected, without distractions, and consciously (mindfully) aware.
2. **Overcoming existential issues** – when we cope with difficult times, transitions, or situations relating to meaning and purpose in life, choice, death, illnesses, and freedom in life.
3. **Connections greater than ourselves** – efforts infused with passion and purpose creating interest, curiosity, exploration, awakening, and perspective for the greater good.
4. **Intentionality** – focus on an object, affirmation, or outcome, setting specific goals for wellness, spiritual renewal, and self-healing, and being aware of thoughts, decisions, and actions.
5. **Ethical and moral practices** – values, attitudes, and actions with integrity, honesty, fairness, respect, accountability, justice, and transparency.
6. **Purpose and life meaning** – awareness and focus of spiritual wellness practices that include mindful processes, cultivation of values, and intentional actions.
7. **Life satisfaction** – a consequence of dedication to something greater than the self, living aligned to core values, practicing gratitude, and seeking ultimate meaning.
8. **High-level wellness** – behaviors and lifestyle processes that go beyond physical health and incorporate all aspects of well-being.

Attribute of Mindfulness and Presence

Mindfulness is a practice and a way of settling into the present moment. It encompasses attention, awareness, acceptance, and being present and includes being grounded or centered without judgment. Presence also means the awareness of the moment, one's personal space, or one's immediate vicinity. It is what we feel, notice, and think and what is happening around us. Centering usually refers to our mental and physical state of mind. Centering meditation is one of the many techniques that has been scientifically proven to relieve symptoms of stress and anxiety while increasing mindfulness. Centering often involves breathing and meditation exercises. Grounding or "earthing" is an immersive process involving deep connections to the ground. Being grounded also means that we are more mindful of respect for our environment.

To Peter Zumthor, implications of mindfulness and presence suggest designing with no comment or meaning but pure construction.[4] Mindful designs promote focus, awareness, and calm, often with connections to nature, soothing colors, multisensory experiences, and designated sanctuary spaces and beautiful sacred spaces. Studies show benefits include improving cognitive ability, reducing stress, achieving emotional balance, and improving life quality. Mindfulness and presence in the moment have positive health and wellness benefits including reduced stress, anxiety, and depression; improved emotional regulation; increased self-awareness; and enhanced cognitive function and attention span. Mindfulness enhances the ability to cope with illness and helps facilitates recovery.[5] It further can reduce negative thinking and distractions and can help with improving emotional regulation. Mindfulness is also related to increase resilience and improved relationships.

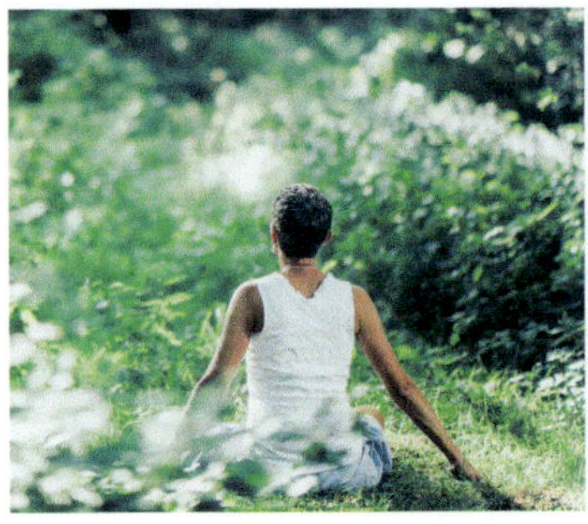

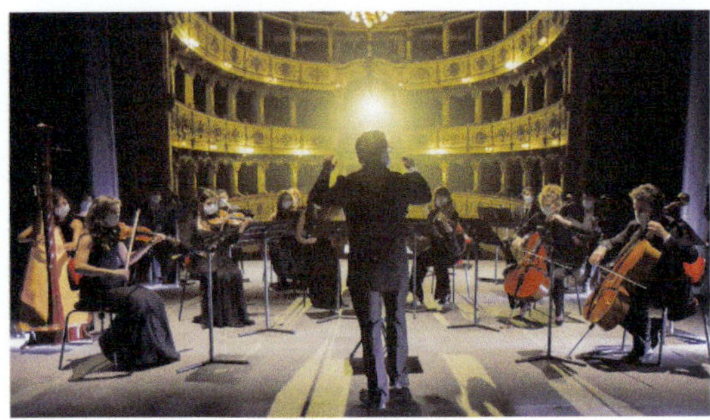

4.1
Mindfulness and Presence: (a) Meditation in Nature, (b) Focus on Conductor by Symphony Orchestra

The spiritual connections include experiences of self-reflection, gratitude, and inner peace; understanding of life purpose; and living in the present moment. Being present can lead to the spiritual wellness experience of things greater than ourselves. They can be experienced in everyday occurrences as well as special processes and events. Meditation, forest bathing, mindful breathwork, activating all the senses, visualization techniques, and reducing temporal density can contribute to the positive spiritual benefits of mindfulness. Figure 4.1a illustrates mindfulness practiced while taking in sounds and fragrances found in nature and simply being present with all the senses activated. Further, mindfulness can help focus attention, such as when performing in a symphonic production, as in Figure 4.1b. This singular performance demonstrates the orchestra's focus on the conductor while the audience focuses on the performance. These images suggest that context and focused attention influence the process of spiritual wellness. In architecture and urban design, there can be a sense of presence that motivates us emotionally and can heighten our everyday experience of living.[6] Thus, this notion of embodied presence is a prime objective of spiritual wellness in architecture and urban planning.

Attribute of Coping with Existential Issues

Spiritual and existential issues are important factors for well-being as well as factors influencing meaning in life and hope or positive emotions.[7] Spiritual experiences can produce opportunities that address perplexing and existential issues in an ensemble of feelings in finding meaning while experiencing pain, physical and psychological limitations, and needs frustration. Questions such as "What is the meaning of life?" or "Is there life after death?" express existential concerns with fear and death, identity and meaning, emptiness and isolation, the unknown, and freedom.[8] According to Koole, Geenberg, and Psyzezynske in 2006, there are five major existential concerns. They are death, isolation, identity, freedom, and meaning.[9] The existential concern for death is the innate anxiety of this knowledge and human reaction to reminders of mortality. Isolation involves disassociation and limited contact with other beings, and social isolation particularly occurs in significant relationships. Existential loneliness affects purpose in life and relates to depression. Lack of identity, freedom, and meaning creates loss of motivation and hope and leads to failing to embrace potentialities. Other existential issues include physical health, financial wellness, and guilt.

Perplexing moments can be filled with difficulty, confusion, and uncertainty, as well as when we deal with issues such as life changes or the climate crisis.

According to the National Institutes of Health, we become aware of the existential dimension of health during times of illness.[10] Places of sanctuary, contemplation, caring, and healing can help ease the anxiety and stress accompanying challenging moments. Existential issues are concerns that arise from distress or questions about difficult subjects, such as death, meaning, freedom, and isolation, and as such do not have direct implications for design. However, design experiences that inspire, are ineffable, or are full of light might relieve the anxiety around these questions.

Such experiences contribute to spiritual wellness by helping people to connect with others, nature, or their own creative abilities. Furthermore, spiritual wellness has the capability to empower one's choices and decisions in a way that such decisions become easier and, more importantly, makes one grounded during phases of change or adversity. Such groundedness enables one to progress resiliently, peacefully, and gracefully.[11]

Spiritual wellness can reverse existential crises and can be a catalyst for understanding, change, and growth. This can be triggered by everyday events such as a walk in the woods or along a beach, working in a garden, enjoying the company of friends, or engaging in physical activity. The image in Figure 4.2a illustrates the fear of death or of chronic illness. Figure 4.2b illustrates a person who appears to be isolated or lonely. And Figure 4.2c illustrates a person seemingly experiencing poverty. Spiritual wellness is effective through coping with existential issues that positively impact the lessening of anxiety, depression, loss of purpose, physical health, and isolation from family, friends, and community. Spirituality can provide

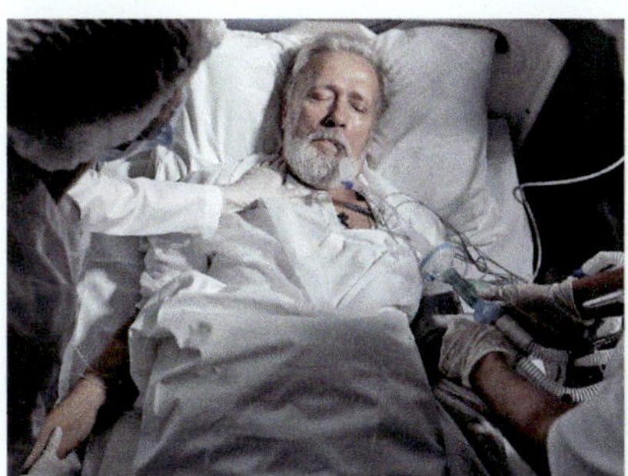

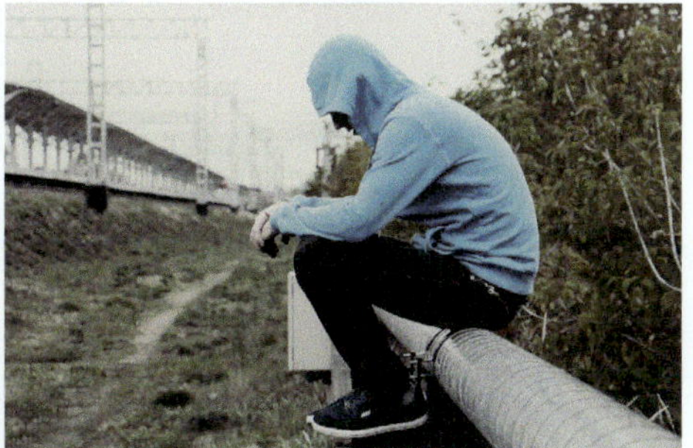

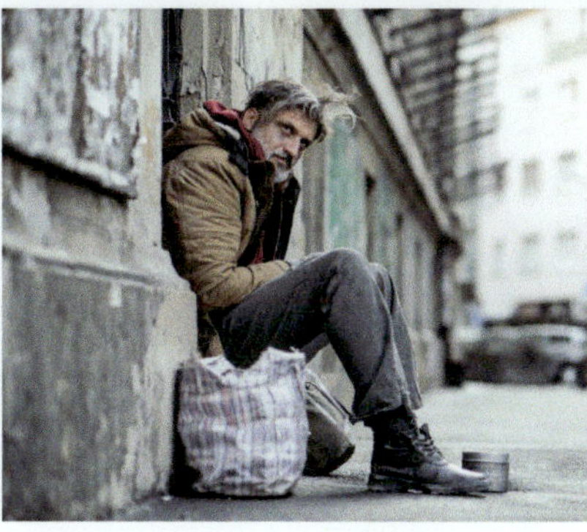

4.2 Existential Issues: (a) Chronic Illness, (b) Feeling Lonely, (c) Experiencing Poverty

processes for understanding and coping with life's big questions, offering a sense of meaning, purpose, and connection.

Attribute of Connections to Things Greater than Ourselves

Going beyond personal contrivances, levels of comfort, making mistakes, personal distractions, and risklessness is considered selfless behavior. This includes even going beyond reciprocal altruism, with its give-and-take relationship. Spiritual altruism or moral altruism involves helping others when it is risky and without reward. Such benevolence and wellness behaviors and lifestyle practices can expand our viewpoints and lifestyle activities. The emotion of "elevation" appears to inspire altruism and, in the context of the built environment, could reference acts of heroic design. Common among things larger than ourselves are our sense of the universe, a high, towering mountain, the vastness of the ocean, a large group of people, or even our families. Huge buildings and vast cities are also larger than ourselves. Extraordinary people and works of art can appear elevated. Furthermore, powerful spiritual, philosophical, or poetic ideas can also appear larger than ourselves. Characteristics such as size, vastness, and perspective contribute to a diminished self-importance and an increase in prosocial and pro-environmental behaviors.[12] This attribute is central to spiritual wellness.

The attribute of connection to things greater than ourselves is generally elicited by two factors. The first is the nature of awe experiences. According to Keltner and Haidt, awe is an emotional response to perceptually vast stimuli that transcend current frames of reference.[13] Further, their definition includes what they call the need for accommodation. Moreover, accommodation is common among emotional responses associated with spiritual experiences; it is the process of adjusting or making sense out of pre-existing mental structures that were unable to be assimilated in current awe experiences. The experiences challenge our concept of ourselves and the world around us through awe-inspiring emotions that require us to adjust our cognitive schema to accommodate them. According to Murray Stein, the crossing back and forth between ordinary and extraordinary experiences is where links or insights can lead to deeper perspectives on life through the transfer from one state (the spiritual) to another (the secular).[14]

The second factor that elicits a sense of connection to things greater than ourselves is the scale of the place, from large, impressive buildings and cities to vast landscapes and night skies. By contrast, these places, while inspiring, diminish the sense of self. One can feel so small in comparison with these cityscapes. This self-diminishment is not a source of low self-esteem but rather a process of perspective and transcendence. It is an understanding of the grandeur of many of the places we experience and our relationship to them.

The design implications take on many forms, including planning and design works that are client- and public-centered, socially conscious, aware, and just. They include those with spatial generosity, those eliciting awe, and designs with universal designs and an outward focus to others and the environment. Often unique, spectacular, or even unusual examples of architecture can elicit a small-self

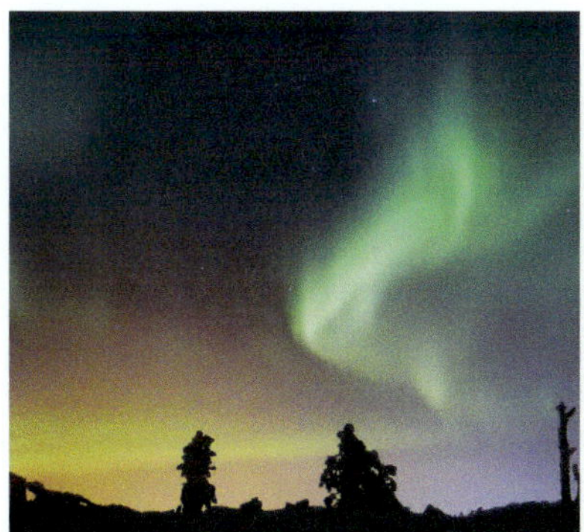
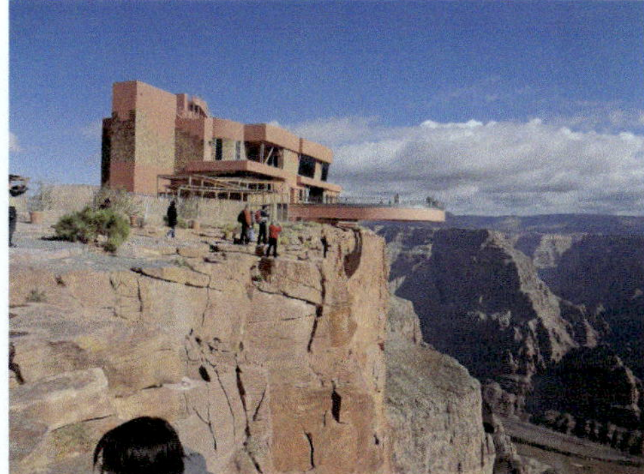
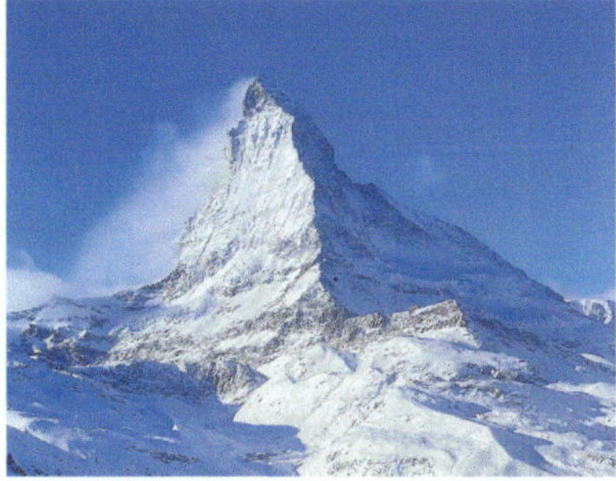
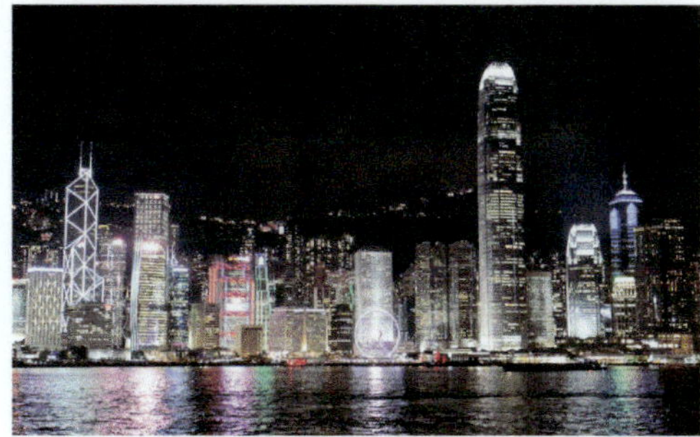

4.3 Connections Greater than Ourselves: (a) Northern Lights, (b) Grand Canyon West Skywalk, (c) the Matterhorn, Switzerland, (d) Hong Kong Cityscape

perspective. The images in Figure 4.3 illustrate varying scales of vastness that prompt connections with things larger than ourselves. Flying over the coastline of Iceland, experiencing the skywalk precariously hovering over the Grand Canyon, or taking a train in the Swiss mountains all give us a perspective of vastness or something unusual. Even large cityscapes, such as Hong Kong, are inspiring and often overwhelming (Figure 4.3d). The spiritual wellness outcomes of connections greater than ourselves include physical benefits of reduced stress, greater resilience, an increased sense of belonging, and prosocial and pro-environmental behaviors. These are positive relationships between ourselves and the places we inhabit, our social networks, and the natural and physical environments.

Attribute of Intentionality

Intentionality involves the projection of awareness, with purpose and efficacy, toward some object or outcome, such as wellness and self-healing. Intentionality involves setting specific goals, affirmations, and designs toward improved well-being, including increased effectiveness, self-awareness, and gratitude practice. It is about making conscious choices and efforts of being aware of thoughts, decisions, and actions. The spiritual nature of intentionality informs one's spiritual journey. Our spiritual journey, in part, can be facilitated by our curating our personal sacred place, creating spiritual wellness routines, daily journaling, and having time for regular reflection. Living a life of intention helps us realize that we have control over where our lives go and who we become. The spiritual wellness attribute of intentionality is linked to purpose in life and life satisfaction. Further, service to others plays an important role in spiritual wellness intentionality.

Intentionality involves goals particularly directed toward high-level activities. Intention toward right livelihood involves behaviors and lifestyle choices that involve work that is ethical and does not harm others and foster growth through each of the wellness pillars, including spiritual wellness. Since this is a process-based dimension, it suggests a strong connection to stewardship and the goal of high-level wellness. In Wayne W. Dyer's book *The Power of Intention* (first published in 2004), he explores intention not as something you do but as energy of which you are a part.[15] Bruce Lipton posits that a large percentage of physical health is determined not by genetics but by our beliefs about life and our stress levels, suggesting that intention can influence beliefs.[16] Goal and objective setting, creation of positive affirmations, visualization, and self-inquiry facilitate this attribute. Intentionality, like a compass, guides these affirmations into positive action and, like a lodestar, such as the North Star, guides us in the right direction.

Figures 4.4a and 4.4b illustrate the intentionality associated with the Palio race in Siena, Italy, or that of planting a tree. Both suggest having focused attention, being deliberate, and cultivating a sense of purpose. A by-product of this is reduced stress, increased productivity, increased presence, and improved relationships. Two ends of spiritual wellness intentionality are positive affirmations that reinforce spiritual beliefs and intentions, and gratitude practice, fostering a sense of abundance and contentment. Attending wellness and spiritual retreats is another example of intentionality. Nestled on the banks of the Ayung River, Fivelements Retreat Bali is an award-winning eco-conscious wellness retreat deeply rooted in the ancient

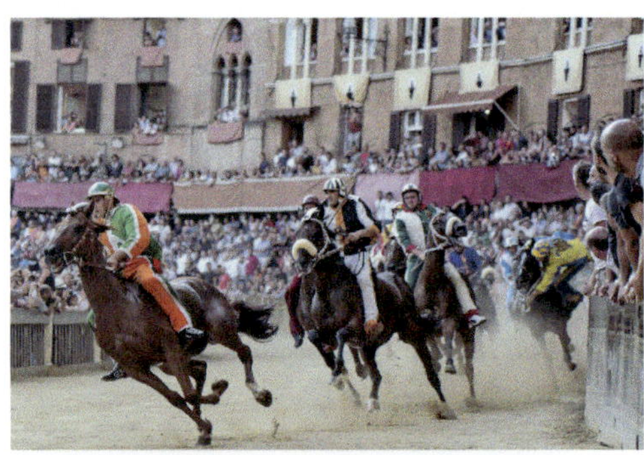
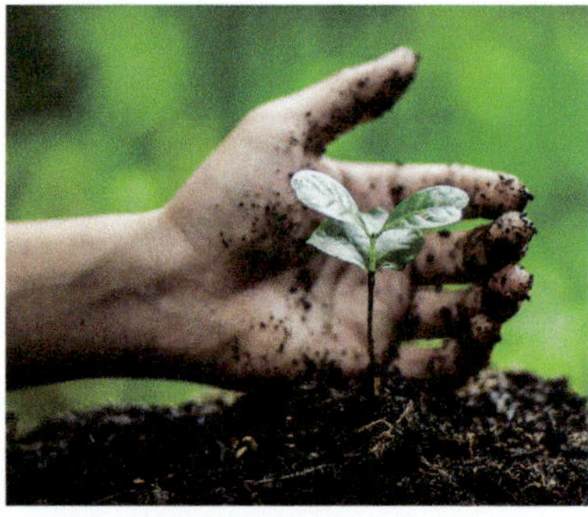
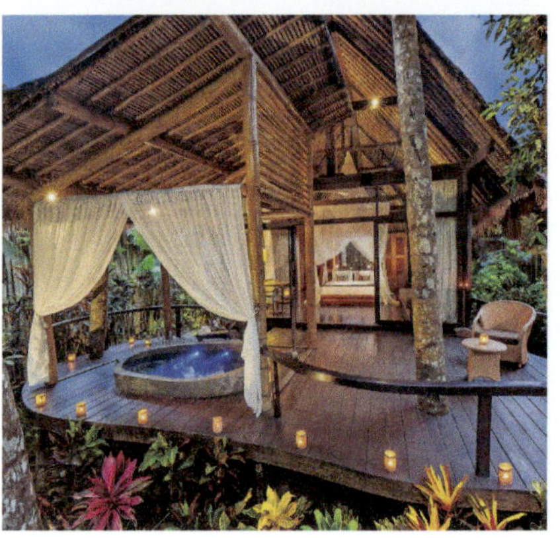
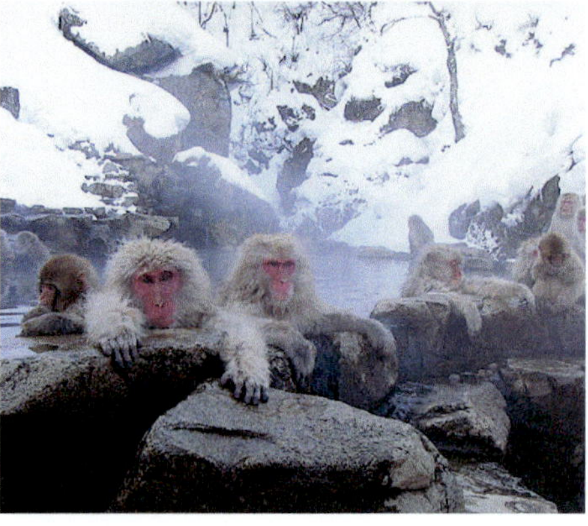

4.4
Spiritual Wellness Intentionality: (a) the Palio Race, Siena, Italy, (b) Planting a Small Tree, (c) Fivelements Retreat Bali, (d) Nagano, Japan, Hot Springs

traditions of Bali. It is a peaceful, rejuvenating sanctuary in which to embrace authentic Balinese healing and wellness rituals, regenerative plant-based cuisine, and transformative sacred arts practices (Figure 4.4c). The Jigokudani hot springs in Nagano, Japan, are an example of wellness hot springs and spas that facilitate healing even for wild snow monkeys, as in Figure 4.4d. The ultimate attribute of intentionality is actualizing spiritual experiences and high-level wellness within our lifestyle choices and the places within which they occur.

Attribute of Ethical and Moral Practices

Ethics and morals are values, attitudes, and actions with integrity, honesty, fairness, respect, accountability, justice, and transparency. Living with purpose and aligning positively with the larger world often result in honesty and accountability. The wellness benefits of ethical and moral behavior include increased self-esteem, greater sense of purpose, improved relationships, and reduced stress. In the built environment, this means designing with integrity, authenticity, and transparency; user focus and public input; universal design; and functional considerations such as safety, privacy, accessibility, usability, and affordability. In addition, ethical design considers the well-being of all people throughout the planning and design processes. Ethical design goes beyond personal beliefs, considering a framework of collective wellness principles, while moral design focuses on values, such as designing for inclusivity, sustainability, responsibility, justice and social equity, and beneficence. Further, ethical design is a harmonious blend of aesthetics, functionality, and well-being.[17]

Ethical principles and moral values influencing design do not necessarily generate specific design languages or urban forms; however, they do possess certain characteristics. Transparency suggests how products, buildings, and urban design should function. Privacy and security are important safeguards. Considering the broader social impacts of planning and architectural solutions should include the effects of economic inequality, political polarization, or environmental harm that can result from the designs.

Specific examples are difficult to cite because many building types and urban settings are designed specifically for protection, isolation, or control, such as penitentiaries, hospitals, or corporate research laboratories. However, some examples better illustrate the ethical and moral design principles. At the planning scale, the town center is made up of shops, offices, housing, and the public domain, which are interwoven to create a communal "home" where people feel welcome. Designed in 2018, the Oodi Helsinki Central Library has a friendly entrance; peaceful open-plan reading room on the upper floor that has been nicknamed "book heaven"; and facilities including a café, restaurant, public balcony, movie theatre, audio-visual recording studios, and a makerspace. The building is accessible and transparent, offering many choices, with light-filled spaces (Figure 4.5a). Another ethical issue involves solar access for projects that want to utilize solar energy. Solar access means that adjacent buildings cannot cast shadows on the solar collector surfaces of a building (south façade and roof). Finally, it is ethical for buildings to accommodate universal design standards for all users, especially those with disabilities.

The Singapore Park Connector Network (PCN) ties together six loops with a network of jogging, cycling, skating, and walking pathways. It is a linear urban network capable of utilizing existing greenery, improving conservation, offering recreation space and habitat for wildlife, providing greater access and linkages to other urban districts, and contributing to a stronger sense of place (Figure 4.5b). What makes it an ethical plan is its accessibility, inclusiveness, and regenerative principles that reach large percentages of Singapore's population. The benefits include physical, mental, social, and environmental wellness. While the PCN is not intentionally spiritual, it does support immersive connections to nature, peaceful activities, and respect for residents and visitors to the park network. The ethical principles of Singapore's PCN are expressed through stewardship of the land, mindfulness, and respect for all living things.

Ethics in architecture also extends to form–function relationships, structural integrity, and honesty of material use. Each requires clarity, honesty, and goodness, resulting in public safety and well-being. This is to suggest that a building's form should honestly reflect its function and not confuse or mislead. The expression of and design for structural integrity support confidence and safety. Material honesty is the idea that a building's material or substance should be sincere and true to itself, rather than mimic something else. Place types that lend themselves to ethical and moral practices include public parks, affordable housing, housing for the poor, sanctuary camps, community centers, and designs for buildings used by people with disabilities. Habitat for Humanity illustrates ethical architecture at an international scale. It is a nonprofit organization founded in 1976 that helps families and communities with affordable housing. The organization operates in more than 70 countries. Habitat for Humanity builds new homes and improves existing homes for families with limited resources and the need for housing. This is accomplished through volunteer labor, including that of Habitat homeowners through the practice of sweat equity, as well as paid contractors for certain construction or infrastructure activities.

Ethical design in the form of affordable housing can be found in post-Katrina housing, Habitat for Humanity, and Copenhagen floating affordable housing (Figures 4.5a–4.5c). The original Sandy Hook Elementary School building in Newtown, Connecticut, is an example of the ethical values of a community. The original school was torn down after the tragic mass shooting that occurred on December 14, 2012. The redesign features a winding entrance tucked away from the main road, myriad surveillance cameras, and floor-to-ceiling windows. While some critics think the large amount of natural light is distracting, the school feels the openness benefits students and can even boost performance. The school's roof is shaped like an undulating wave to blend in with the landscape, as well as to replicate the hills of the Newtown region. Svigals + Partners, architects for the project, designed the school so it does not look like a security fortress but rather a friendly, inviting place for students. The building is a symbol of the enduring spirit of the community and expresses the ethical values of a caring community while also being designed to meet the security needs of the students and teachers. The new school opened in 2016. These project examples illustrate

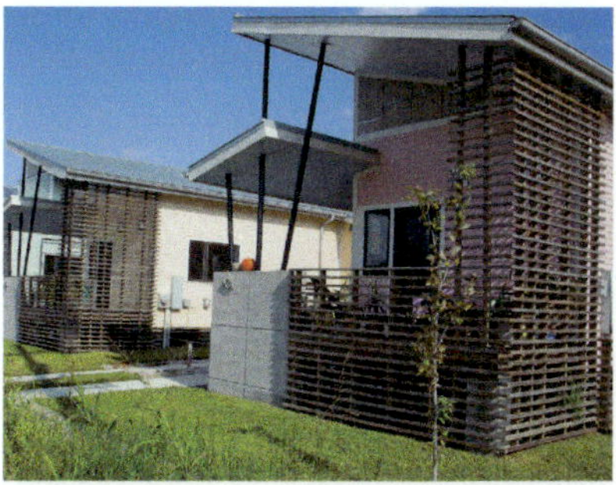
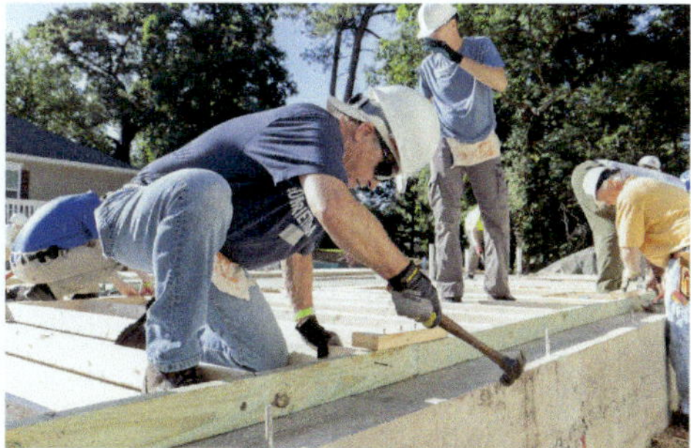
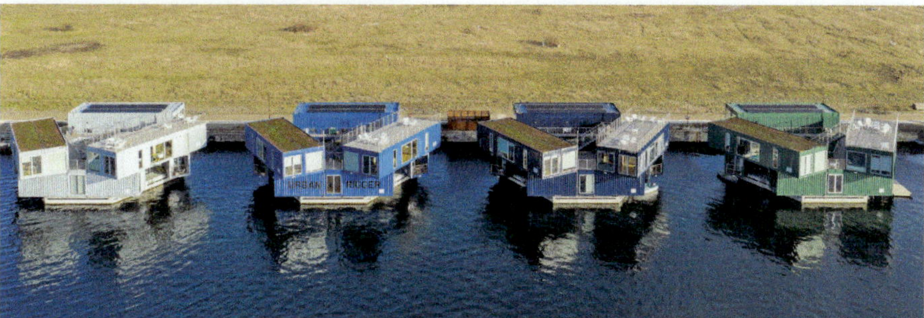
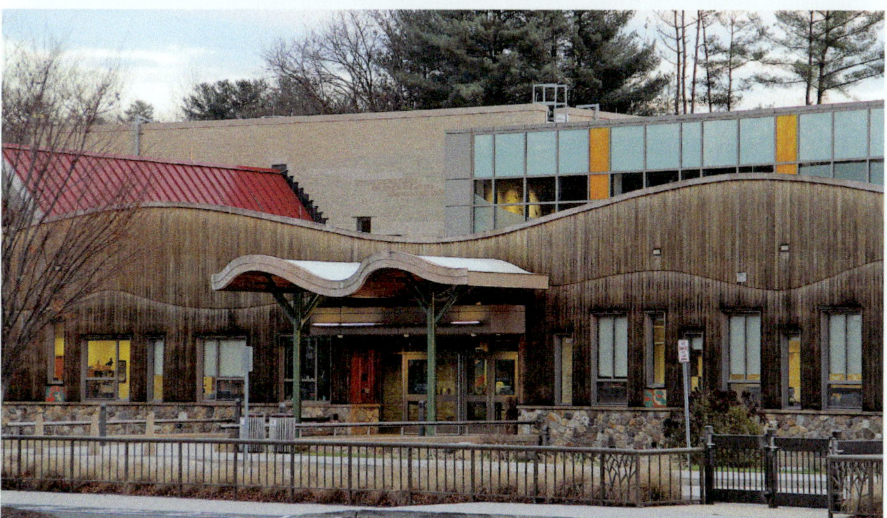

4.5 Ethics and Morals: (a) Post-Katrina Housing, New Orleans, (b) Habitat for Humanity, (c) Copenhagen Floating Affordable Housing, (d) Sandy Hook High School, Connecticut

many attributes of spiritual wellness. Refer to Figure 4.5 for examples of ethical architecture.

Attribute of Purpose and Meaning in Life

Purpose and life meaning affect each of the wellness pillars of physical, mental, emotional, social, financial, and environmental well-being. Spiritual wellness is also affected and influenced by positive goal setting, life direction, and increased life motivation. Meaning in life can be viewed from certain angles: comprehension/coherence, purpose, and mattering/significance.[18] Direction in life suggests setting goals, exploration, and an alignment with values. Further, it enhances self-esteem,

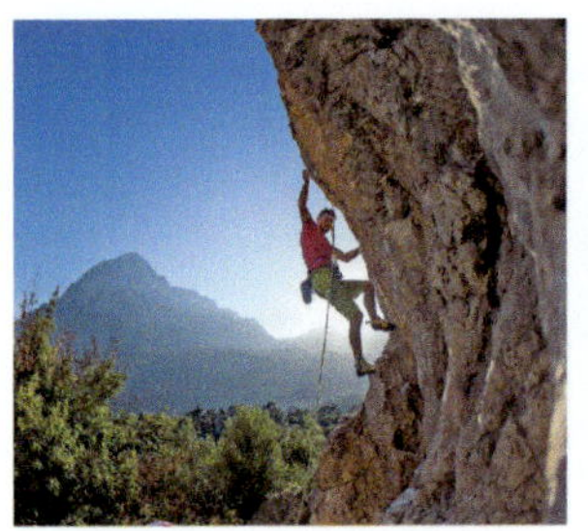

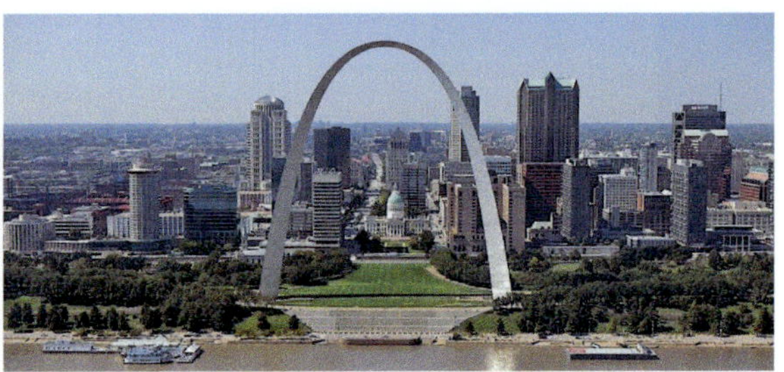

4.6
Purpose and Meaning: (a) Rock Climbing, (b) St. Louis Gateway Arch, Missouri

increases resilience, and can reduce stress and anxiety. Research suggests that people with increased meaning appear happier, exhibit increased life satisfaction, and report lowered depression.[19] How the physical environment supports purpose in life is important and is reflected in architect Louis I. Kahn's words that a city is the place where one may see something that will inform one's purpose for one's whole life.[20]

It is difficult to find images that illustrate purpose in life as it is such an individual and personal process. Sunrises, creating something beautiful, a sports competition, helping others, or climbing a mountain evoke a sense of purpose (refer to Figure 4.6a). In design within the built environment, meaning can be expressed in several ways, such as through a concept, program, function, or form language. Architecture and urban design can foster a strong sense of identity and sense of belonging. The design of healthy public spaces can encourage social interactions. They also can contribute to cultural expressions. Examples include historic city centers, modern sustainable communities, and spiritual buildings and sites. Certain designs also contribute to placemaking and identity, such as the St. Louis Gateway Arch, designed by Eero Saarinen in 1965 (refer to Figure 4.6b). The archway is a portal symbolic of Thomas Jefferson's vision of the purpose of westward expansion and a transcontinental United States in the 1803 Louisiana Purchase. Meaningful and purposeful planning and design processes can help in integrating spiritual sensitivities, wellness objectives, sustainability and regenerative technologies, and biophilic, environmental, and climate-oriented strategies, as well as socially responsible designs.

Meaning and purpose in life are integral to our well-being. According to Eric Berne, we all need to be touched and recognized and to engage in activity which we think is of consequence.[21] And, according to Donald Ardell, it is essential to develop means of self-expression that fit your unique talents and skills. An aim in life can be directed to balance and fulfillment.[22] From a spiritual wellness point of view, the physical environment can shape purpose and meaning through the framework of lifestyles, and experiences. Meaning can be emplaced within historic places and buildings, sacred sites and religious buildings, public places and civic buildings, and urban renewal and revitalization projects. This particular attribute is important to spiritual wellness, even though it does not necessarily possess specific planning or design strategies owing to its personal and subjective nature. In addition, it extends to the purpose and function of certain places and cities within the overall mosaic of planetary development. Meaning and life purpose do have general considerations for overall well-being.

Attribute of Life Satisfaction

Life satisfaction is a subjective measure influenced by positive relationships, meaningful work life, physical health, and overall well-being. Life satisfaction occurs through dedication to something greater than the self, living aligned to core values, practicing gratitude, and seeking ultimate meaning. Research shows that higher life satisfaction is associated with better physical, psychological, and behavioral health.[23] Life satisfaction is formed by genetics, social factors, and changing life circumstances, but also can be influenced by the built environment. Life satisfaction is a form of subjective well-being and, therefore, is primarily a result of inherited and learned predispositions to perceived and interpreted life circumstances and events.[24]

Recent research asserts that it consists of two main components: an emotional component and a cognitive component.[25] Life satisfaction and emotional well-being refer to being able to manage emotions effectively, to cope with life challenges, and to experience positive emotions such as joy, happiness, and gratitude. Life satisfaction and cognitive well-being deal with our thoughts, beliefs, and perceptions in relation to how we interpret our life experiences and events. Life satisfaction is influenced by physical, mental, and emotional health and well-being, family life, social wellness, financial security and stability, and environmental wellness in both the home and easy access to the natural environment. When we are satisfied with our lives, we tend to experience more positive emotions. Conversely, a lack of life satisfaction can lead to feelings of dissatisfaction, unhappiness, and even depression.

Cities and the buildings they contain shape everyday experiences, thereby affecting the degree to which we can access nature, feel safe, have a sense of belonging. They are able to support positive social interactions and give access to life-support functions, services, and products (healthy food, clean water and air, and energy). Through wellness design, they can reduced commuting and congestion with increased public transport systems and achieve economic well-being. Other factors that affect life satisfaction include climate, cost of living, employment opportunities, culture, and lifestyle. According to an Oxford University analysis, the global cities well-being evaluation cites Helsinki, Finland, Aarhus, Denmark, Wellington, New Zealand, Zurich, Switzerland, and Copenhagen, Denmark, as the cities with the highest ranking.[26]

To illustrate, Zurich, Switzerland (see images in Figure 4.7), possesses many of the characteristics of cities that enhance life satisfaction. Like many countries, Zurich has a higher average national income.[27] Switzerland in general and Zurich specifically have an integral connection to nature, a history of wellness and world-class healthcare, a robust economy, and a keen environmental awareness resulting in clean water and air. The Swiss have come to expect happiness as a human right. Zurich's central location makes it a hub for many destinations in Switzerland. In addition, Zurich is blessed with scenic views, beautiful parks, a preserved old town, centuries-old churches, a robust nightlife, and numerous cultural venues (see Figures 4.7a–4.7c).[28] Transport in Zurich combines trains, trams, bicycles, automobiles, and pedestrian streets (Figure 4.7a).

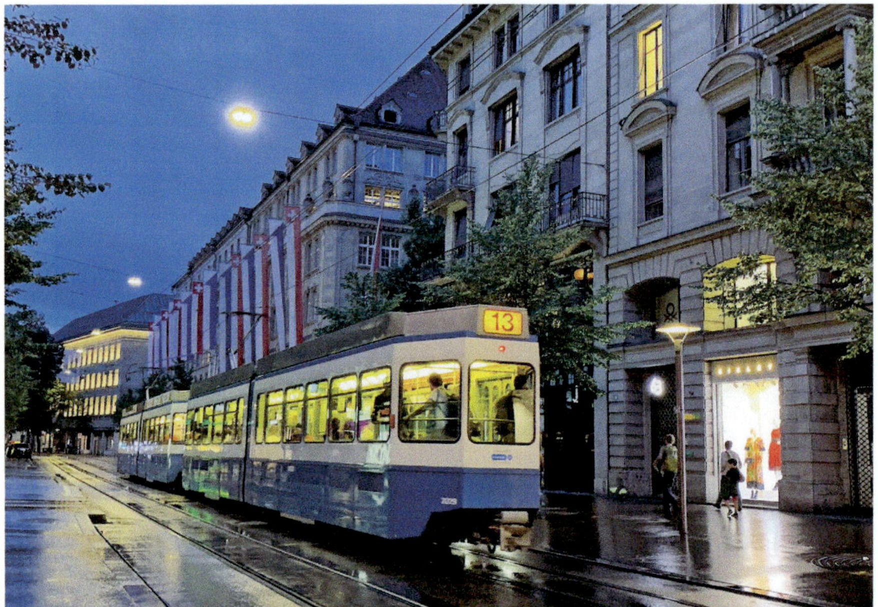

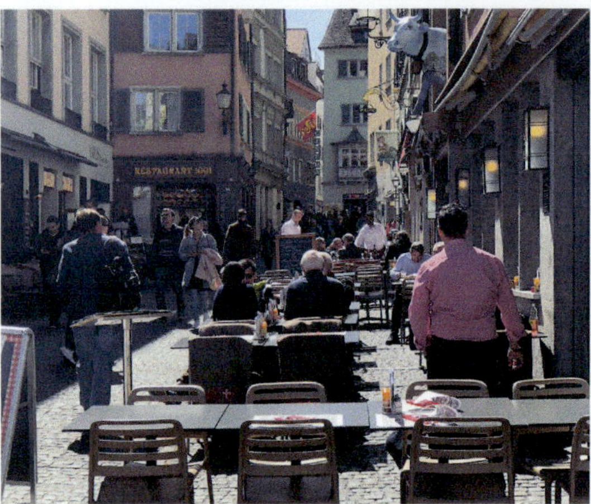

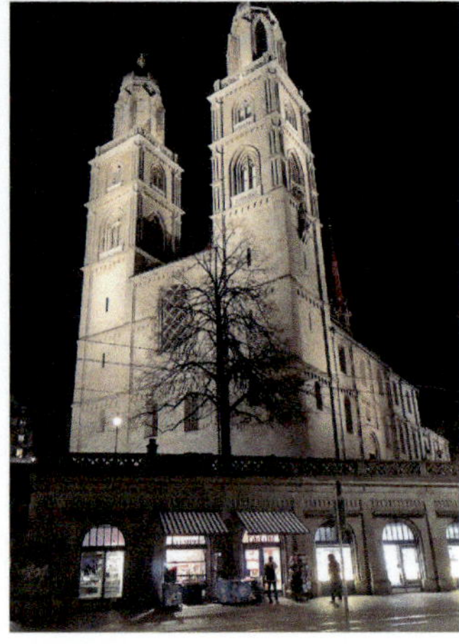

4.7
Life Satisfaction: (a) Night View, Zurich, Switzerland, (b) Pedestrian Street and Café, Zurich, (c) Grossmünster Monastery Church, Zurich

The attribute of life satisfaction is important to spiritual wellness. However, owing to its broad and subjective nature, the attribute of life satisfaction does not possess specific planning or design strategies. Some cities and buildings, however, have more general expressions with spirit of place, beauty of form, inclusion of nature, and connectivity that contribute to life satisfaction. Nonetheless, it does have general considerations for overall well-being, especially related to the quality of urban life and urban environments.

Attribute of High-Level Wellness

High-level wellness transcends the mere absence of disease and wellness in general and suggests a wellness process much more elevated, amplified, and encompassing. Spiritual high-level wellness further delves into a deep sense of purpose, transcending fulfillment and a world far beyond ourselves. Characteristics of high-level wellness include flourishing, attaining purpose and meaning in life, experiencing life satisfaction, having a perception of mastery and optimism, and having a positive effect on one's life. *Human flourishing* is a state of optimal functioning and well-being across our individual lives.[29] According to Haugan and Dezutter, *purpose and meaning* are mediating variables in psychological health and they contribute to vitality and motivational forces for survival.[30] *Life satisfaction* is associated with lower mortality and risk of hospitalization and is an influence on wellness behaviors.[31] *Mastery* is associated with a better physical and mental quality of life.[32] *Positive effects*, including experience of happiness, longer lives, and positive responses to chronic diseases, occur across a wide range of health outcomes.[33] According to Donald Ardell, high-level wellness requires taking care of the physical self, being mentally constructive, channeling stress energy positively, expressing emotions effectively, being creative with others, and connecting to the environment.[34]

High-level wellness is broad in its application, extending from organizations, buildings, and communities to nations, eco-regions, and humankind as a whole. Here, the discussion of high-level wellness must include the health of the Earth's biosphere and natural systems. This includes the wellness determinants directed toward infectious diseases, harmful lifestyle behaviors, human population growth and migration patterns, and the irresponsible use of natural resources. This includes planetary health, defined by the Rockefeller-Lancet Commission of Planetary Health as "the health of human civilization and the state of the natural systems on which it depends."[35] High-level wellness impacts the spatial realm in the ways in which both natural and built places encourage, organize, elicit, and materialize spiritual and wellness connections in their designs.

High-level wellness also includes spiritual dimensions and outcomes with concepts of whole health, including physical fitness, good nutrition, flourishing, longevity, positive family and social interactions, and relations to nature. The wellness implications of high-level wellness include holistic harmony along with the other pillars (physical, mental, emotional, social, and environmental) of wellness. Experiencing high-level spiritual wellness can amplify transformation and enhance the wellness benefits. The benefits include aging younger, meaning improving health as one ages through high-level wellness. This can occur through taking responsibility for personal health and wellness, being aware of and improving nutrition, reducing and managing stress, improving or maintaining physical fitness, nurturing and supporting social connections, stewarding the home and work environments, and participating in quality connections to spiritual events, experiences, and moments.

High-level wellness is generated from many, diverse sources. Figure 4.8a shows an assortment of fruit and vegetables, implying high-level wellness as a function of good nutrition. An alpine hideaway, hotel, and spa with a two-Michelin-star restaurant is seen in the image of the Tschuggen Grand Hotel with Bergoase spa. Both were designed by the Swiss architect Mario Botta (see Figure 4.8b). They represent high-level physical, emotional, and spiritual wellness experiences. The Santa Maria de Poblet Cistercian Monastery in Spain was founded in 1149 and is a

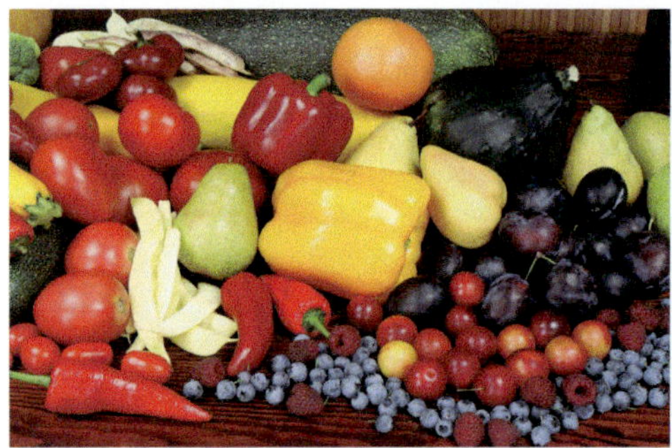

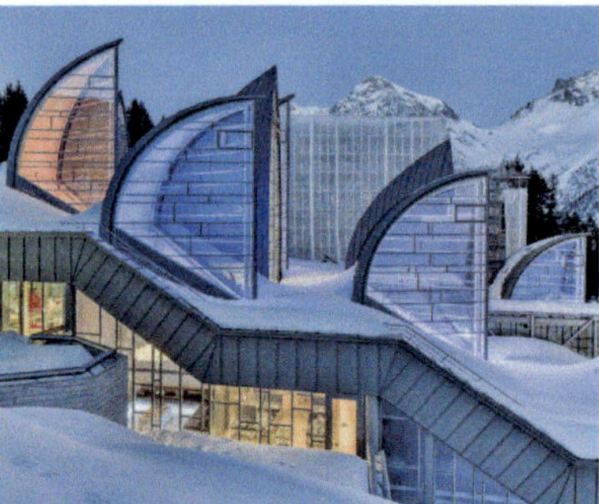

4.8
High-Level Wellness: (a) Good Nutrition, (b) Tschuggen Grand Hotel, Switzerland, (c) Santa Maria de Poblet Monastery, Spain

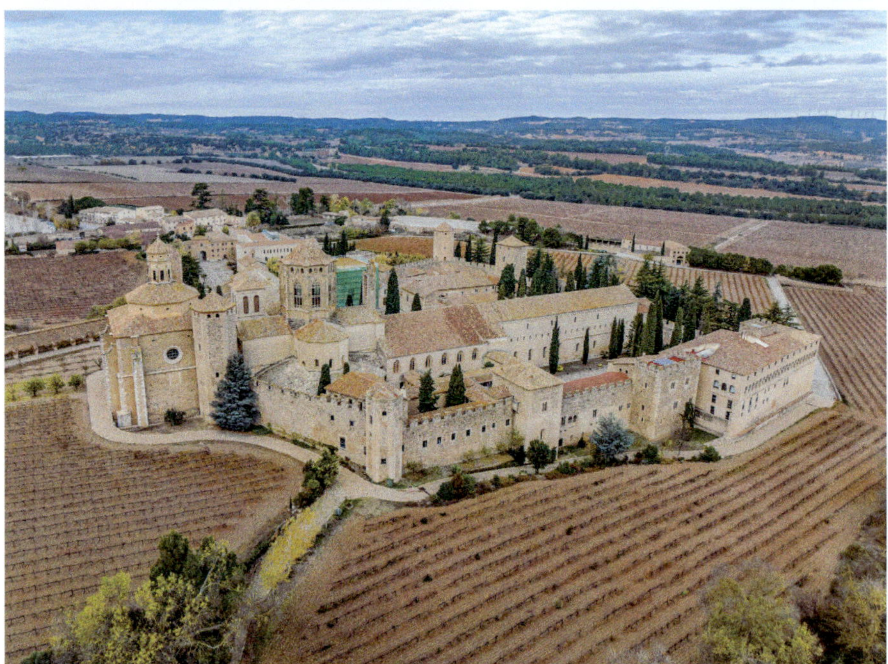

good example of flourishing wholeness and spiritual practices with cloistered living surrounded by agriculture and a small rural community. The monastery is peaceful and beautiful and is designated one of the most important abbey complexes in Europe. It was declared a UNESCO World Heritage Site in 1991 (see Figure 4.8c). Monastic environments are good models. Their integrated qualities and practice of spiritual wellness places, experiences, and processes can serve as models for larger, more secular contexts.

SUMMARY

Spiritual wellness is an ongoing process of self-discovery and active participation shaping the deepest part of us, including our beliefs, values, feelings, behaviors, and lifestyle practices. The wellness benefits are in part achieved through design as the dimensions inform the design opportunities in the built environment. Many of the attributes have a more direct impact upon design opportunities in the built environment, while some have secondary effects on attitudes, convictions, and sensibilities that can influence planning and design decisions. The experience-based attributes provide multiple connections to transcendent experiences.

The attributes described in this chapter relate to wellness and spiritual wellness characteristics or dimensions. Although some are practices and processes, they may not have direct application to physical designs. Importantly, it must be remembered that spiritual presence is not human-created and not guaranteed to occur. However, many do have direct application to the built environment as in form, function, and materiality. The place-oriented attributes have direct application to design at all scales. The experience-based attributes describe multiple connections to transcendent experiences and well-being. And process attributes occur over time and address more wholistic and deeper personal issues. These attributes have derived directly from definitions and research and reflect a broad view of spiritual wellness. A list of the eight attributes from the practice- and process-based dimensions follows:

1. **Presence and mindfulness** – the state of being physically connected, without distractions, and consciously (mindfully) aware.
2. **Coping with existential issues** – coping with difficult times, transitions, or situations and. addressing big fundamental questions in life such as death and mortality, meaning and purpose, and freedom and choice.
3. **Connections greater than ourselves** – infuse efforts with passion and purpose creating interest, curiosity, exploration, awakening, and perspective for even the greater good.
4. **Intentionality** – awareness and focus of spiritual wellness practices and spiritual journey that include mindful processes, cultivation of values, and intentional actions.
5. **Ethical and moral practices** – values, attitudes, and actions with integrity, honesty, fairness, respect, accountability, justice, and transparency.
6. **Purpose and life meaning** – spiritual wellness is affected and influenced with positive goal setting, life direction, and increased motivation.
7. **Life satisfaction** – through dedication to something greater than the self, living aligned to core values, practicing gratitude, and seeking ultimate meaning.
8. **High-level wellness** – behaviors and lifestyle processes that go beyond physical health, aging younger, flourishment, and incorporation of all aspects of well-being.

Chapters 5–7 address the implications of the spiritual wellness dimensions and their attributes as well as wellness outcomes at various scales of the built environment. They are applied at three scales – personal space, architecture, and urban design – and are intended to provide the largest scope for wellness planning and design pathways. The spiritual dimensions and attributes contribute to or inform specific outcome strategies at these varying scales.

NOTES

1 Gesler, Wilber M., *Healing Places* (Lanham, MD: Rowman & Littlefield, 2003).
2 Dunn, Halbert L., *High Level Wellness* (Pitman, NJ: Charles B. Slack, 1977).
3 Ardell, Donald, *High-Level Wellness: An Alternative to Doctors, Drugs, and Disease* (Emmaus, PA: Rodale Press, 1976), p. 57.
4 Merin, Gigi, Peter Zumthor: Seven Personal Observations on Presence in Architecture (accessed June 30, 2024), https://www.archdaily.com/452513/peter-zumthor-seven-personal-observations-on-presence-in-architecture.
5 Ackerman, Courtney E., 23 Amazing Health Benefits of Mindfulness for Body and Brain (accessed October 9, 2024), https://positivepsychology.com/benefits-of-mindfulness/.
6 Cruz, Marlon Guitirrez, Searching for Embodied Presence in Architecture (accessed October 9, 2024), https://digital.lib.washington.edu/researchworks/items/10a57c45-0d3c-434d-aff0-2a52e1f43698.
7 Health, Relig, Beneficial Effects of Spiritual Experiences and Existential Aspects of Life Satisfaction of Breast and Lung Cancer Patients in Poland: A Pilot Study (accessed November 24), pp. 20–23, https://www.ncbi.nlm.nih.gov/pmc/articles/PMC9569296/#:~:text=Spiritual%20experiences%20can%20have%20a,emotions%20(Galen%2C%202018).
8 Kretschmer, Madeline, & Lance Storm, The Relationship of the Five Existential Concerns with Depression and Existential Thinking (accessed January 24, 2024), https://www.meaning.ca/web/wp-content/uploads/2019/10/216-13-513-4-10-20180704.pdf.
9 Koole, Sander, Jeff Greenberg, & Tom Pyszczynski, Introducing Science to the Psychology of the Soul Experimental Existential Psychology (accessed November 12, I2024), https://www.researchgate.net/publication/242251661_Introducing_Science_to_the_Psychology_of_the_SoulExperimental_Existential_Psychology.
10 National Institutes of Health, Suffering a Healthy Life – On the Existential Dimension of Health (accessed September 24, 2023), https://www.ncbi.nlm.nih.gov/pmc/articles/PMC8830493/.
11 Rao, Preeti, Comprehending the Spiritual Dimension of Wellness and its Importance in One's Life (accessed September1, 2024), https://www.weljii.com/blog/comprehending-the-spiritual-dimension-of-wellness-and-its-importance-in-ones-life/.
12 Allen, Summer, The Science of Awe (accessed July 20, 2024), https://ggsc.berkeley.edu/images/uploads/GGSC-JTF_White_Paper-Awe_FINAL.pdf.
13 Keltner, Dasher, & Jonathan Haidt, Approaching Awe, a Moral, Spiritual, and Aesthetic Emotion (accessed October 10, 2022), https://www.tandfonline.com/doi/abs/10.1080/02699930302297.
14 Stein, Murray, Importance of Numinous Experience in Alchemy of Individualism (accessed October 12, 2022), https://jungchicago.org/blog/murray-stein-on-the-importance-of-numinous-experience-in-the-alchemy-of-individuation/.
15 Dyer Wayne W., The Power of Intention (accessed October 7, 2024), https://www.healthandwellnesscoaching.org/tools/12Chpts/1RM/WellnessChapter_RMcLean.pdf.
16 Lipton, Bruce, Embracing the Immaterial Universe: Toward a New Noetic Science. Shift: At the Frontiers of Consciousness (accessed October 7, 2024), https://www.healthandwellnesscoaching.org/tools/12Chpts/1RM/WellnessChapter_RMcLean.pdf.
17 Rethinking the Future, The Ethical Implications of Architectural Design (accessed July 20, 2024), https://www.re-thinkingthefuture.com/architectural-community/a11267-the-ethical-implications-of-architectural-design/#:~:text=Ethical%20architects%20carry%20the%20responsibility%20of%20creating%20a,of%20cultural%20heritage%2C%20and%20advocacy%20for%20social%20equality.
18 King, Laura, & Joshua Hicks, The Science of Meaning in Life (accessed July 21, 2024), https://pubmed.ncbi.nlm.nih.gov/32898466/.
19 Sutton, Jeremy, 15 Ways to Find Your Purpose of Life & Realize Your Meaning (accessed July 21, 2024), https://positivepsychology.com/find-your-purpose-of-life/.

20 Lobell, Robert, *Between Silence and Light: Spirit in the Architecture of Louis I. Kahn* (Boulder, CO: Shambhala, 1979), p. 44. This is a paraphrase of Lobell's book.

21 Ardell, Donald, *High-Level Wellness: An Alternative to Doctors, Drugs, and Disease* (Emmaus, PA: Rodale Press, 1976), p. 54.

22 Ardell, Donald, *High-Level Wellness: An Alternative to Doctors, Drugs, and Disease* (Emmaus, PA: Rodale Press, 1976), p. 99.

23 Kim, Eric, High Life Sanctification Linked to Better Overall Health (accessed July 21, 2024), https://www.sciencedaily.com/releases/2021/03/210303091405.htm#google_vignette.

24 Maddux, James E., Subjective Well-Being and Life Satisfaction (accessed August 27, 2024), https://www.taylorfrancis.com/chapters/edit/10.4324/9781351231879-1/subjective-well-being-life-satisfaction-james-maddux.

25 Andrews, F.M., & S.B. Withey, Social Indicators of Well-Being: America's Perception of Life Quality (accessed August 24, 2024), https://positivepsychology.com/life-satisfaction-scales/.

26 De Neve, Emmanuel, Cities and Happiness: A Global Ranking and Analysis (accessed July 21, 2024), https://worldhappiness.report/ed/2020/cities-and-happiness-a-global-ranking-and-analysis/.

27 Ortiz-Ospina, Esteban, & Max Roer, Happiness and Life Satisfaction (accessed July 21, 2024), https://ourworldindata.org/happiness-and-life-satisfaction.

28 From 2018 to 2022, I visited my son and his family in Zurich a half dozen times and was able to experience it firsthand from an expat's point of view. I was impressed with its vitality and the train and tram system. On occasion, we used Uber, but mostly used the tram. The tram was so accessible and easy to use. For Switzerland's largest city, it was remarkably clean.

29 Logan, Alan, Brian Berman, & Susan Prescott, Relevance to Personal and Public Health (accessed November 8, 2023), https://www.mdpi.com/1660-4601/20/6/5065#:~:text=Human%20flourishing%2C%20the%20state%20of%20optimal%20functioning%20and,in%20the%20context%20of%20health%20and%20high-level%20wellness.

30 Haugan, Gorill, & Jessie Dezutter, Chapter 8, Meaning-in-Life: A Vital Salutogenic Resource for Health (accessed November 8, 20923), https://www.ncbi.nlm.nih.gov/books/NBK585665/.

31 Bi, Kaiwen, Shuquan Chen, Paul Yip, & Pei Sun, Domains of Life Satisfaction and Perceived Health and Incidence of Chronic Illness and Hospitalization (accessed November 8, 2023), https://bmcpublichealth.biomedcentral.com/articles/10.1186/s12889-022-14119-3#:~:text=As%20a%20promising%20health%20asset%2C%20life%20satisfaction%20has,intake%20restriction%29%20%5B%204%2C%205%2C%206%2C%207%20%5D.

32 O'Kearney, E.L., C.R. Brown, G.A. Jelinek, S.L. Neate, K.T. Taylor, W. Bevens, A.M. De Livera, S. Simpson Jr., & T.J. Weiland, Mastery Is Associated with Greater Physical and Mental Health-Related Quality of Life in Two International Cohorts of People with Multiple Sclerosis (accessed November 8, 2023), https://pubmed.ncbi.nlm.nih.gov/31756608/.

33 Pressman, Sarah, Brooke Jenkins, & Judith Moskowitz, Positive Affect and Health: What Do We Know and Where Next Should We Go? (accessed November 8, 2023), https://www.annualreviews.org/doi/10.1146/annurev-psych-010418-102955.

34 Ardell, Donald, *High-Level Wellness: An Alternative to Doctors, Drugs, and Disease* (Emmaus, PA: Rodale Press, 1976), p. 10.

35 Haines, Andy, Addressing Challenges to Human Health in the Anthropocene Epoch - an Overview of the Finding of the Rockefeller-Lancet Commission on Planetary Health (accessed November 6, 2023), https://link.springer.com/content/pdf/10.1186/s40985-016-0029-0.pdf.

5 SPIRITUAL WELLNESS AT THE PERSONAL SCALE

INTRODUCTION

Wellness strategies are a mutually supporting set of design approaches that serve as prime actionable elicitors of wellness benefits promoting individual physical health, positive emotional responses, mental clarity, prosocial behaviors, spiritual renewal, and environmental reparation. Most of these strategies have a basis in science, health and wellness, and spirituality and are informed by the fields of public health, health sciences, religious and spiritual theology, and environmental psychology. The design implications and strategies include an understanding of the basic needs of human beings and an understanding of potential opportunities at varying scales of the built environment. The strategies describe design approaches, patterns, and elicitors and offer several examples that show the ways in which spiritual wellness has been effectively responded to and applied in previous works.

In what ways can planning and design solutions contribute to human and environmental health and wellness? It goes without saying, health and wellness benefit both human beings and the environments they inhabit, including both natural and built places. Human-centered benefits are directed to the dimensions of wellness, including our physical bodies, mental health, emotional well-being, social connections, and spiritual growth, as demonstrated with illness and joy. Financial health is also seen as a wellness benefit. The environment-centered benefits are directed to the natural environment around us and the cities and buildings we occupy. The contrast between these two environmental conditions is moving – one is polluted, and the other is endowed with clean air. The spatial implications of spiritual wellness are influenced by biophilic principles, sacred geometry, physical materiality, and place patterns. As further discussed, they are applied at three scales: the personal scale, the architecture scale, and the urban design scale. These scales are intended to provide the largest scope for wellness planning and design pathways.

Design considerations or strategies are intended to help elicit spiritual wellness benefits at any scale. They share DNA, or inherent information and characteristics, with healthcare, sacred space design, biophilia, and thin places. Furthermore, they are intended to respond to both spiritual dimensions and wellness outcomes. A series of works by the architect and architectural educator Michael Brill and his students at the State University of New York at Buffalo showed that a sacred – or,

DOI: 10.4324/9781003546085-5

in their words, a "*charged*" site – could contain a common set of fundamental characteristics or patterns by which the sacred was revealed.[1] The planning and design determinants and characteristics are generalized below from these sources but are more specific to each of the applicable scales.

SPIRITUAL WELLNESS ATTRIBUTES AND OUTCOMES

The spiritual wellness attributes and outcomes represent dimensions from places, experiences, and processes influencing our behaviors and lifestyles. These dimensions can become goals, desired outcomes, or planning and design strategies. The designs occurring at each scale will be based on different attributes that generate differing sets of outcomes. The following lists are a recap of the dimensions of spiritual wellness from Chapters 2–4. Place-based attributes and outcomes are as follows:

1. **Spirit of place and original cause** – represent distinctive and cherished qualities of a place that sometimes are thought to possess guardians, spirits, or creation myths.
2. **Biophilia and love of nature** – are the innate tendency for connections to nature and life processes.
3. **Thin places** – are locations where a thin veil exists between the earthly world in which we live and the heavenly, spiritual world that is qualitatively different.
4. **Third places** – are locations away from home and work that serve as places for frequent encounters and social interactions.
5. **Sanctuary places** – refer to physical locations that provide a sense of peace, security, refuge from the stresses of daily life, and rejuvenation; they also refer to passive survival spaces advantageous for survival in an emergency situation.
6. **Healing landscapes** – are used to produce medicinal plants and are considered therapeutic landscapes for recovery, restoration, and spiritual renewal.
7. **Religious places** – are places that focus on spiritual and wellness practices, such as monasteries, ashrams, spiritual retreats, and pilgrimage sites.
8. **Ritual and ceremonial places** – stimulate through active participation and transformative routines of awe experiences, meditation practices, forgiveness, and gratitude.

Experience-based attributes and outcomes are as follows:

1. **Numinous experiences** – have an engaging power and are typically momentary and associated with fascination, wonder, mystery, tranquility, and even terror.
2. **Awe experiences** – are human emotions associated with vastness, diminished focus on self, changing time perception, and the need for accommodation; they can be overwhelming.
3. **Serenity experiences** – are sustained inner peace, tranquility, calm, trust, sedation, and freedom from anxiety; they need accommodation for cognitive and emotional readjustments.

4. **Synchronicity and coincidences** – occasions when circumstances and personal experiences have meaning connections.
5. **Noetic experiences** – reference the notion that spiritual experiences reveal an otherwise hidden or inaccessible knowledge and feelings of connections to something beyond ourselves.
6. **Transcendence and spiritual renewal** – are experiences of moving beyond ordinary limitations, including connections to spiritual wellness.
7. **Experiences of the unknown** – are experiences that cannot be described through other experiences; we can feel their special character without being able to give it clear conceptual expression.
8. **Unity experience, sense of oneness** – a profound experience encompassing a deep sense of interconnectedness, harmony, and oneness with the world around us. It dissolves the illusion of division and separateness.

Practice- and process-based attributes and outcomes are as follows:

1. **Presence and mindfulness** – are the state of being physically connected, without distractions, and consciously (mindfully) aware.
2. **Coping with existential issues** – is coping with difficult times, transitions, or situations and addressing big, fundamental questions in life such as death and mortality, meaning and purpose, and freedom and choice.
3. **Connections greater than ourselves** – infuse efforts with passion and purpose creating interest, curiosity, exploration, awakening, and perspective for even the greater good.
4. **Intentionality** – is an awareness and focus on spiritual wellness practices and the spiritual journey, including mindful processes, cultivation of values, and intentional actions.
5. **Ethical and moral practices** – are values, attitudes, and actions with integrity, honesty, fairness, respect, accountability, justice, and transparency.
6. **Purpose and life meaning** – affects and influences spiritual wellness with positive goal setting, life direction, and increased motivation.
7. **Life satisfaction** – is experienced through dedication to something greater than the self, living aligned to core values, practicing gratitude, and seeking ultimate meaning.
8. **High-level wellness** – comprises behaviors and lifestyle processes that go beyond physical health and incorporate all aspects of well-being.

SCALES OF APPLICATION

Where the dimensions and attributes, described in the previous chapters, derive from research and definitions of spiritual wellness, the planning and design strategies provide specific guidelines across several scales constituting the built environment. It is important to view these scales independently but also to see them as nested domains. Three scales that span from personal space to architecture and finally to urban design are used for the purpose of this work.

- **Personal space scale** – includes intimate, small, personal, and well-defined spaces that serve a variety of wellness functions and spiritual practices for individuals or small groups.
- **Architecture scale** – includes building sites, buildings, climatic form responses, envelope design, building elements, material choices, building systems, and indoor–outdoor relationships.
- **Urban design scale** – includes city planning, town planning, neighborhoods, mixed-use development, water systems, urban parks, pastureland, agriculture, and infrastructure design.

PERSONAL SPACE SCALE STRATEGIES

Personal space is generally defined as the space with physical, psychological, and emotional boundaries surrounding a person, an encroachment into which feels threatening or uncomfortable. Personal space can also be open and inviting. Entering somebody's personal space is normally an indication of familiarity and, sometimes, intimacy. Personal is the smallest scale for spiritual wellness.

The size of personal space varies depending upon the relative relationship between people. Edward T. Hall asserts that personal spaces can range from intimate distances of several inches to social and public distances between 4 and 25 feet (1.2 and 7.6 meters).[2] The personal space scale includes intimate, soulful, normative, domestic, authorless, serene, and everyday lived places. Generally, these places create a personal, subjective, and interior experience. Fundamental characteristics at this scale include centering, bounding, spatial intimacy, discriminating views, natural light, sanctuary, less formal geometry, peaceful connections to nature, inclusion of personal objects or symbols, and silence.

At the smallest and most intimate scale, the eliciting personal space can be subtle, serene, and momentary. Spiritual wellness is extremely personal. This personal space scale offers both inside and outside integration of interior space, and landscape eliciting wellness dimensions and spiritual experiences. The personal scale offers the opportunity for inclusion of sacred elicitors, such as comfortable and safe spaces; access to nature, either physically or visually; openings to pollution-free views of nature or the night skies; placement of significant symbols; and silence. Figure 5.1 illustrates several ways to experience personal spaces, from resting in a chair to hanging out in nature or fly fishing alone in a beautiful river. Figure 5.1a is an image of a woman sitting in a chair enjoying a quiet moment. Figure 5.1b is an image of Ledro Land Art, which is an environmental art park where artistic creativity meets nature through the reinterpretation of spaces and interaction with existing elements. And, finally, Figure 5.1c is a man fly fishing in in middle of a small river. Each of these depict a personal space experience.

Designing for Personal Scale

Personal scale is smaller and more intimate than the architecture and urban design scales. Personal spatial scale is accessible, even reachable, and is related to human anatomy. In this regard, scale creates a sense of closeness, comfort, safety, and

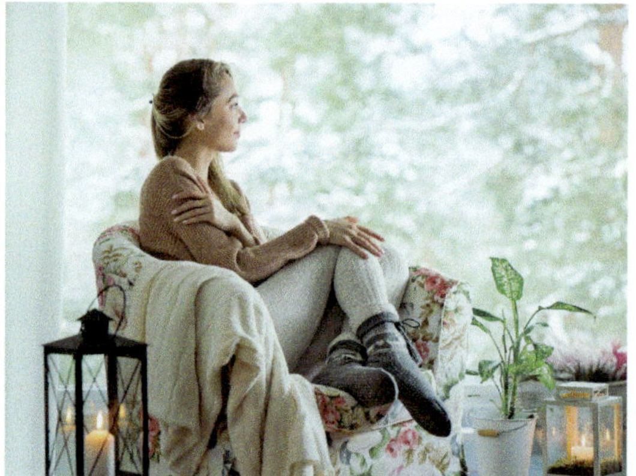

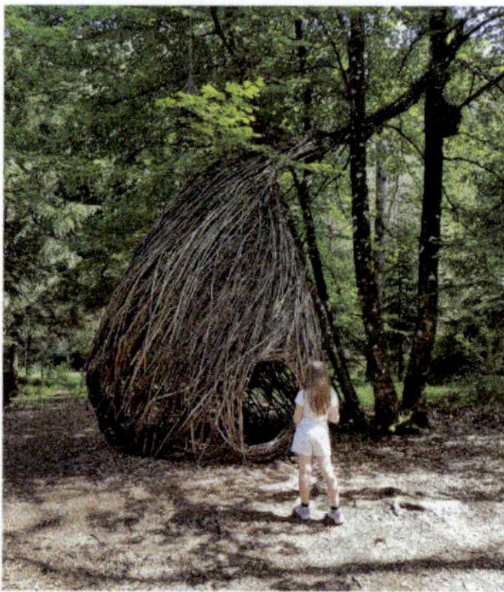

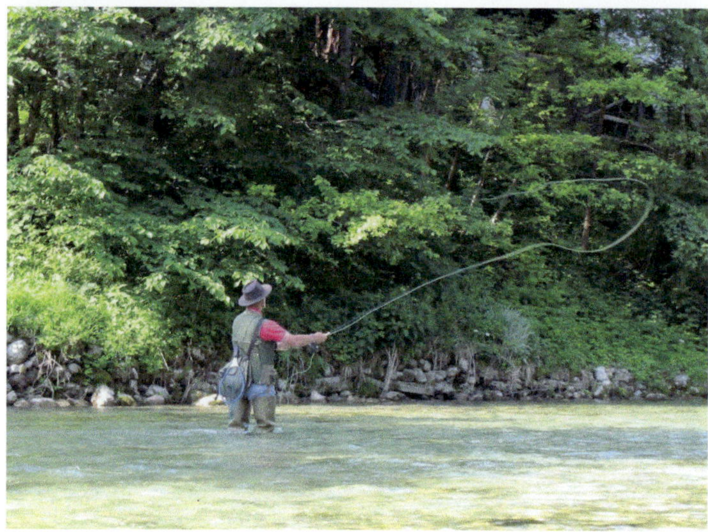

5.1
Personal Space Scale: (a) Comfortable Chair as Personal Space, (b) Land Art Installation Ledro, Italy, (c) Serene Moments Fly Fishing

shelter. It is accessible through all our senses. Elements are arranged in proximity and often have soft edges. Moreover, intimate spaces can occur both in nature and within architecture and urban design settings. In the urban design context, personal scale is a function of accessibility, especially when walking. Design elements within an intimate space have human-centered dimensions. Spiritual intimate spaces are typically sanctuary spaces fostering connections to self, others, and the divine. These spaces are usually minimalist, full of natural light, and quiet. Such spaces are designed to promote relaxation, rejuvenation, intimacy, and overall well-being. Further, these are spaces with minimal clutter and visual noise, and discriminating views. Often, they are very personal.

Nature can provide a context for intimate spiritual wellness experiences. Where vast landscapes elicit awe emotions, more intimate natural settings create serene and peaceful moments. Serenity and its relationship to emotion theory, health and wellness, and spirituality first appeared in the nursing literature in the mid-1960s when it was identified as an important factor for terminally ill patients. Serenity is defined as sustained inner peace. The positive benefits of serenity include appreciation of the moment, formulation of a more refined sense of self, a strong sense of groundedness, and the sense of congruence and gratitude.[3] Personal scale often takes the form of nooks, alcoves, inglenooks by a fireplace, a quiet corner or office in the workplace, or a quiet bench in a park. Typically, these spaces have smaller, more proxemic dimensions, especially regarding their height. Designing for personal space includes the following:

1. **Accessibility** – is easily accessible throughout the day and within a variety of building types, functions, and activities.
2. **Response to scale** – is intimate, small and inviting, safe, and based on human-centered dimensions and proportions.
3. **Ability to be personalized** – has the ability to be changed, used in different ways, and personalized through interior design elements.
4. **Safety and protection** – is typically bounded, sheltered, clearly defined, and quiet.

There are several spiritual wellness attributes and desired outcomes associated with intimate personal scale spaces. They include experiences such as the numinous, unity, and transcendence. They include serenity and awe emotions and spiritual renewal. Further, these can be elicited by thin places, third places, sanctuary places, and healing gardens; they are biophilic, with connections greater than ourselves. The spirit of a place can be amplified by the sensory character of the space. Many forms and examples of personal space exist. Figure 5.2 shows a baby in a crib and a man in his campground tent; both are well defined and protected spaces.

Accessibility to Everyday Sacred Wellness Spaces

Accessibility and everyday practice are important in maintaining spiritual wellness. This includes sustaining benefits of personal growth and community building. Accessibility plays a critical part in being able to sustain positive behaviors and lifestyles related to wellness, and this incudes spirituality as well. Both accessibility and spiritual wellness prioritize inclusivity, ensuring holistic experiences and community building that are accessible to everyone.

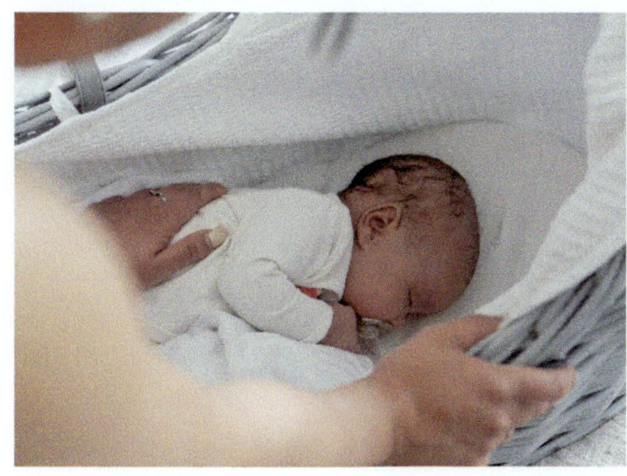

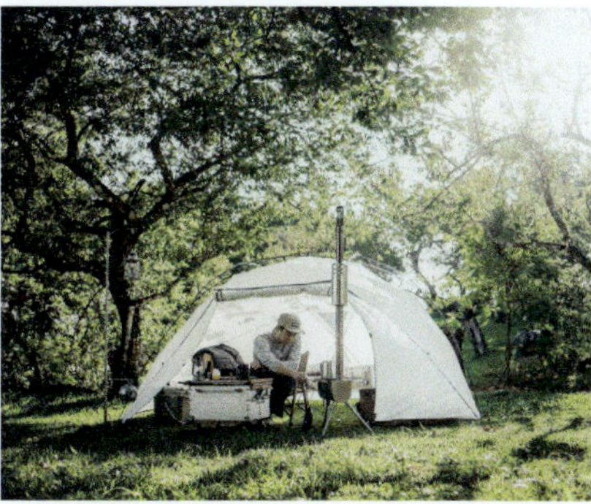

5.2 Intimate Scale Spiritual Wellness: (a) Baby in a Crib, (b) Quiet Moment in a Campground Tent

In his 2008 book *The Blue Zones*, Dan Buettner documented geographic areas where people are said to live longer than they do in other places. This claim, although not completely verified, is based on the residents' ability to maintain healthy lifestyles.[4] Residents in blue zones share lifestyle characteristics that reduce stress: less cigarette smoking, moderate caloric intake, moderate alcohol intake, increased social engagement, semi-vegetarian diet, moderate physical activity as part of everyday life, and some form of spiritual engagement. Thus, they engage in places and activities that support spiritual wellness, and most of the residents live within tight-knit communities. Moreover, these activities are accessible and practiced daily.

Familiar everyday domestic activities exist that provide opportunities for spiritual wellness. These include bathing, preparing a family meal, working in the garden, taking time to relax in a favorite chair, tidying up clutter, and even nursing an infant. Meditation, journaling, or other reflective activities can also elicit spiritual wellness. Although it may be more difficult at work than at home to engage in activities that elicit spiritual wellness owing to the focused activities and social interactions necessary to accomplish the work, it is still important to find moments and safe places to collect yourself and rejuvenate.

Designing for accessibility involves the following:

1. **Spatial considerations** – relate to the physical proximity to spiritual wellness places, activities, and events, assuming that physical, informational, and technological spaces are available and reachable.
2. **Temporal considerations** – relate to accessibility through time (daily and seasonally) and assurance that the time is available and uninterrupted.
3. **Safety considerations** – relate to the accessibility of the spiritual wellness functions and the safety of spaces without potential harm or universal design restrictions (i.e., the Americans with Disabilities Act requirements).

There are several spiritual wellness attributes and desired outcomes associated with access to everyday sacred spaces. They importantly include experiences such as personal thin places, third places, sanctuary places, and healing places. They include biophilic places, safe places, and those with connections that are greater than ourselves. Such spaces need to be accessible, protected, and safe in order to for us to fully experience the spiritual wellness benefits. Figure 5.3 shows an extremely personal space activity of bathing, available to nearly everyone. Preparing a special meal can also be personal, activating all the senses.

Creating Sanctuary Spaces

Sanctuary spaces exist in varying forms, sizes, and locations, from special alcoves in a bedroom or a home office to a favorite hiding place in the woods or vacation spot. They can be used throughout everyday experiences or on special occasions. They are nurturing and they are personal. Children's treehouses and forts are favorite sanctuary spaces that allow for intimacy, comradeship, creativity, and solitude. Google is known for its unique and varying workspaces that serve to provide

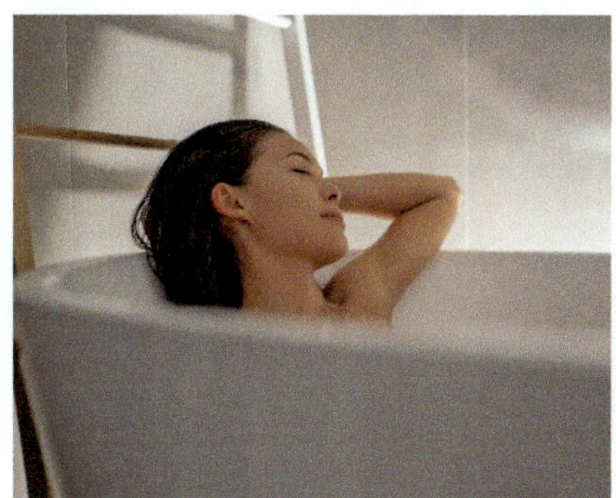

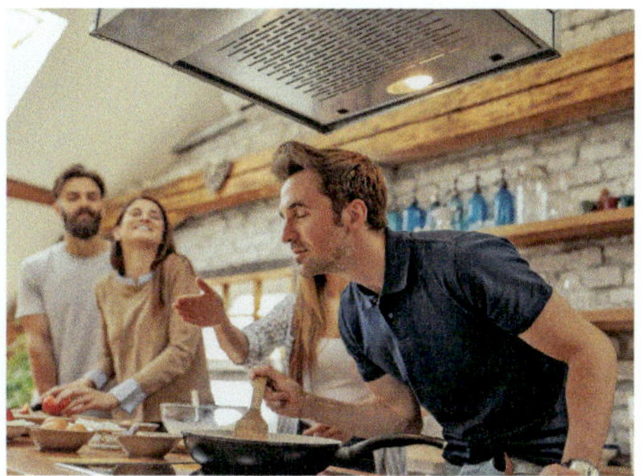

5.3
Everyday Spiritual Wellness: (a) Taking a Hot Bath, (b) Preparing a Homecooked Meal

privacy, focus, and an opportunity to recharge. Sanctuary spaces are also found in natural beauty spots, spiritual and thin places, therapeutic environments, and wellness retreats. During COVID-19, sanctuary spaces allowed for isolation and limited physical contact with fellow employees. The impact of infectious diseases is not new, yet the coronavirus has presented new challenges in a highly connected global community. The wellness benefits of such interesting environments include sources of renewal, relaxation, and quiet. Experiences within them can reduce stress and overstimulation, can strengthen the immune system, and can improve mood and positive feelings.

The sanctuary spaces health benefits for individuals include mental clarity, decreased stress, lower blood pressure and heart rate, reduced cortisol, improved sleep, and increased focus and positive moods. Sanctuary spaces are places that are safe, nurturing, and therapeutic. They provide protection and a haven from negative environmental, social, and political conditions, and they support social healing. Moreover, sanctuary spaces can be sacred. They are familiar spaces and can include workshops, storm shelters, bedroom alcoves, treehouses, children's forts, bathtubs, and even baby cribs. The moments of silence experienced in such spaces can be transitions to transcendent experiences of spiritual wellness. An integral function of a sanctuary space is its ability to support prospect and refuge. Prospect creates discerning views of distant objects, changes in weather, intruders, and potential sources of danger. Refuge provides a secure, safe, and protected setting at both the urban design and architectural scales. Sanctuary spaces:

1. **Offer shelter and safety** – they are places of shelter and safety and are essential to sanctuary spaces; they function in secular or spiritual ways and can produce strong wellness emotions of awe and serenity.
2. **Offer prospect and refuge** – they are places that offer prospect and refuge; prospect allows for surveillance and the identification of danger, and refuge provides safety from potential intruders and suspicious activity, and protection from inclement weather.
3. **Support introspection** – they are places that are nurturing, comforting, and therapeutic and provide protection and a safe haven. They support silence, facilitating deeper, more self-reflective, peaceful moments.

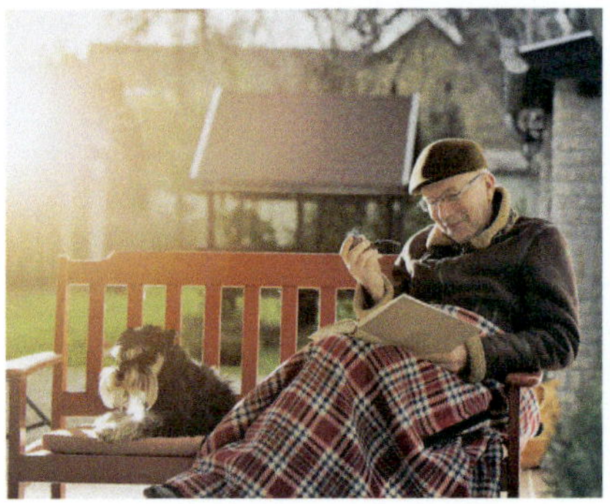

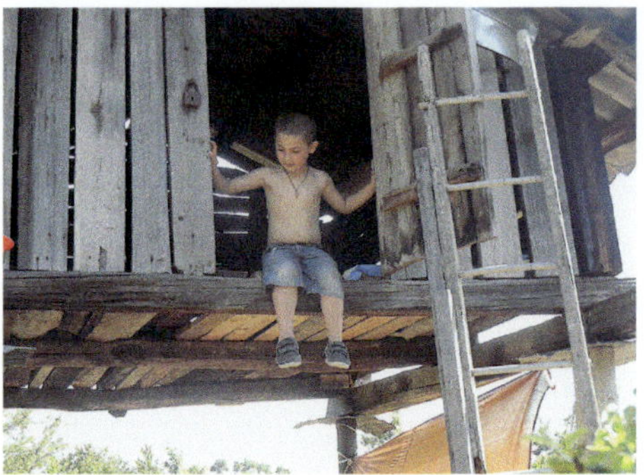

5.4
Sanctuary Wellness Spaces: (a) Person Reading on a Porch Bench, (b) Boy in Treehouse

There are several spiritual wellness attributes and desired outcomes associated with sanctuary spaces. They include numinous, serenity, and awe experiences, transcendence and spiritual renewal, unity experience, a possible third place, a sanctuary. They can include healing garden experiences that are biophilic and enable connections greater than ourselves. They support social healing, can be sacred, and can include workshops, storm shelters, bedroom alcoves, treehouses, children's forts, bathtubs, and even baby cribs. Depending upon geographic location, the spirit of place can create identity and be experienced. Figure 5.4a shows a man on a back porch bench quietly reading a book next to his dog, and Figure 5.4b shows a young boy hanging out in a treehouse.

Bounded Safe Places

Bounding is extremely important in personal places. The boundary of a place has a comprehensible surrounding edge with a fixed relationship to the spatial domain and center, giving the place a sense of enclosure, containment, clarity, and identity of form. Bounded spaces are inwardly focused and thus facilitate more introverted experiences. Bounding can be solid, permeable, and defined by either natural or built forms. Its circumscription can be complete, porous, or partially defined around a healing place and serves to contain the sacred or charged energy. A differentiated boundary does not remain the same around its perimeter but rather has elements that reflect and define entrance/exit, direction, orientation, and other special meanings or features of the place.[5] The boundary must help maintain the sanctity and charge of a sacred place within the context of the secular space. Bounding examples are plentiful and include walls, fences, buildings, tree lines, rock formations, dramatic elevation changes, water, landforms, or other natural features. Courtyard buildings, compounds, monasteries, prisons, urban plazas, and walled cities are other bounding examples.

Spiritual bounding takes the form of a veil. Veils are defined beyond their literal associations as garments with ceremonial significance and serve as something that covers, conceals, or disguises. Veils bound sacred spaces, protecting them from secular space. Initially, veils maintain a certain sense of separation, as well as concealment and closeness to something magical, unknown, sacred, or divine. As veils become thinner, more transparent and accessible, they can allow for a source experience. The three primary forms are veil as *edge*, veil as *passage*, and veil as *encompassing space*. A veil can be a membrane, wall, window, or doorway. Lionel Corbett suggests that the whole veiled place is like a container or cauldron that cooks the sacred ingredients, facilitating the transformative process.[6] Bounded spaces function in several ways:

1. **Comprehensible edge** – serves to create containment within, protection from without, and porosity and control of natural systems flowing through. It can contribute to community building and identity.
2. **Containment** – serves to protect and contain the sacred or charged energy of the place, giving it enclosure, clarity, and identity.
3. **Differentiated articulation** – serves as a perimeter that reflects and defines entrance/exit, direction, orientation, or other special meanings.

Boundaries can be personal. Personal boundaries are individualized limits that delineate the borders of personal comfort in interpersonal relationships; they also are physical and spatial. Several spiritual wellness attributes and desired outcomes are associated with bounded spaces. They include numinous, serenity, and awe experiences, transcendence and spiritual renewal, unity experience, a possible third place, a sanctuary. They can include healing garden experiences that are biophilic and enable connections greater than ourselves. The spirit of place can be charged by bounding and containing other spiritual wellness attributes and the sensory character of the space. Other wellness effects include reduced stress, improved relationships, and heightened self-esteem. Additional spiritual effects include minimizing distractions, cultivating a sense of the sacred, promoting mindfulness, and creating a safe sanctuary. In Figure 5.5a, the bounded building, Saynatsalo Town Hall in Finland, contains the green courtyard in its center that acts as a central open space for the town, a public plaza where people can meet and interact. The civic offices and library open onto this courtyard, enhancing its role as a community hub. The Zen garden in Figure 5.5b illustrates the carefully designed elements for contemplation, focused attention, and encouraging healing of the mind and body. Both protect and create a safe haven.

Sensory Connections

Our senses provide an endless amount of information, yet, unless we pay attention, their input can be easily overlooked. Personal and intimate spaces create an interiority of experience with all our senses, and exposure to nature produces positive effects. The classic senses are visual, auditory, olfactory, haptic, and gustatory. There are other perceptions that could be considered senses – including proprioception or the sense of movement in space, balance, and temperature – which contribute to this experience. Although humans are dominantly visual, the other senses are important in biophilic design. Natural sounds restore moods, and natural olfactory sensations are important for memory, language, social attraction, and reproduction. Tasting food can be transformative. Haptic touch is experienced in gardening and enjoying horticulture activities, a walk in the rain or snow, and playing with domesticated animals. Balance, or equilibrioception, is considered another

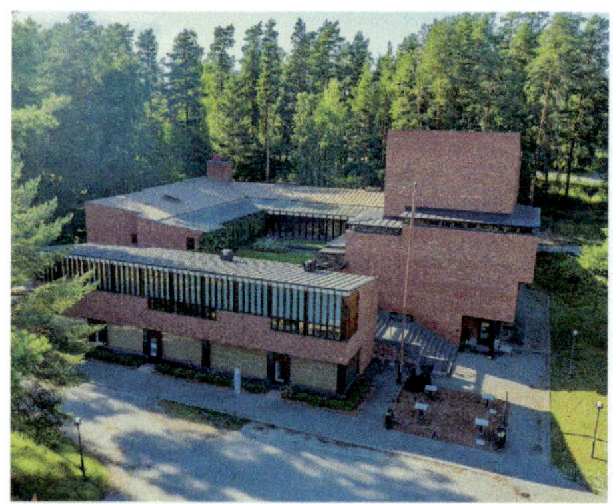

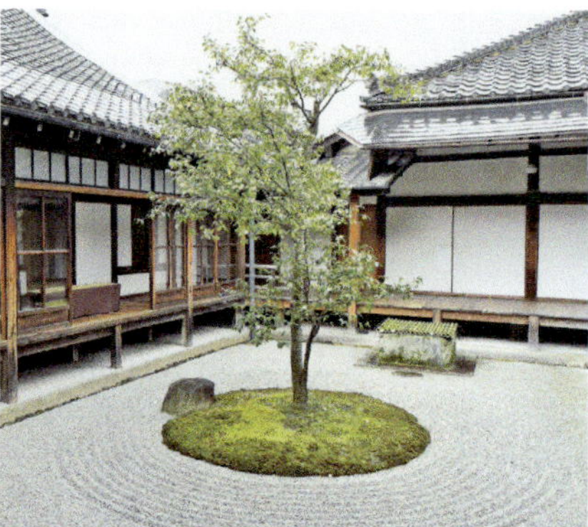

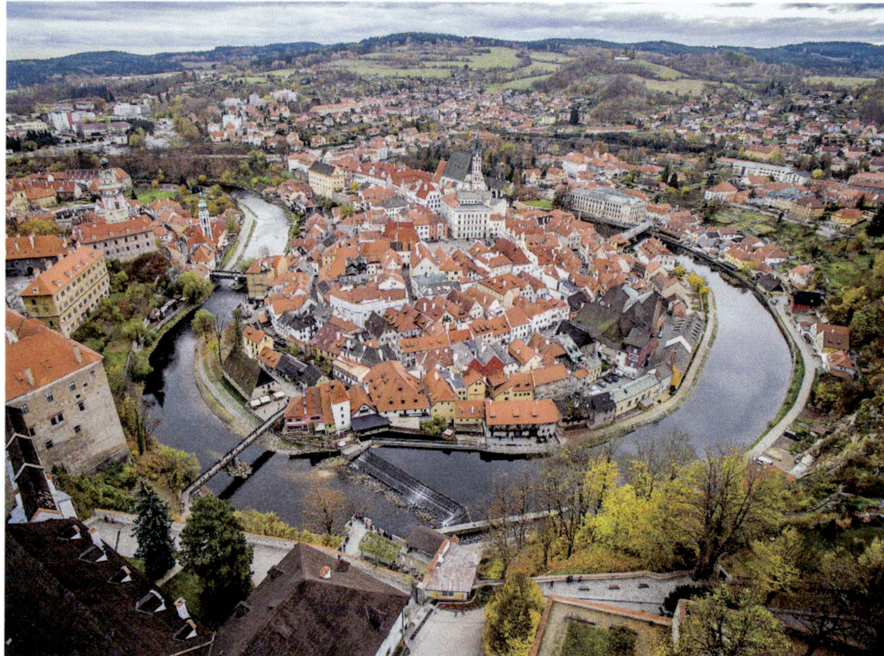

5.5 Bounded Places: (a) Civic Space Bounding in Saynatsalo Town Hall, Finland, (b) Spiritual Space Bounding in Zen Garden, (c) Bounded Old City, Czech Republic

sense; moving through varying spaces, either spatially intimate or generous, affects our experience of wellness. According to John Steele, the combination of senses creates enhanced perception and more focused memory.[7]

Another sense is identified as the "spiritual sense." The spiritual sense offers a deeper perception of the world around us, as well as understandings of moral, existential, and even metaphysical questions. The spiritual sense has five attributes, including the sense of intuition, connection, inner knowing, transcendence, and the spiritual sense.[8] Several spiritual wellness attributes and desired outcomes are associated with sensory connections. They include numinous, serenity, and awe experiences, transcendence and spiritual renewal, unity experience, a possible third place, a sanctuary. They can include healing garden experiences that are biophilic and enable connections greater than ourselves. Exposure to nature produces positive effects as experienced by all our senses. Paying attention to what we see, hear, smell, touch, and taste can bring us deeper into the present moment, evoke meaningful memories, and help us connect with other people in our lives. Furthermore, the spirit of place can be amplified by the sensory character of the space. Sensory connections for place function in several ways:

1. **Enhance perception** – they convert external-world information received through the senses to perceptions that lead to our experiences, especially for spiritual wellness.
2. **Focus memory** – sense-based information serves as the initial staging area for incoming information from our environment, and, according to John Steele, the combination of senses creates enhanced perception and more focused memory.[9]

Sensory perception is especially important for older adults and those experiencing dementia or cognitive decline. What we see and hear deeply influences our thoughts, actions, and moods. Classic examples of the wellness effects of sensory perception include enjoying the stillness and beauty found in nature or the elevating effect of ephemeral architecture. Figure 5.6a shows a woman smelling garden flowers, activating touch, sight, and smell, and Figure 5.6b depicts a mother and daughter engaged in preparing breakfast.

Experience of Color

Humans are visual creatures, and, as a result, color expresses a visible and vital element of life. Color plays a tremendous role in how we react and respond to things around us. It can affect the way we feel, how we think, and how we interact with one another. Natural color is activated by varying qualities of light and can produce numinous experiences. Color is experienced as properties of surfaces that change color over the course of a day. Morning light tends to be yellow, with mid-level electromagnetic wavelengths; the light becomes bluer at midday, with shorter wavelengths, and shifts to red with even longer wavelengths in the late afternoon.[32] The rich color of an iris or rose petal, the intricate and vibrant colors of a butterfly's wings, and the fiery colors of a midsummer sunset are all living colors.

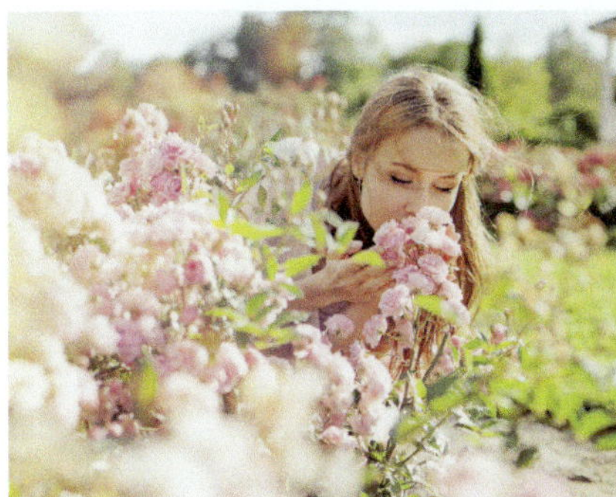

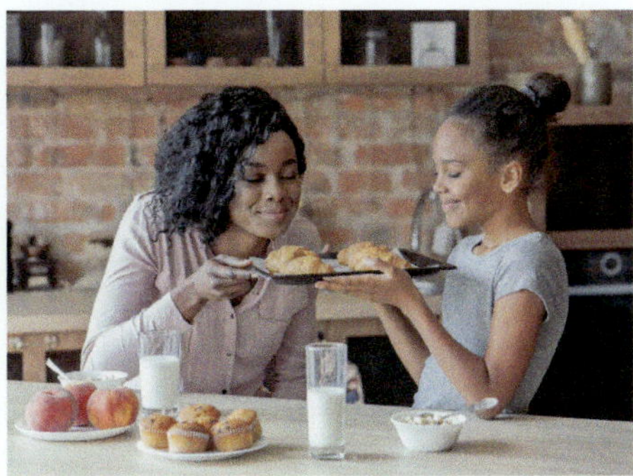

5.6 Sensory Connections: (a) Woman Smelling Garden Flowers, (b) Mother and Daughter with Kitchen Smells

Color has been used extensively in feng shui as a notion of *living color*, invoking a transcendent dimension with regenerative powers. In intimate spaces, stained glass that is activated by the changing qualities of light can produce transcendent effects. Colors also can have symbolic associations and elicit certain emotional responses, such as the color red representing passion and fire, blue associated with the calmness of water, and green associated with nature and the plant world.[10] The color goal of feng shui is to create balance and the correct color placement thought to improve vital energy.

The healing benefits vary by color. Even though not all colors possess the same meaning and impact across cultures, they do have some overall emotional commonalities. The warmer colors tend to be more passionate and stimulate the senses and energy, while cooler colors calm the nervous system, influencing mood and state of mind. Simply put, red is stimulating, orange is uplifting, yellow is cheerful, green is soothing, blue is calming, and purple is transforming. Color is used to raise awareness and to enhance safety – for example, to signal physical hazards, such as danger, warnings, caution, and biological hazards. Color, in concert with textures, lighting, and ambiance in physical spaces, helps define a sense of space and impacts moods, thoughts, and productivity.

The healing benefits of color include fostering the numinous, serenity, and awe experiences, transcendence and spiritual renewal, unity experiences, and possibly third places and sanctuary places. They can include healing garden experiences that are biophilic, and enable connections greater than ourselves. The spirit of place can be amplified by the sensory character of the space. The use of color benefits spiritual wellness as follows:

1. **Aesthetic experiences** – specific colors and combinations of colors enhance mood, relate to biophilic experiences, and can contain or curate cultural and symbolic meaning.
2. **Emotional connections** – warmer colors tend to be more passionate and stimulate the senses and energy, while cooler colors calm the nervous system, influencing mood and state of mind.
3. **Living color** – living color has connections to alive, vital, and natural color, whether from plants, animals, or minerals. Human-made colors from natural pigments also represent living color.

The design implications for the use of color are plentiful. They occur at all scales, from cities and buildings to interiors and furnishings. At the personal space scale, color appears as an intimate, emotive quality. Subdues and white color and light reflect the immeasurable and unknown. Figure 5.7a is a photograph of a lavender field in the south of France, and Figure 5.7b is a photograph of Luis Barragan's colorful horse ranch home, Casa Cuadra San Cristóbal, in Mexico, built in 1968.

Subtle and Dramatic Use of Light

Light is integral to spiritual wellness and manifests in so many ways. Daylight affects both our eye functions and our inherent circadian rhythms. Light expresses in many

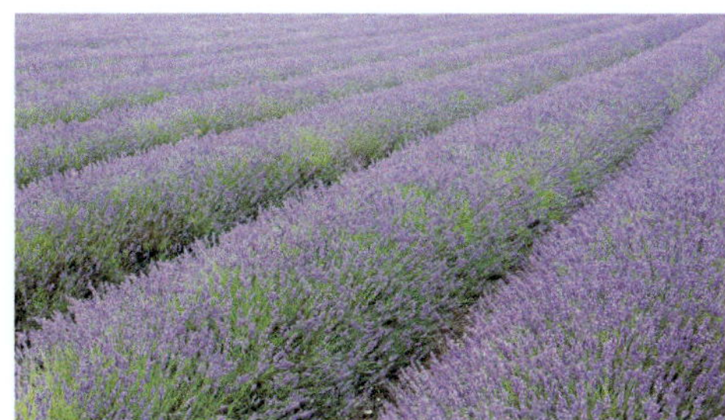
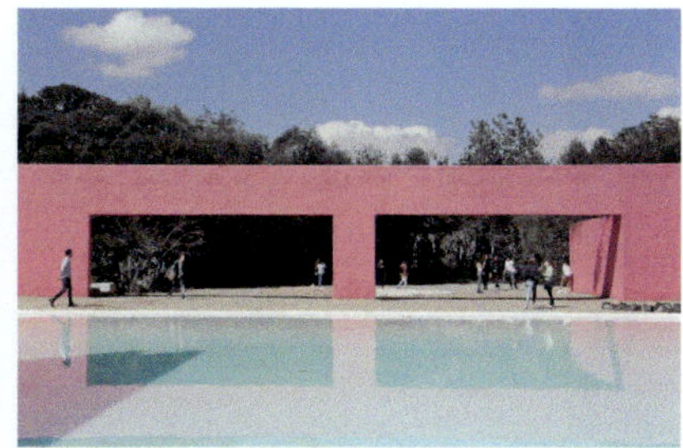

5.7 Experiences of Color: (a) Lavender Field in Provence, France, (b) Luis Barragan's Equestrian House, Mexico

forms and is related to luminosity, the ethereal, inspiration, and the numinous. Light is natural, dynamic, and can be direct, filtered, diffused, or reflected. Twilight, occurring at dawn and dusk, expresses as three types – civil, nautical, or astronomical twilight – depending upon its position relative to the horizon. Light elicits both awe and serene emotions, often in very differing ways. These differences express through their quality of light, from more stimulating sunlight and storm light to moonlight and starlight. Very focused and intense light can elicit awe experiences, while soft, translucent light can foster a more serene and contemplative mood. Light in concert with shadow gives definition, giving cues about depth and position. Further, moving light and shadow can create fractals facilitating de-materialization and transcendent experiences.

Fluid luminosity refers to the changing qualities of light, whether due to fluctuating conditions, source, color, or architectural design. Fluid luminosity has a co-existing dance with shadow to give expression to form. Light can also derive from moon- and starlight, campfires, fireplaces, and candles. Artificial light produces glare, skyglow, light trespassing, and cluttered light. Personal spaces should be designed to reduce the impact of night light pollution. For example, night light pollution creates a barrier to clearly viewing the night sky. Stargazing, an important night activity, is said to create connections to nature, inspire stillness, and promote new perspectives on life. When planning outside spaces, steps should be made to reduce the impact of street and automobile lights. Downward-directed light and use of lower wattages will help reduce night light pollution.

Light brings visibility to places of well-being. *Luminosity* is measure of radiant power and, in thin places, it relates to the emittance of light or emanation from a source (stars, sun, campfire, or candle) and can be facilitated by frames or openings such as a natural clearing or a building's window, skylight, cupola, or oculus. Light communicates levity and joy as its radiance has a quality of silence. Light in concert with shadow gives definition, giving cues about depth and position. Light also marks the passage of time from the changes of seasons to the daylight hours of the day. There are several spiritual wellness attributes and desired outcomes associated with both the subtle and dramatic use of light. The health benefits of daylighting are reduced eyestrain, increased vitamin D production, improved circadian rhythms and sleep patterns, forestalled seasonal depression, enhanced mental clarity, increased focus and productivity, and increased positive moods. Careful use of light prevents seasonal affective disorder, improves sleep and circadian

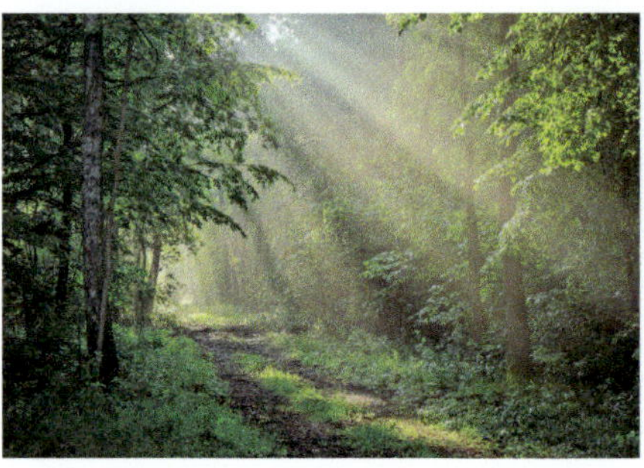

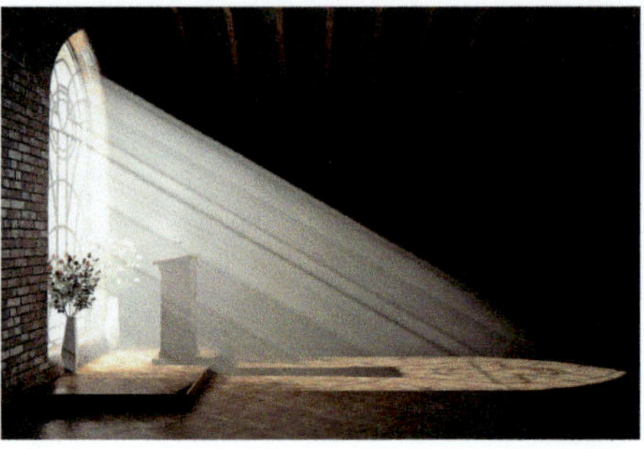

5.8
Sacred Natural Light: (a) Light Shafts in the Forest, (b) Light Shining through Church Window

rhythms, improves mood, and enhances the spirit of place. There is now limited but convincing evidence that moderate sunlight exposure is capable of modulating the immune system and improving health. The healing benefits of light include fostering the numinous, serenity, and awe experiences, transcendence and spiritual renewal, unity experiences, and possibly third places and sanctuary places. They include healing garden experiences that are biophilic and enable connections greater than ourselves. The spiritual qualities of light are well documented, and light that radiates, glows, streams, washes, or highly contrasts is particularly potent. The use of light supports spiritual wellness as follows:

1. **Daylighting** – creates healthy, natural ambient lighting, illuminates soft forms, or creates glowing space.
2. **Special effect lighting** – refers to directed light beams and streams creating ethereal and mystical effects.
3. **Fluid luminosity** – refers to the changing qualities of light, whether it is due to fluctuating outdoor conditions, source, color, diurnal or seasonal changes of sunlight, play of light and shadow, or architectural design.

The design implications for the subtle and dramatic use of light include the intentional directing of light washes or streams highlighting significant geometric, spatial, or architectural features of a building. The light quality in Figure 5.8 is highly inspirational in both natural and built contexts – light that evokes a spiritual experience, sense of transcendence, and something larger and more mysterious, beyond ourselves.

Wellness Stewardship

Stewardship is an ethical value and conduct that embodies nurturing and care of, and responsibility for, resources and places, both natural and built, entrusted to us and on which we depend. These include our personal spaces, buildings, communities, cities, and the natural environments that surround these places. Moreover, wellness stewardship extends to the personal dimensions of wellness – physical, mental, emotional, social, financial, and environmental wellness. And, in particular, it includes a focus on the spirituality and health behaviors with high-level effects. This suggests maintenance, closeness, and connections to a higher power or purpose.[11] Stewardship behaviors suggest a proactive process that is trustworthy, mindful, diligent, responsible, sustainable, and equitable.

There are several spiritual wellness attributes and desired outcomes associated with wellness stewardship. They include noetic and serenity experiences, presence and mindfulness, transcendence and spiritual renewal. There are emotional benefits as well, with self-satisfaction for the attendance to the experiences, wellness processes, and the places within which they occur. The benefits of stewardship also extend beyond the self to include social, community, public lands, and environmental stewardship. Given the need to protect the planet, environmental stewardship results in significant benefits. Environmental stewardship means protecting natural resources and preserving delicate eco-systems through lifestyle choices and behaviors. These efforts lead to our saving energy, reducing waste, incorporating renewable systems, and lowering our carbon footprint. Spiritual wellness stewardship goes beyond corporeal and pragmatic processes as responsibility to personal physical, mental, emotional, social, and financial health and include being open and present. When we realize that wellness stewardship efforts contribute to something greater than ourselves, we experience the transformative power of the stewardship moment.

The Findhorn eco-community is a good example of a steward lifestyle in the creation and maintenance of a spiritual garden and intentional community. Findhorn was established in the early 1960s by Peter and Eileen Caddy and grew into a community because of the remarkable garden they first created there.[12] They prepared the barren, sandy soil of coastal Scotland, planted with care and phenomenal success, and became wonderful stewards of the place, which evolved from a garden to an eco-community. Within a year of its planting, the garden grew 65 different types of vegetables, 21 kinds of fruits, and 42 different herbs and was overflowing with life. Today, the community is a constantly evolving demonstration of the spiritual, social, ecological, and economic dimensions of life. Concurrently, the community extends also to individuals, businesses, and organizations within a 50-mile (80-kilometer) radius of the Park and to the islands of Iona and Erraid on the west coast of Scotland. Figure 5.9a shows the Findhorn residents in front of their eco-community. Stewardship is an important supporter of spiritual wellness, as follows:

1. **Intentional stewardship** – minimizing waste of materials, spaces, buildings, and urban enclaves and carefully conserving natural resources.
2. **Nurturing care** – maximizing conscious cleaning, tidying, repairing, reusing, and maintaining spaces, buildings, urban places, and the natural environment.
3. **Attention to order** – referring to the spatial order supporting efficiency, organization, resiliency, use of resources, and things having their own place.

The design implications for wellness stewardship suggest spaces that are loved and cared for and that possess a kind of thriving vitality, which contributes to spiritual wellness. Characteristics of strong stewardship environments indicate that they are usually tidy, clean, and ordered and tend to be clutter-free. Further,

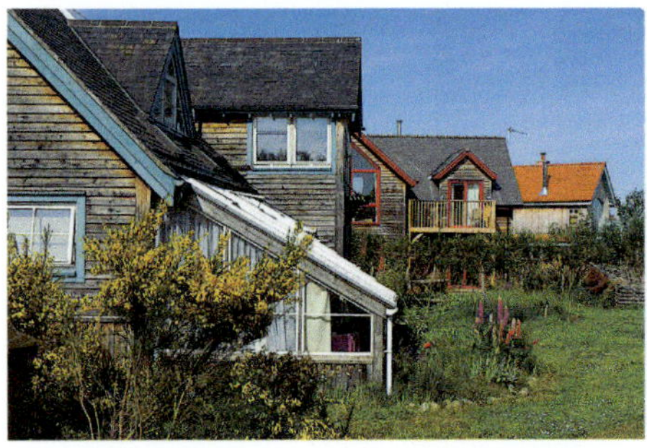

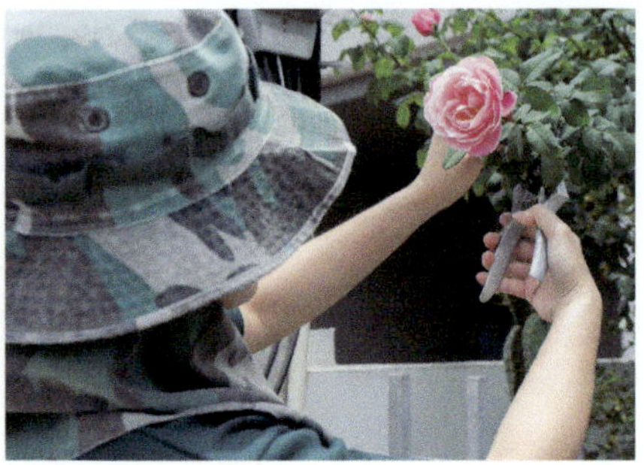

5.9
Designing for Self-Stewardship: (a) Findhorn Eco-Community, Scotland, (b) Pruning the Garden

they are flourishing, vital, and managed and tended on a regular basis. The quality of stewardship directly influences the realization of biophilic reciprocity, as mindful care and responsible interaction with the natural world are essential for cultivating a mutually beneficial and thriving relationship between humans and the environment. Figure 5.9b shows a woman pruning roses in her garden, depicting another example of stewardship.

Encouraging Personal Expression

Self-expression is the action of expressing yourself, communicating ideas and feelings, or creating forms of representing these expressions. It is a way of sharing one's unique perspective and connecting with others on a deeper level. Moreover, it is a way of expressing values. In the personal domain, one intra-relates with oneself with regards to meaning, purpose, and values in life. Self-awareness, a possible outcome of self-expression, is the driving force or transcendent aspect of the human spirit in its search for identity and self-worth.[13] From a wellness point of view, self-expression is crucial to emotional well-being. Further, it adds to mindfulness, a sense of presence, identity, familiarity, support, and nurturance. With regard to self-expression, Carol Venolia suggests that we do not need more symbols, especially those that depersonalize and fragment, but, rather, we need symbols that express continuity, wholeness, community, and self-worth.[14]

Self-expression can take a wide variety of forms, from the clothing you wear or car that you drive to the design or decoration of your home. Self-expression on an individual or personal level can take the form of how we present ourselves to others in terms of how we act or the clothing, hairstyle, and even sunglasses we choose. Personal expression in the form of creative outlets such as painting, drawing, writing, photography, filmmaking, gardening, cooking, and home design allows us to explore innermost thoughts and feelings in ways that are both therapeutic and spiritual. According to Filipe Bastos, true self-expression comes from within and reflects an individual's unique thoughts, feelings, and beliefs. It is crucial for overall well-being.[15]

Self-expression as a strategy for wellness can reduce stress, enhance relationships, enhance creativity, increase happiness, and boost self-esteem. In addition, self-expression plays a vital role in maintaining and improving mental health. It serves as a bridge between our inner world and the external environment, allowing us to communicate our thoughts, feelings, and experiences in ways that go beyond verbal communication.[16] The process of creative expression gives the ability to transition out of negative thoughts and patterns in constructive ways. It helps in sourcing the present by creating spaces that are familiar and safe. Self-expression authentically and freely promotes connections to others and the places within which we live. One's home, in particular, can be an expression of self and family. From a spiritual viewpoint, personalizing space can create a sanctuary and haven that help enhance grounding and centering. Such spaces may contain meaningful symbols and objects that help facilitate transformative experiences.

The design implications for personal expression suggest that spaces be allocated for individual creative self-expression. Within the home, for example, there should be spaces for each family member to self-express, including room color, symbols, posters, photographs, furnishings, and music. This allows each family member a safe, familiar, and heart-felt space that expresses their personality, interests, values, stories, and aspirations. Such spaces become a reflection of who they are and a sense of belonging. Taken together, they provide a canvas and place of memories for spiritual wellness. Our homes are more than financial assets, as they have deep emotional meaning. Other spaces can also elicit these kinds of meaning, such as our workplaces, third places, treehouses, and natural places such as gardens.

The wellness benefits of self-expression include creative expressions and developing new skills, helping cope with emotions, contributing to feelings of belonging, and improving mental health.[17] Further, self-expression can positively affect mood, function, cognition, and behavior.[18] Additional wellness benefits of self-expression include the creative expressions developing new skills, helping cope with emotions, contributing to feelings of belonging, and improving mental health.[19] Encouraging personal space supports spiritual wellness as follows:

1. **Self-expression** – creating meaning and preference through design, personal furnishing, decorations, color choices, symbols, and landscape elements.
2. **Mirror of self** – personalizing rooms or homes as an expression of personal taste, values, stories, and soulful qualities, especially at the domestic scale.[20]
3. **Identity** – creating a personal identity through design.

Figure 5.10 shows several examples of spaces with personal expression. The first example shows a rather cluttered room full of laptops, computer games, and soft drinks. It is complex, with "things" everywhere in sight. The second image shows a couple hanging a photograph that celebrates their wedding on their bedroom wall. And the third image shows a young boy painting a rainbow on his window as a form of self-expression.

Design for Silence

Noise is unwanted or harmful outdoor sounds created by human activity, typically caused by air, rail, and automobile traffic; railroads; loud construction and industrial sounds; sirens; street repairs; and even recreational activities. Such noise has been negatively linked not only to measures of mental well-being but also to more corporeal health consequences. The negative effects include sleeplessness, raised

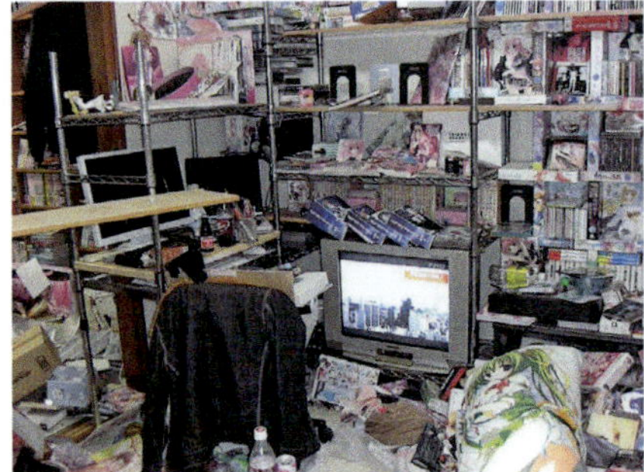

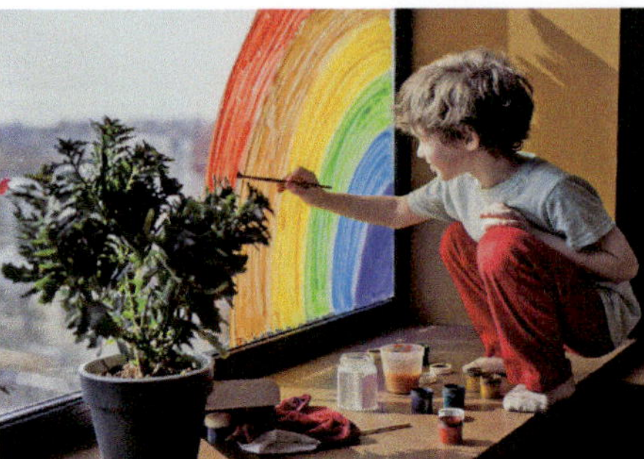

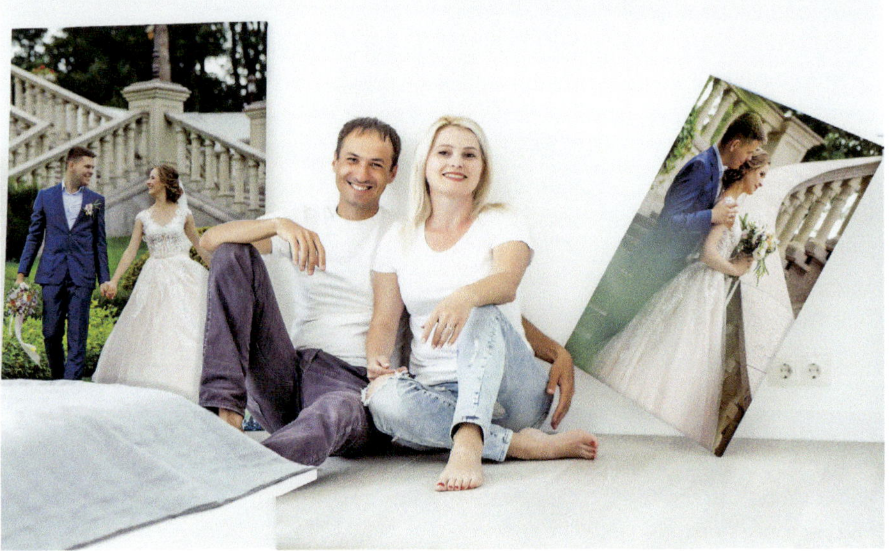

5.10 Personalizing Space: (a) Teenager's Room, (b) Child Painting a Rainbow on a Bedroom Window, (c) Couple Hanging Wedding Pictures

blood pressure, increased heart rate, hearing loss, nonauditory physiological effects, increased occurrence of hypertension, cardiovascular disease, negative moods, depression, cognitive fatigue, increased stress, and high levels of annoyance.[21] Yet the spirit of place can be amplified by the sensory character and sound of the space.

The relationship between acoustical design and spiritual wellness is complex and has the power to evoke emotions, influence thoughts, and even induce altered states of consciousness. In spiritual contexts, sound has long been used as a tool for meditation, prayer, and healing. According to Anne Kulinski, "Acoustics play a vital role in the health and success of space." Further, Kulinski suggests there are a myriad of health implications associated with noise and poor acoustics, including headaches, increased stress and anxiety, reduced quality of sleep, and possibly hearing loss.[22] Acoustical design refers to the strategic planning and design of building elements to achieve optimal sound quality and control. In very general terms, acoustical design is influenced by the following parameters:

1. **Reverberation and reverberation time** – sound source, sound waves, and time for reflections to decay, to avoid echo and to create a sense of awe and mystery, while shorter times can promote clarity and focus.

2. **Reflection** – sound distribution and reflection within a space using baffles, isolated ceilings, geometry, and reflective materials.
3. **Material absorption** – sound energy reduction through contact with absorbing materials and regulation with insulating and soundproofing materials, allowing for more peaceful and contemplative environments.

The term "soundscape" is currently credited to Michael Southworth who, in 1969, studied the sonic environment in cities. Natural sounds can be generated by biospheric and human sources. Research has found that natural soundscapes produce decreased stress annoyance and improved health outcomes (decreased pain, lower stress, improved mood, and enhanced cognitive performance).[23] Sound bathing, involving certain vibrations and frequencies, provides distinct somatic experiences.[24] And acoustic ecology is a movement started in the late 1960s by musician R. Murray Schafer that promoted mediated sound between animals, humans, and nature. His work also included the idea of *soundwalks*, with a focus on tuning into and listening to the environment.[25] Soundscapes can offer acoustic environments generally consisting of natural sounds (geophony) and animal vocalizations (biophony). They can also include pleasant sounds produced by human activity (anthropophony). Natural sound sources comprise ocean surf, waterfalls, rain, gentle breezes in trees, or wind-blown grasses. Sources also include animal vocalizations and calling behaviors, such as certain insect chirps, grazing sheep, songs of humpback whales, and cooing and birdcalls as might be imagined being produced by the songbird in Figure 5.11b.

There are several spiritual wellness attributes and desired outcomes associated with designs for silence. Soundscapes reduce stress, lower blood pressure, reduce cortisol, encourage mindfulness, promote self-awareness, and slow heart rates. They include numinous, serenity, and awe experiences, transcendence and spiritual renewal, unity experience, a possible third place, a sanctuary. They include healing garden experiences that are biophilic and enable connections greater than ourselves. According to Zorn and Marz, the deepest silence is not just absence but is also a presence. It is a "presence that can center us, heal us, and teach us."[26] It is an awakening. Furthermore, the spirit of place can be amplified by the sensory character of the space in which silence is important. Silence in spiritual wellness can be aided by the following:

1. **Design for silence** – reducing outdoor noise, using sound-absorbing materials, reducing reverberation, and creating harmonic spatial order.
2. **Soundscapes** – providing bird feeders for songbirds, small bells, water features, and windchimes masking unwanted noise.
3. **Soundwalks** – engaging in forest bathing and taking contemplative walks in nature with silence or only natural sounds.

The design implications for designing for silence and soundscapes suggest eliminating noise-generating technologies – for example, using geothermal heat pumps instead of noisy condensers in air-conditioning systems, or planning for

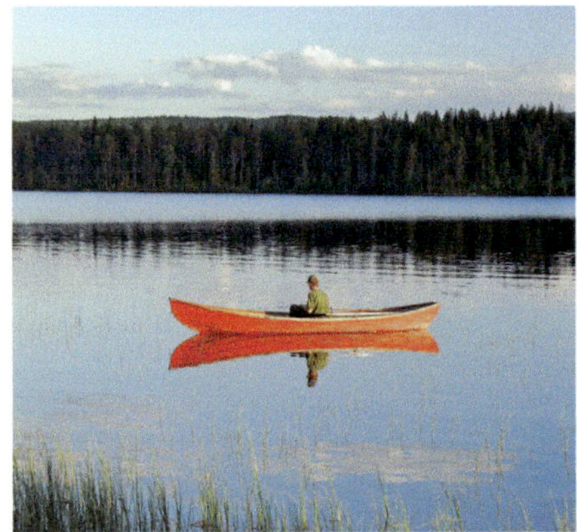

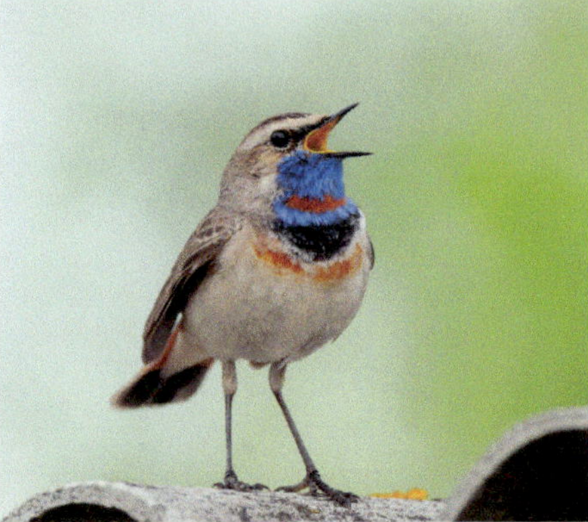

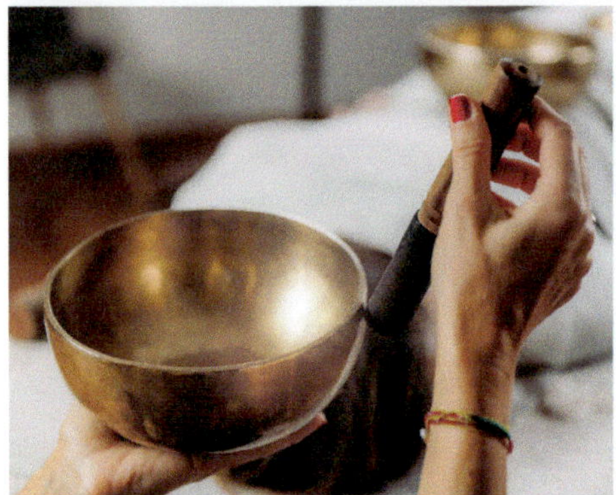

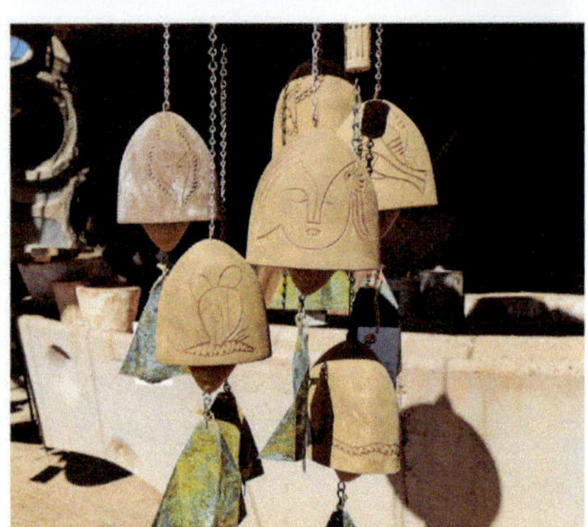

5.11
Sounds of Silence and Soundscapes: (a) Canoe in a Lake, (b) Songbird, (c) Sound Bathing, (d) Paolo Soleri Bells, Arizona

pedestrianization, thereby reducing automobile traffic and associated noise. Building fenestrations are other areas where noise can be reduced, such as by double and triple glazing, using insulating window inserts, or simply by incorporating shutters or curtains. The use of various soundscapes can also mask noise and provide pleasant sounds that contribute to spiritual wellness. Refer to Figure 5.11 for varying sources of soundscapes.

SUMMARY

Spiritual wellness is an ongoing process of self-discovery and active participation shaping the deepest part of us, including our beliefs, values, feelings, behaviors, and lifestyle practices. The wellness benefits are in part achieved through design as the dimensions inform the design opportunities in the built environment. Many of the attributes have a more direct impact upon design opportunities in the built environment, while some attributes have secondary effects on attitudes, convictions, and sensibilities that can influence planning and design decisions. The challenge at the personal scale is to protect intimacy, to flourish with individual well-being, and to simultaneously co-exist, cooperate, and participate in planetary stewardship and health.[27] A list of planning and design strategies for the personal scales follows:

1. Designing for personal scale.
2. Accessibility to everyday sacred wellness spaces.
3. Creating sanctuary spaces.
4. Bounded safe places.
5. Sensory connections.
6. Experience of color.
7. Subtle and dramatic use of light.
8. Wellness stewardship.
9. Encouraging personal expression.
10. Design for silence.

NOTES

1 Brill, Michael, *Using Place-Creation Myth to Develop Design Guidelines for Scared Space* (Self-published, September 25, 1985), p. 22.
2 Hall, Edward T., A System for the Notation of Proxemic Behavior (accessed July 30, 2024), https://www.jstor.org/stable/668580.
3 Roberts, K., & T. Messenger, Helping Older Adults Find Serenity. *Geriatric Nursing,* 1993, 14. Roberts, Kay, & Cheryl Aspy, Development of the Serenity Scale. *Journal of Nursing Measurement*, 1993, 155–156.
4 Buettner, Dan, *The Blue Zones: 9 Lessons Learned from the People Who've Lived the Longest*, 2nd edition (Washington, DC: National Geographic, 2012).
5 Brill, Michael, *Using Place-Creation Myth to Develop Design Guidelines for Scared Space* (Self-published, September 25, 1985), p. 22.
6 Corbett, Lionel, *The Sacred Cauldron: Psychotherapy as a Spiritual Practice* (Ashville, NC: Chiron, 2015), p. xi.
7 Steele, John, *Geomancy: Consciousness and Sacred Sites* (New York, NY: Trigon Communications, 1985).
8 The 5 Spiritual Senses: A Complete Guide (accessed September 2024), https://relaxlikeaboss.com/what-are-the-5spiritualsenses/#:~:text=The%20three%20primary%20spiritual%20senses%20are%20intuition%2C%20connection%2C,of%20interconnectedness%20with%20all%20beings%20and%20the%20universe.
9 Steele, John, *Geomancy: Consciousness and Sacred Sites* (New York, NY: Trigon Communications, 1985).
10 Shepard, Roger, Perceptual Organization of Colors: An Adaptation to Regularities of the Terrestrial World? in *The Adapted Mind: Evolutionary Psychology and the Generation of Culture*, Jerome H. Barlow, Leda Cosmides, & John Tooby (Eds.) (New York, NY: Oxford University Press, 1992), P. 496.
11 Bozek, Agnieszka, Pawel Nowak, & Mateusz Blukacz, The Relationship between Spirituality, Health-Related Behavior, and Psychological Well-Being (accessed September 2, 2024), https://www.ncbi.nlm.nih.gov/pmc/articles/PMC7457021/.
12 Findhorn Community, *The Findhorn Garden: Pioneering a New Vision of Man and Nature in Cooperation* (New York, NY: Harper & Row, 1975).
13 Fisher, John, The Four Domains Model: Connecting Spirituality, Health and Well-Being (accessed September 2, 2024), https://www.mdpi.com/2077-1444/2/1/17.
14 Venolia, Carol, *Healing Environments* (Berkeley, CA: Celestial Arts, 1988), p. 48.
15 Bastos, Filipe, Finding Your Unique Path: Exploring the Importance of Self-Expression (accessed September 4, 2024), https://mindowl.org/self-expression/.
16 Pennock, Seph Fontane, Unleashing the Potential of Self-Expression in Mental Health (accessed September 2, 2014), https://quenza.com/blog/mental-health-tool-for-self-expression/.

17 Wu, Ren, 5 Reasons Why We Need Self-Expression (accessed September 22, 2024), https://maniology.com/blogs/maniology-blog/why-is-self-expression-important?srsltid=AfmBOopgn_BBYn1FAvT16gl6vUy6YfWKbvMlayewRY1ftG5J17-HES_Y.

18 Cortese, Giuliana, & Georgetown University Medical Center, Creating Space for Self-Expression at "What Makes You?" (accessed September 22, 1224), https://gumc.georgetown.edu/gumc-stories/creating-space-for-self-expression-at-what-makes-you/.

19 Wu, Ren, 5 Reasons Why We Need Self-Expression (accessed September 22, 2024), https://maniology.com/blogs/maniology-blog/why-is-self-expression-important?srsltid=AfmBOopgn_BBYn1FAvT16gl6vUy6YfWKbvMlayewRY1ftG5J17-HES_Y.

20 Marcus, Clare Cooper, *House as a Mirror of Self: Exploring the Deeper Meaning of Home* (Berkeley, CA: Conari Press, 1995).

21 Buxton, Rachel, Amber Peterson, Caludia Allou, & George Wittemyer, A Synthesis of Health Benefits of Natural Sounds and Their Distribution in National Parks (accessed December 14, 2023), https://www.pnas.org/doi/10.1073/pnas.2013097118.

22 Kulinski, Anne, Acoustics 101: Best Practices Designing Healthier Sounding Spaces (accessed November 7, 2024), https://carnegiefabrics.com/resources/carnegie-convo-acoustic-design-101-best-practices-for-designing-healthier-sounding-spaces.

23 Krause, Bernie, The Voice of the Natural World (accessed December 15, 2023), https://www.ted.com/talks/bernie_krause_the_voice_of_the_natural_world/transcript.

24 Weis, Haley, Tuning in to Your Most-Ignored Sense Can Make You Happier (accessed September 4, 2024), https://time.com/6244162/how-sound-can-improve-happiness/#:~:text=Tuning%20into%20and.

25 Schafer, R. Murray, *The Soundscape: The Sonic Environment and the Tuning of the World* (Rochester, VT: Destiny Books, 1993).

26 Zorn, Justin, & Leigh Marz, *Golden: The Power of Silence in a World of Noise* (New York, NY: Harper Collins Publication, 1022), p. 5.

27 Ichioka, Sarah, & Michael Pawlyn, *Flourish: Design Paradigms for Our Planetary Emergency* (Axminster, UK: Triarchy Press, 2021), p. 50.

6 SPIRITUAL WELLNESS AT THE ARCHITECTURAL SCALE

INTRODUCTION

Wellness strategies are a mutually supporting set of design approaches that serve as prime actionable elicitors of wellness benefits promoting individual physical health, positive emotional responses, mental clarity, prosocial behaviors, spiritual renewal, and environmental reparation. Most of these strategies have a basis in science, health and wellness, and spirituality informed by the fields of public health, health sciences, religious and spiritual theology, and environmental psychology. The design implications and strategies include an understanding of the basic needs and opportunities at varying scales of the built environment. They describe design approaches, patterns, elicitors, and several examples that show the ways in which spiritual wellness has been effectively responded to and applied in previous works.

In what ways can planning and design solutions contribute to human and environmental health and wellness? Health and wellness benefit both human beings and the environments they inhabit, including both natural and built places. Human-centered health, as experienced within the continuum of illness-to-high-level wellness is defined by the dimensions of wellness, including our physical bodies, mental health, emotional well-being, social connections, and spiritual growth. Financial health is also seen as a wellness benefit. The environment-centered benefits are directed to the natural environment around us and the cities and buildings we occupy, as exemplified with air pollution. The contrast between these two environmental conditions is stark – one is polluted, and the other is endowed with clean air. The spatial implications of spiritual wellness are influenced by biophilic principles, sacred geometry, physical materiality, and place patterns. They are applied in three scales – personal space, architecture, and urban design – and are intended to provide the largest scope for wellness planning and design pathways.

Design considerations or strategies are intended to help elicit spiritual wellness benefits at any scale. They share DNA or characteristics with healthcare, sacred space design, biophilia, and thin places. And they are intended to respond to both spiritual dimensions and wellness outcomes. A series of works by the architect and architectural educator Michael Brill and his students at the State University of New York at Buffalo showed that a sacred – or, in their words, a "charged" – site could contain a common set of fundamental characteristics or patterns by which the sacred was revealed.[1] The planning and design determinants for spiritual

DOI: 10.4324/9781003546085-6

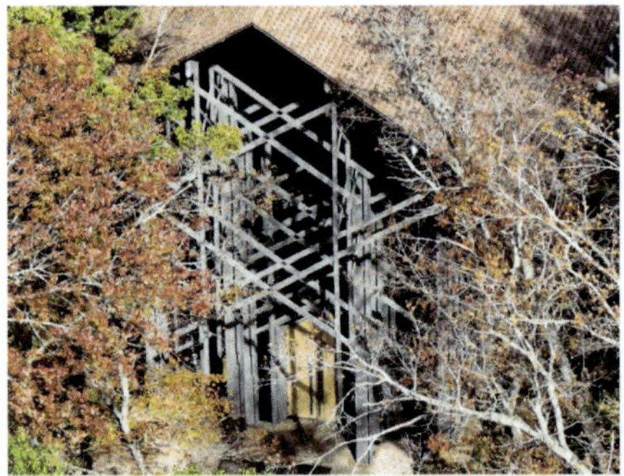

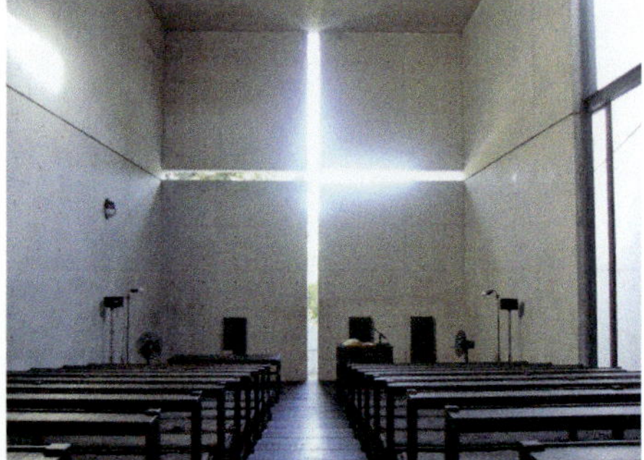

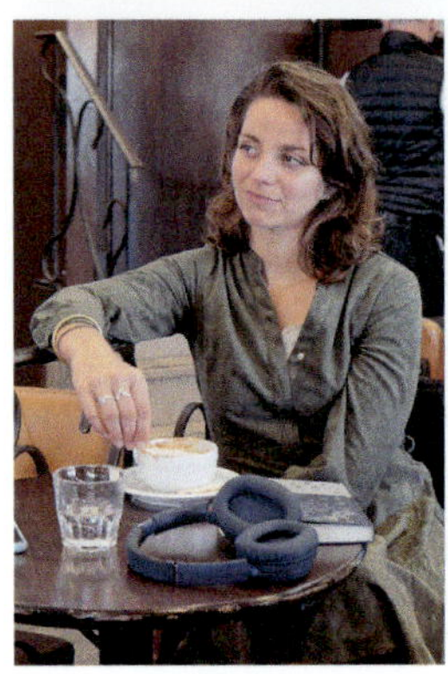

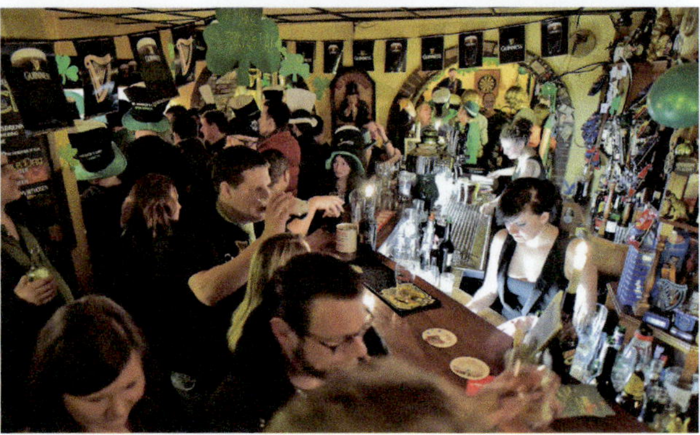

6.1 Spiritual Wellness: (a) Thorncrown Chapel, Arkansas, (b) Ibaraki Kasugaoka Church, Osaka, Japan, (c) Coffee in a Paris Café, (d) Dublin Pub, Ireland

wellness, although generalized below from these sources, are more specific to each of the applicable scales. Building types also vary in their ability to support spiritual wellness according to location, building form, and function or the architectural features and details. Figure 6.1 shows a variety of building types, from chapels in Arkansas and Japan to coffee in Paris and a pub in Ireland.

ARCHITECTURAL SCALE DESIGN STRATEGIES

Architecture is an intermediate scale under consideration for spiritual wellness. This scale also considers interior design and landscape features associated with buildings. Architectural scale includes building sites, building forms, use of light, spatial sequencing, building elements, material choices, on-site resources, and indoor–outdoor relationships.

Fundamental characteristics at this scale include centering, passage, bounding, spatial generosity, natural and luminous light, discriminating views, more formal geometry, balance and proportionality, intentional interactions with nature, and celestial, solar, and biospheric connections. Further, the formal characteristics may include symbolism if appropriate to the function, natural and unusual materials, as well as the incorporation of soundscapes. The architectural scale is composed of building types, sizes, functions, and forms that vary greatly, from a small wayfarers woodland chapel in Rancho Palos Verdes, California to a biophilic high-rise in Milan, Italy, to the Google Bay View building in Mountainview, California (Figure 6.2).

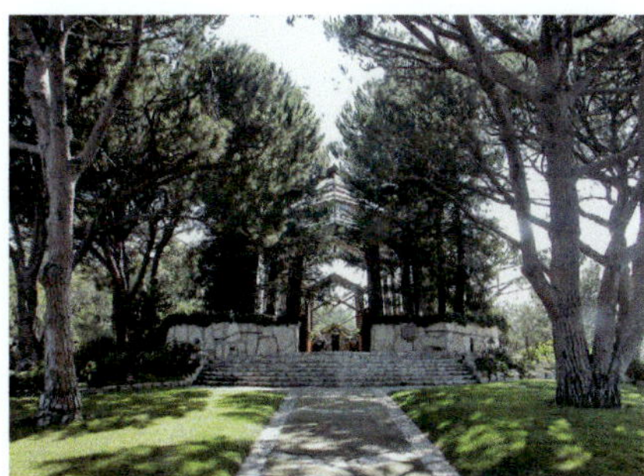

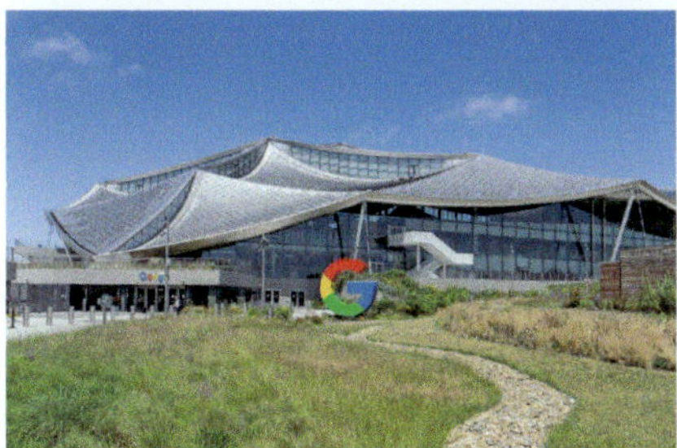

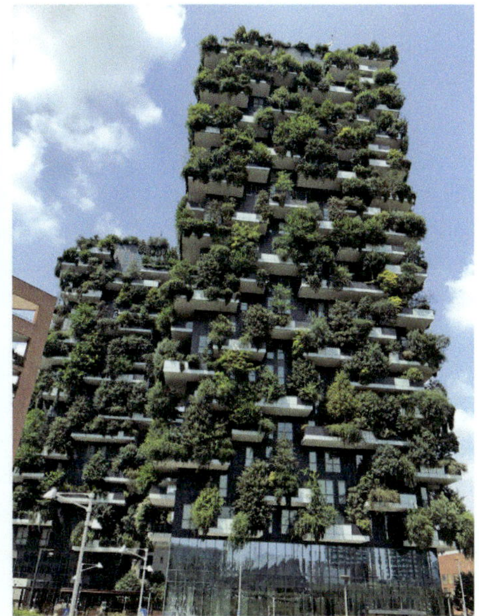

6.2
Biophilic Architecture: (a) Wayfarers Chapel, California, (b) Bosco Verticale, Milan, (c) Google Bay View Campus, California

Architecture offers many opportunities to respond to both spiritual and wellness design considerations. Together, these considerations produce power, health, wellness, and financial benefits. At this scale, there seem to be responses to three different types or contexts of architectural spiritual wellness. There are places that are sacred, those that are spiritual, and those that are soulful. Each of these types of spiritual space offers different qualities and physical characteristics.

- **Sacred architecture** – suggests places that are important, extraordinary, and have special meaning and symbolic content, whether they are religious, historic, cultural, or even personal. They support ceremonial or ritual participation.
- **Spiritual architecture** – suggests buildings that display spirited qualities and are uplifting, awe-inspiring, and transcendent through building form, spatial generosity, and light qualities. There are universal sacred principles and an energy within the places.
- **Soulful architecture** – suggests places that are loved, used, cared for, personal, emotional, introspective, highly resonating, and materially grounded. They tend to be older and complex, and sometimes darker in nature.

The architectural responses to both wellness and spiritual attributes require detailed considerations. The following pages describe ten different architectural-scale strategies that support sacred, spiritual, and soulful architecture that elicits spiritual wellness. The architectural scale includes building siting, exterior form, envelope and details, and interior design considerations. Architectural strategies can offer physical, psychological, mental, social, spiritual, economic, and environmental benefits. Spiritual wellness strategies include passage in and out of buildings, the incorporation of sacred geometry, beneficial building orientations, design for weather and climate, and the concept of spatial generosity. Additional strategies include designing for light and luminosity, incorporating water in special ways, responding to celestial phenomena, designing to create dematerialization of form, and reinforcing biophilic connections.

Spatial Sequencing and Passage

Spatial sequencing is the organization of spaces for approach, anticipation, pausing, entering, and then experiencing a charged or spiritual space. Passage is the transition from ordinary space or the secular realm into a sacred or religious realm. A veil separates the two wherein the sacred becomes a spiritualized place. Passage both is a means of accessing and entering these places and serves as a place of pause and orientation.[2] This passage not only represents physical movement between the two but also suggests a conscious and emotional transition. Passage as a pattern has physical and spatial characteristics and is considered a neutral space, separate from the secular or sacred spaces. This neutrality serves both the crescendo of anticipating, preparing, and entering and the decrescendo of departing, accommodating, and reassimilating a thin place experience. The passage pattern is a distinct and separate space or moment, with implicit or implied thresholds. Examples of spatial sequencing and passage include landscape entrances, pinch points, doorways, foyers, forecourts, vestibules, and passageways. Over time, how we approach and enter a building is important and helps facilitate a spiritual or wellness experience.

Passage patterns serve unique functions in religious architecture. For example, in some rural churches, there are intimate entrance structures that house benches for momentary seating before entering or leaving the churchyard. Part of the function of the passage pattern is to aid one to let go of stress and reduce temporal density before entering a sacred place. Although the spatial sequencing from outside to inside might require a number of spaces, there are three categories of spaces typically created for spiritual and religious architecture. In its simplest form, this sequence is "A" (exterior space), "B" (exterior portal and entrance), and "C" (interior foyer). This ABC sequence helps prepare participants for transformation that may come from the overall experience. This transformation is also highly influenced by the participant's state of mind. The spatial sequencing often follows what is termed an "A, B, and C" sequence of spaces, as follows:

1. **Exterior entrance space (A)** – a larger outdoor space, such as a plaza or courtyard, that leads to the building's entrance. These spaces serve an anticipatory and focusing function.
2. **Passage space (B)** – the veil and transition space that functions as a pause between the secular and sacred experiences.
3. **Interior spiritual space (C)** – the emersion into and experience of the sacred space within the building.

There are several spiritual wellness attributes and desired outcomes associated with spatial sequencing and passage. Spatial sequencing and passage contribute

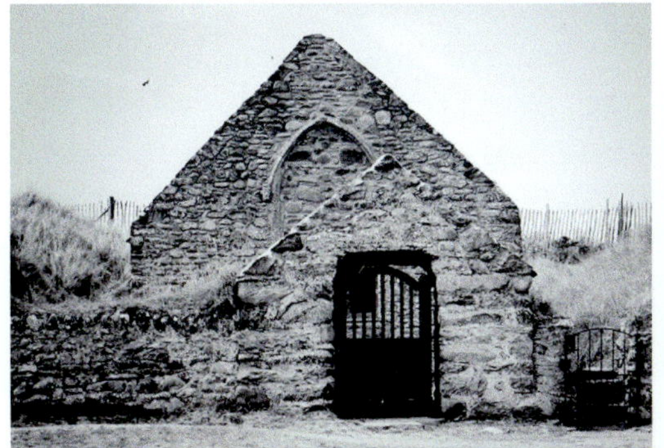
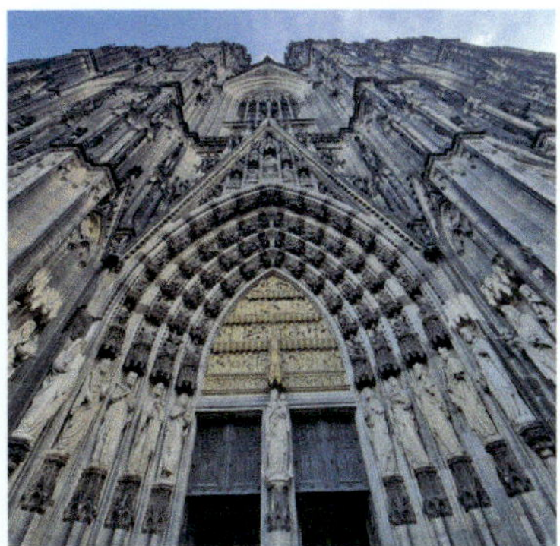
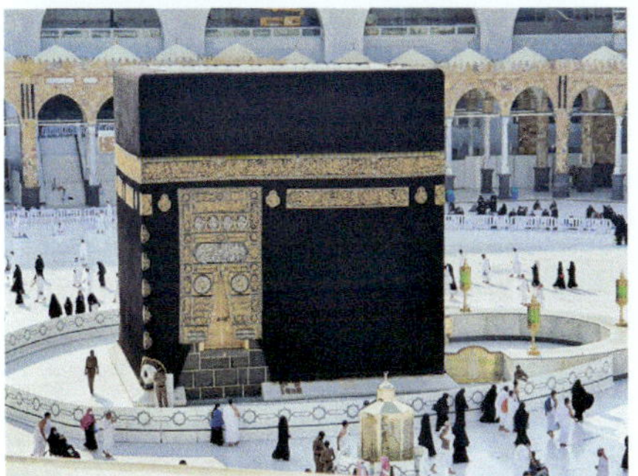
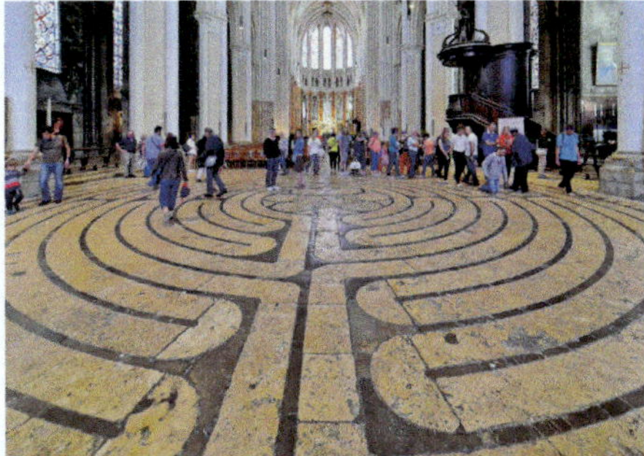

6.3 Spatial Sequencing: (a) Rural Welsh Chapel Entrance Structure, United Kingdom, (b) Cologne Cathedral Entrance Portal, Germany, (c) Pilgrimage around the Ka'ba, Mecca, Saudi Arabia, (d) Chartres Cathedral Labyrinth

to numinous, serenity, and awe experiences, transcendence and spiritual renewal, and unity experiences. They include connections greater than ourselves. The spatial sequence for spiritual wellness building is a process or journey of both entering, where there is a build-up or developmental crescendo, and exiting, or gradual reentry into a secular space and consciousness. Figure 6.3a is a photograph of a rural church along the coast in north Wales that clearly shows the bounded stone wall, the entrance structure with its gate and places to sit and pause, and the church beyond it. Figure 6.3b is a photograph of the entrance portal of Cologne Cathedral showing the archway corbeling that creates a place which is focused on the physical entranceway. The portal creates a space of pause, eliciting both serene and anticipatory feelings. The massive doors likely take an effort to actually be opened. The corbeling, massive doors, and vestibule create a thin place veil between the secular and sacred. Once within the cathedral, the interior space is exhilaratingly beautiful, eliciting awe experiences.

Figure 6.3c is a photograph of the Ka'ba or "black stone" in the center of the Great Mosque in Mecca, Saudi Arabia. In Islam, the Ka'ba is considered the most sacred spot on Earth and a most sacred pilgrimage destination. If they are able, at least one time in their lives, pilgrims gather and circumambulate the stone counterclockwise seven times. The wellness benefits include spiritual purification and growth, physical and mental wellness, both social and emotional connections, experiences of grace and gratitude, and connections to something greater than ourselves. The temporal dimension of these examples frames the sequence and procession of spaces that support transformational passage and sacred experience.

Use of Sacred Geometry

Sacred geometry supports spiritual wellness. According to dictionary definitions, sacred geometry ascribes symbolic and sacred meanings to certain geometric shapes and proportions. These meanings have personal, spiritual, and religious significance. Moreover, sacred geometry organizes material space and contains the space, enabling transcendent triggers. All buildings employ some form of geometry to organize spaces, such as structural systems, envelope designs, proportioning building elements, and organization of building materials. Sacred geometry goes further by eliciting transcendent experiences. Etymology elucidated the sacred further. The sacred qualities of the dimensions of things suggested that "breadth," from the Greek *platos*, meant great extent, "length," from *mekos*, meant foreshowing greatness, "depth," from *bathos*, meant hidden above human scrutiny, and "height," from *hypsos,* meant a metaphor for heaven.[3] These physical dimensions are the context for the embodiment of intentional sacred, wellness, and inclusive concepts, forms, and designs. The particular design and emphasis on any or all of these dimensions contribute to transformative experiences.

There appears to be a resonance between a person and geometric form or space. And, in the case of use of golden mean geometry, this resonance is intensified because our bodies are organized by this same proportional system. Further, when buildings are balanced and well proportioned, they tend to be more beautiful than other buildings. This experience of beauty can lead to spiritual wellness. The use of sacred geometry can be further described by the types and contexts as follows:

1. **Celestial or calendrical geometry** – is time-based and has to do with celestial movements of the galaxy, planets, and the Moon and the rotation of the Earth about its axis. These movements create patterns and rhythms that give structure and meaning to our lives – day and night, changes of the seasons, and direction of the sun.
2. **Terrestrial geometry** – is nature-based and not only finds expression in the land, geography, and other natural sciences but also in living organisms. Morphological growth and living organisms embody beautiful geometric patterns, from leaf and flower patterns to shapes of insects, fish, and other animals.
3. **Intrinsic geometry** – is mathematically based and has inescapable principles, rules, and meanings which are specific to the nature and character of various number and geometric systems. It seeks patterns whether they are found in numbers, space, time, form, or other abstractions.

Geometry and building types can express meaning. Circular and spherical buildings are fairly uncommon and usually are designed to embody important community ideals and aspirations. The use of this kind of geometry is special and evokes a strong sense of unity. Rectangular and square buildings are common, representing the majority of buildings in the world. The use of this kind of geometry lends itself to modular materials and construction methods, and multiplication in the urban environment. Triangular and angular buildings are somewhat rare and usually

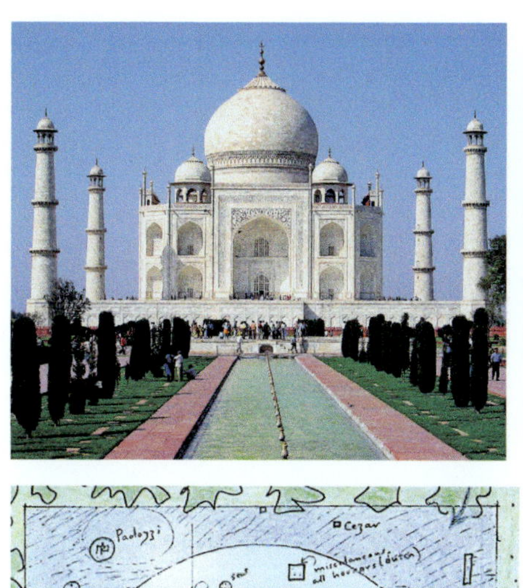
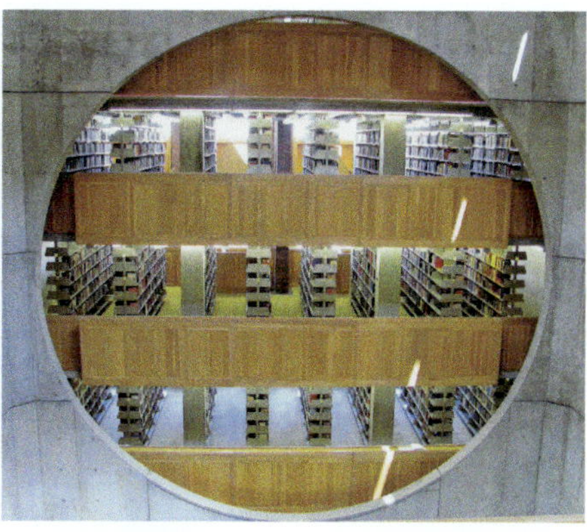
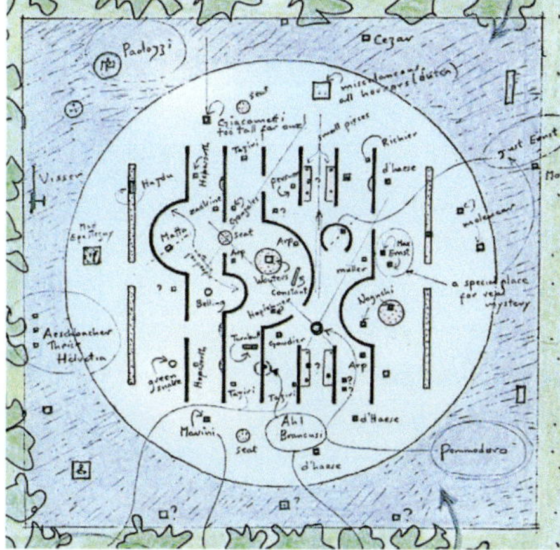
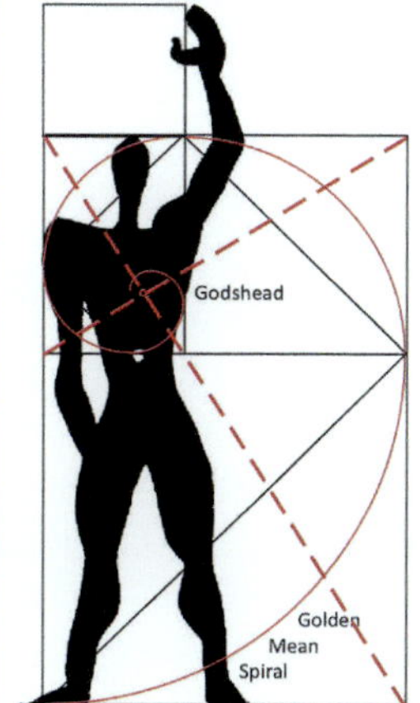

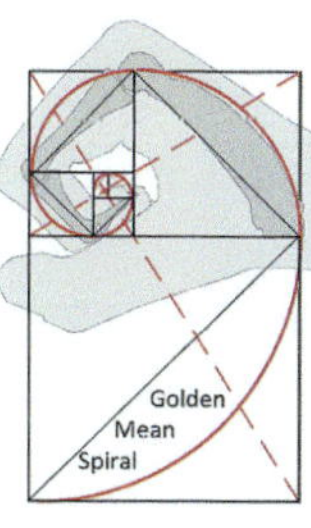

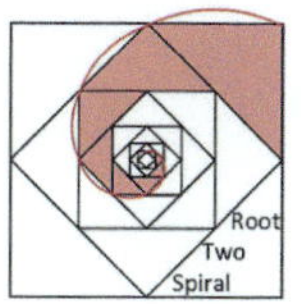

6.4 Sacred Geometry: (a) Taj Mahal, India, (b) Phillips Exeter Academy Library, New Hampshire, (c) Kröller-Müller Museum, Arnhem, the Netherlands, (d) Le Corbusier Man Geometry

are designed to accommodate special site conditions or are more dominantly expressed in section (elevation). Pentagonal buildings are fairly rare and usually are designed to accommodate unique functional needs or special requirements. Having said that, many current building designs using parametric software tend to be more curvilinear, using ambiguous forms and designed for one-off sites. As discussed in Chapters 9 and 12, opportunities exist for sacred geometry to be incorporated in everyday buildings. Space-filling geometry is used at the urban scale, delineating street and circulation patterns using square and rectangular grids (most common), octagon-square grids, as in Barcelona, and hexagonal or radial grids, as in Paris and Washington, DC.

The images in Figures 6.4a–6.4c show the Taj Mahal, considered one of the most beautiful buildings in the world, Louis Kahn's Phillips Exeter Academy Library interior, and Aldo van Eyck's pavilion at the Kröller-Müller Museum, all highly geometric. Figure 6.4d shows the relationship between the human body (Le Corbusier's proportional man), a hand, and golden mean geometry. There are several spiritual wellness attributes and desired outcomes associated with sacred geometry. They include awe, noetic, and thin place experiences through ritual and ceremonial sequences, transcendence and spiritual renewal, and connections greater than ourselves.

Orientation Responses

The orientation of a building responds to many external factors. They include the urban context within which it exists, the nature of the topography of the site, the shape of the property, possible views that are negative or positive, the relation to the sun and cardinal directions, or specific symbolic orientations. Orientation was more important to ancient builders than it is today. In his book *Dwellings: The House across the World*, Paul Oliver discusses Sakalava houses in Madagascar, where inside elements and activities, such as hearth, utensils, household head, guests, winnowing, and animals, are located in specific places that correspond to the surrounding stellar constellations.[4] The internal dwelling functions were not seen as being separate from the outside world beyond.

The practice of feng shui is connected profoundly to orientation responses in building siting, building design, and interior rooms. While feng shui was born out of a philosophical system, it had practical applications as well, which are still in play today. Historically, feng shui was used to site and situate buildings in the most auspicious ways. Orientation of rooms, furniture, and circulation into and through them were of importance. Further, the design for a building was a terrestrial response to the context and the energetic qualities of the internal spaces and circulation through them. The purpose was to design or place the formal aspects of a building such that *chi*, or life energy, and the health of the occupants were most achievable.

There are several orientation design objectives that include providing optimal positioning in response to surroundings; access to and protection against solar energy; responses to increase natural light and ventilation; protection against dust, noise, and prevailing winds; provision of privacy; and response to negative and positive views. Avebury, in England, built more than 4,000 years ago, is a good example of building in response to the cardinal directions, as can be seen by the crossing roads today (Figure 6.5a). The Baker House, designed by Alvar Aalto, is a serpentine six-story building with major dormitory rooms oriented to the tree-lined street and the Charles River beyond (Figure 6.5b). With the advancement of the biophilia and wellness design movements, orientation to nature and the sun has gained more importance.

There are several spiritual wellness attributes and desired outcomes associated with site and building orientations. They include the experience of spirit of place, the process of centering within larger cosmic connections that are greater than ourselves, awe experiences, transcendence, and spiritual renewal. They also include

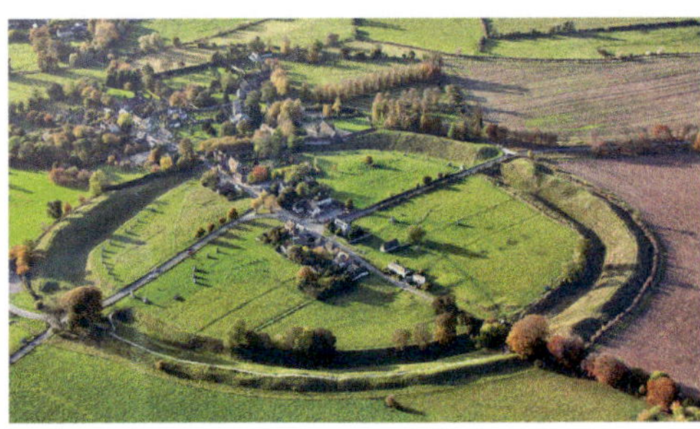

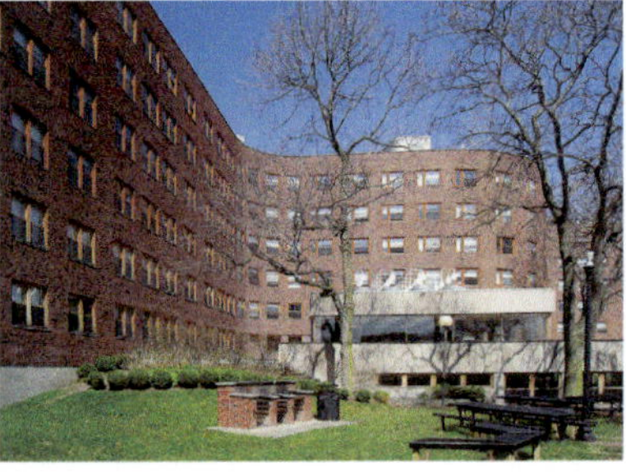

6.5 Orientation Responses: (a) Avebury Stone Circle, UK, (b) Baker House, Cambridge, Massachusetts

biophilic connections as well as possible experiences of the unknown. Further, if oriented to favorable solar energy, natural light, or wind and sound protection, orientation can benefit well-being. The design for specific orientations can respond to both positive and negative forces, as follows:

1. **Positive orientation responses** – allow for maximum natural light, natural ventilation, and desirable solar energy gain or solar masking, adjacencies to natural views and soundscapes, privacy, and orientation to cardinal directions.
2. **Negative orientation responses** – protect from unwanted noise, air pollution, ugly or unwanted views, and too much wind or solar radiation.

There are several spiritual wellness attributes and desired outcomes associated with orientation. These include the process of centering within the larger context, Climate and solar energy in particular have a profound effect on building comfort. Views of and physical access to nature produce positive health, wellness, and spiritual effects. Experiences of the changes of the seasons and sleep are affected by a building's orientation. Taken together, these all contribute to joyful and transformative experiences and experiences of things larger than the self.

Design for Climate

Climatic design determinants vary depending on the location of a building. Extreme locations, such as arctic regions, arid deserts, and tropical forests, require careful consideration of the design of basic architectural elements. The greatest percentage of the human population lives in temperate regions, but this area still requires climatic design responses for high winds, rain, snow, thunderstorms, as well as both over- and under-heating conditions. Much has been published about the negative effects of climate change, natural disasters, and extreme weather events. Real estate websites, such as Realitor.com and Zillow, have included *climate-risk data* to their listings.[5] Home sales in risky climate areas have fallen behind those in safer areas. Risk factors such as storm surges, seismic events, flood, sea level rise, wildfire, extreme wind, air quality, drought, and extreme heat are considered.

Climate change and environmental degradation are also the consequences of our contemporary condition, a situation the public has recently recognized. Climate neutrality and carbon neutrality promote the reduction of emissions-producing activities, improving efficiency, incorporating renewable energy technologies, and phasing out the use of fossil fuels. Design responses to climate can support sustainability and promote health and wellness outcomes.[6] Architecture responses to climate take into consideration seasonality, sun direction (sun path and position), self-shading factors, and environmental factors, such as wind, rainfall, humidity, mildew and mold, under- and overheating, and the destructive hazardous events and vulnerability caused by earthquakes, volcanic eruptions, tornados, cyclones, hurricanes, tsunami surges, drought, wildfires, avalanches, monsoons, and flooding.

Design in response to climate has been a practice from time immemorial, yet more recently it has generally been forgotten, being replaced by other considerations such as abundant fossil fuels, construction costs, and aesthetics. Now it has

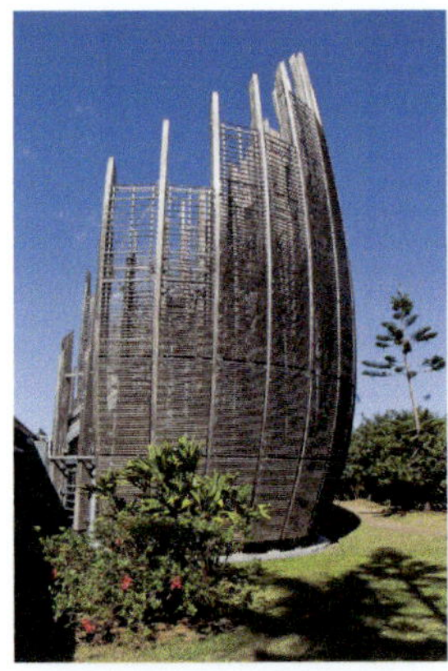

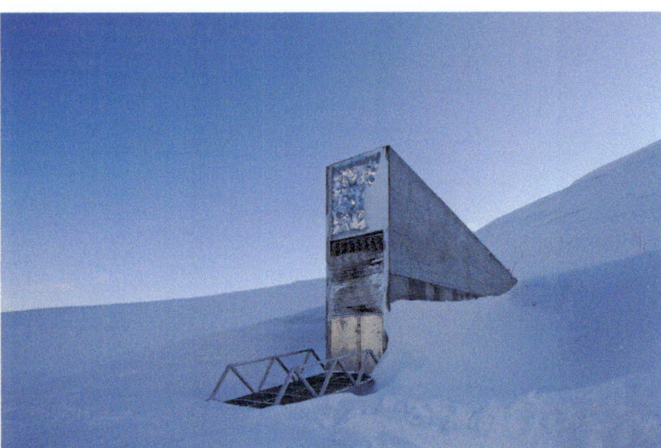

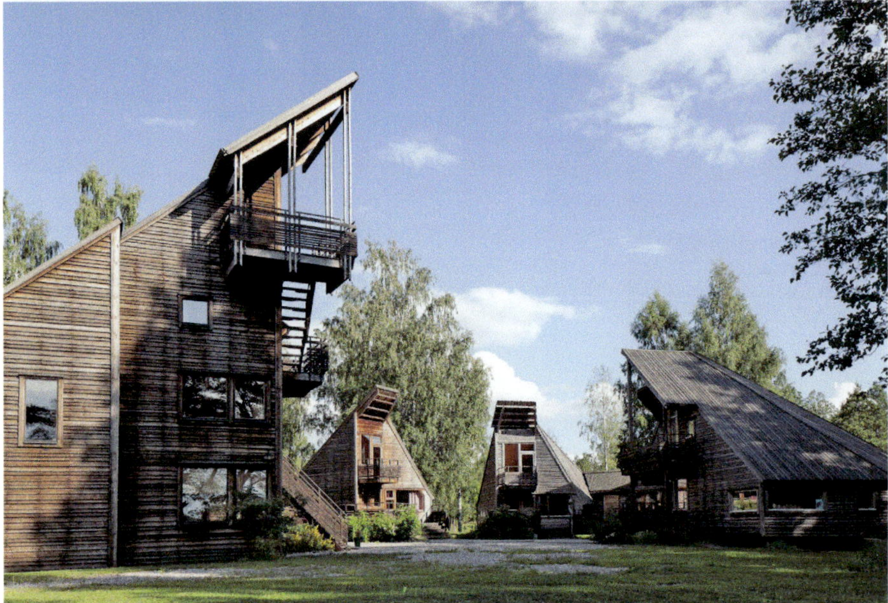

6.6
Climatic Design:
(a) Tjibaou Cultural Center, New Caledonia,
(b) Svalbard Global Seed Vault, Norway,
(c) Hedesunda Housing Cluster, Sweden

re-emerged as an important planning and design determinant primarily targeted for reasons of sustainability and disaster mitigation. In the context of this book, these raise the question, "How can spiritual wellness become a contributing influence on a building's design in response to climate?"

Climatic design considerations at the architectural scale focus on siting; primary, secondary, and tertiary building form responses; and material choices. Three examples of climatic design are illustrated in Figure 6.6. First is the Tjibaou Cultural Center in New Caledonia, designed by Renzo Piano and built in 1998. The design identifies the Kanak culture and identity with links between the landscape and built structures. Located within a subtropical climate zone, the wind-generated forms present a functional, yet symbolic and historic, memory of the place. The second is the Svalbard Global Seed Vault in Sweden. Opened in 2008, it was created to preserve a wide variety of plant seeds that are duplicates of samples already stored in the more than 1,700 gene banks worldwide. Many of them are vulnerable, under threat of civil unrest, lack of funding, flooding, natural disasters, and climate change. The Global Seed Vault is considered the world's largest and most secure seed vault. These examples represent extreme locations, and, therefore, the architectural responses are strong. The third is the housing cluster in Hedesunda, Sweden, which was built in 1989 and employs a dramatic wind protection form concept. The houses have highly insulated shed roofs deflecting the wind over the cluster while, at the same time, having inner vertical façades that are opened up to views of the River Dalalven and south for passive solar energy gain.

Additional spiritual wellness attributes are associated with climatic design. They include the experience of safety from disasters and adverse climate events, comfort, enjoyment of the changes of seasons, transcendence and spiritual renewal, biophilic experiences, and ceremonial participation and connections greater than ourselves. The health benefits are increased energy, mental clarity, decreased stress, lower blood pressure and heart rate, and increased positive moods. The spiritual benefits include connections to things greater than ourselves. With increased exposure to the positive and spiritually beneficial qualities of climate, the other, more negative, consequences, such as the climate crisis and re-occurring natural disasters, may increasingly be addressed. Choosing a place to live in response to climate risk factors and spiritual wellness benefits will become increasingly important. Locations with the greatest survival advantages, vitality, and natural beauty in turn will be most desirable.

Creating Spatial Generosity

The spatial character of a building is important in contributing to the ways in which we experience and function within it. For spiritually oriented architecture, spatial generosity helps facilitate transcendent experiences and well-being. Key architectural elements of spatial generosity include abundant volume of space, emphasis on height, open and fluid circulation, natural light, transparency extending internal space outward, open spatial flow between spaces, and awe-inspired scale. The US Expo 67 pavilion in Montreal, Canada, is a good example of spatial generosity and the use of geometry defining the space (Figure 6.7a). The Hyatt Regency in Atlanta, Georgia, was designed by John Portman and, while controversial because of its "anti-urban" design, introduced an impressive interior atrium space that is daylit by a large skylight (Figure 6.7b). The generous space of this hotel interior might create certain awe emotions owing to its vastness, but may not engender spiritual wellness because of its secular qualities. Other religious and non-religious examples do have explicit spiritual wellness attributes of spatial generosity, such as the Cathedral of Christ the Light in Oakland, California, by SOM, and the Guggenheim Museum in New York City (Figure 6.7c and 3.7d).

In everyday architecture, spatial generosity is more difficult to achieve because of construction budget constraints. However, in residential design, some spaces receive some generosity. For example, foyers, living rooms, dining rooms, great rooms, and sometimes master bedrooms often have high ceilings or are two stories high, affecting the grandeur of the space. Non-residential building types where spatial generosity is employed owing to function include airport terminals, sports stadiums, symphony and opera houses, to name a few. It is the arts venues that

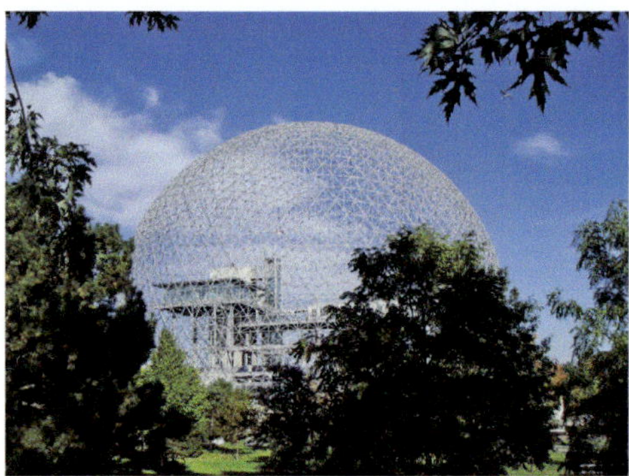
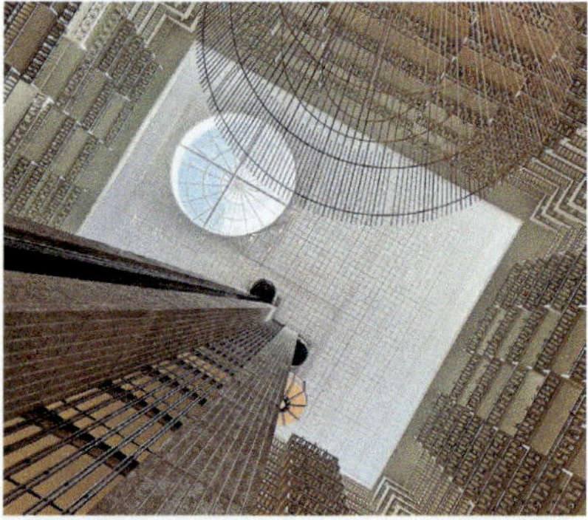
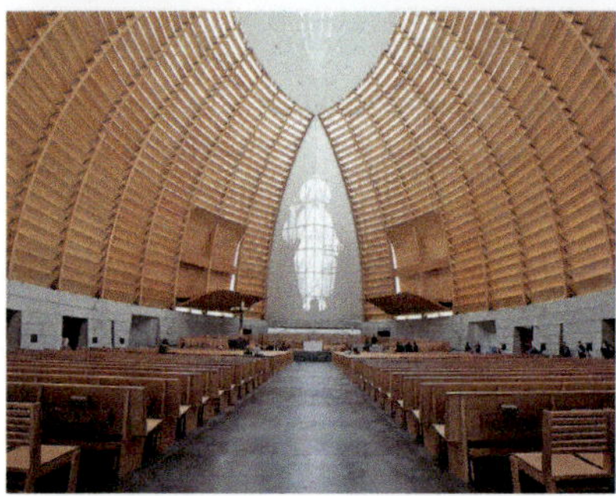
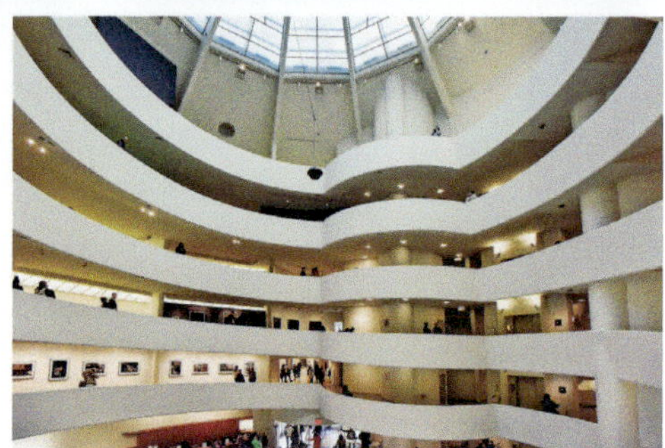

6.7
Spatial Generosity: (a) US Expo 67 Pavilion, Canada, (b) Hyatt Regency Atlanta, Georgia, (c) Cathedral of Christ the Light, Oakland, California, (d) Guggenheim Museum, New York City

most likely elicit spiritual wellness experiences owing to the combination of the spatial quality and the artistic performances. Certain building types are naturally spacious, owing to their functions, such as sports arenas, performance halls, and large churches.

What makes generous spaces spiritual and wellness-oriented is the combination of design elements, including space volume, height, and play with light. Together, these are inspiring and can elicit awe emotions. Such elements associated with spatial generosity contribute to several spiritual wellness attributes and desired outcomes. They include numinous, religious, and awe experiences, transcendence and spiritual renewal, unity and unknown experiences, possible third place experiences, and connections greater than ourselves. Depending upon the actual design, spirit of place can be emphasized through the spatial quality. Spatial generosity can enhance a spiritual experience through:

1. **Vertical space** – characterized by high aspect ratios of vertical space, especially when coupled with streaming natural light, such as the Hyatt Regency Atlanta and the Pantheon in Rome.
2. **Horizontal space** – characterized by terrestrial horizontal expanding spaces in both architecture and urban design, such as Las Ramblas in Barcelona or the Highline Park in New York City.
3. **Volumetric space** – large volumes of space in both the horizontal and vertical dimensions, especially at the urban design scale, such as the Oculus interior in New York City or the Campo in Siena.

At the urban design scale, spatial generosity – characterized by ample public spaces, accessible green areas, and human-scaled environments – can foster a sense of connection and tranquility, contributing significantly to collective and individual spiritual wellness. Within the urban setting, generous spaces promote public physical, mental, emotional, social, and environmental health and well-being. And, lastly, our national park monuments offer immense benefit outcomes that lead to less reliance on medication, fewer trips to the hospital, and lower healthcare costs.

Design for Luminosity

Daylight affects both our eye functions and our inherent circadian rhythms. Light expresses in many forms and is related to luminosity, the ethereal, inspiration, and the numinous. According to the Environmental Protection Agency, the average American spends as much as 93 percent of their time indoors, with 87 percent of that time spent in buildings and 6 percent in automobiles.[7] Night light pollution is a problem for clearly viewing the night sky. It often renders starlight invisible. Artificial light produces glare, skyglow, light trespassing, and cluttered light. According to Wayne Ott, the conclusion of his research on human activity found that, "we are basically an indoor species."[8] With so much time spent indoors, light and its various forms and qualities are essential and, in sacred buildings, are prime elicitors of spiritual wellness. And, according to Louis I. Kahn, silence is immeasurable, while light is the giver of presence.[9]

Light impacts health and performance and is expressed in many forms related to luminosity, inspiration, the ethereal, and the numinous. Fluid luminosity refers to the changing qualities of light, whether due to fluctuating conditions, differing sources, color, or architectural design. Light also marks the passage of time, from the changes of seasons to the daylight hours of the day. Natural light affects both our eye functions and our inherent circadian rhythms. It is natural and dynamic and can be direct, filtered, diffused, or reflected. Natural light can form pools of light, define shapes, and provide warmth. Light in concert with shadow provides definition by giving cues about depth and position.

The two images in Figure 6.8 depict two very different uses of light. The interior of the Pantheon shows the cylindrical beam of light pouring down from the large open oculus above the center of the space (Figure 6.8a). And the interior of Louis Kahn's Kimbell Art Museum in Fort Worth, Texas, shows the vaulted ceiling's subtle spread of diffused light illuminating the museum's walls (Figure 6.8b).

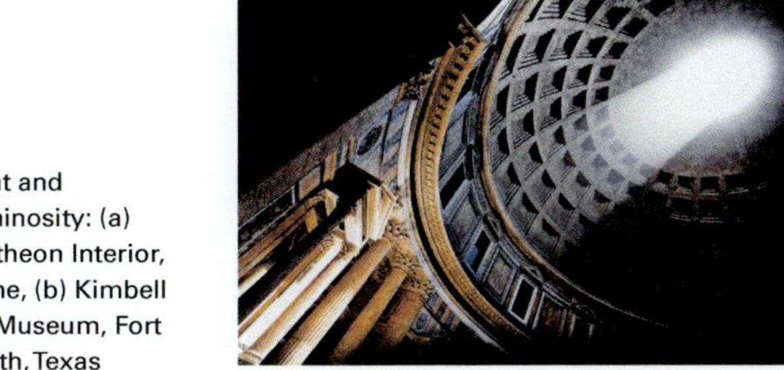

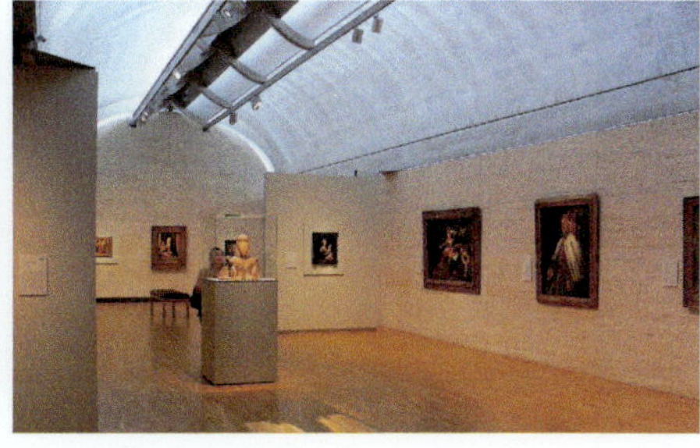

6.8
Light and Luminosity: (a) Pantheon Interior, Rome, (b) Kimbell Art Museum, Fort Worth, Texas

There are several spiritual wellness attributes and desired outcomes associated with light and luminosity. They include numinous, religious, serenity, and awe experiences, transcendence and spiritual renewal, and unity experiences. Other attributes include fostering a sense of presence and mindfulness and effecting connections greater than ourselves. Further benefits include boosting vitamin D storage in the body, aiding dopamine production for healthy eye development, and possibly contributing to higher productivity.[10] Stargazing is said to create connections to nature, inspire stillness, and promote new perspectives on life. Depending upon the actual design, the use of light can be amplified or directed in such a way as to create ethereal effects and help cope with existential issues and experiences of the unknown.

Incorporating Water and Blue Spaces

Water is indicative of life's beginning and inception and is, thus, prominent in creation stories. According to Celeste Ray, "Fresh waters are not only sites of creation, but are prototypical symbols of renewal during life."[11] Water is necessary for life. Elizabeth McAnally explains, "given an ample amount of water that is clean and pure, life flourishes."[12] Water is the most abundant molecule and is necessary for life. Furthermore, water is needed extensively for commercial, industrial, agricultural, and electrical production, and domestic uses. While rivers, lakes, and waterways once served as areas of transport and exchange, today they form borders that separate territories from one another. Water in architecture is both a blessing and a curse. And, according to Abby Phon, the health benefits of water for the human body include increasing energy, flushing out toxins, promoting weight loss, improving skin complexion, maintaining regularity, boosting the immune system, and preventing cramps and sprains.[13]

Water creates blue spaces. While blue spaces are most common outdoors, it is possible to integrate them indoors where people spend most of their time. Views and physical access to outdoor blue spaces is also important. These include views of ocean beaches, rivers, lakes, ponds, and water features such as fountains and rain chains. As explained by Neil deGrasse Tyson, tides are created by hemispheric water bulges that move owing to the rotation of the Earth and the pull of the Sun and Moon, thereby creating lowering and rising tides.[14] So, it is from the dynamic movement of water that its relationship to emotions is derived. Water is commonly associated with emotions, feelings, compassion, empathy, and intuition.

Water has pragmatic benefits. High-quality water improves the efficiency of home appliances, such as washing machines and dishwashers. Water is useful in fire control and fire suppression control systems. And, finally, water features such as fountains, waterfalls, ponds, and other aquascapes evoke tranquility, promote mindfulness, and foster a deeper connection with the natural world, thereby nurturing spiritual wellness. Ecosystems are linked and maintained by water which provides permanent habitat for many species. And, at the urban scale, rainwater can be managed through harvesting, swales, infiltration gardens, porous surfaces, climate responsive landscaping, and retention ponds. The three images in Figure 6.9 illustrate profound integrations of water with architecture.

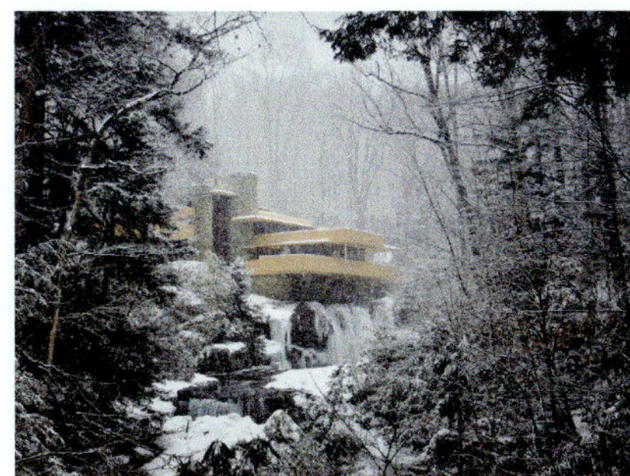

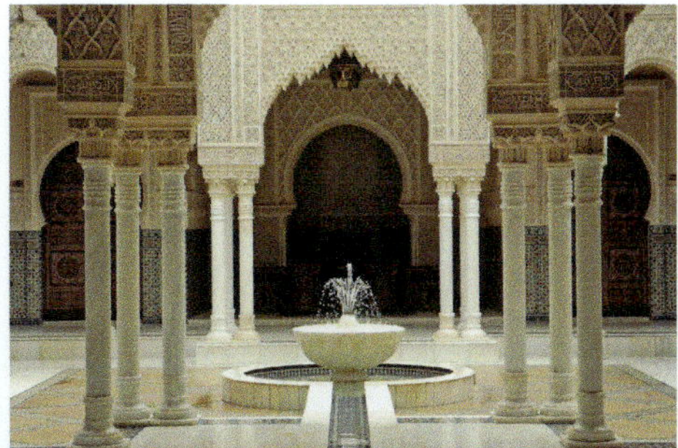

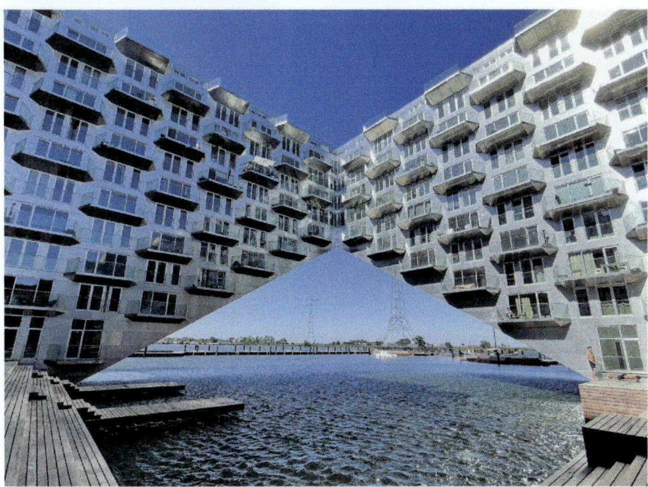

6.9
Presence of Water: (a) Kaufman House, Pennsylvania, (b) Moroccan Interior Fountain, (c) Sluishuis, Amsterdam

From a wellness perspective, water is essential for plant growth and is considered to possess healing power. Water has additional healing qualities when one washes out flesh wounds or immerses oneself or bathes in it, thereby removing toxins and reducing stress. There are several spiritual wellness attributes and desired outcomes associated with the presence of water. They include numinous, serenity, and awe experiences, transcendence and spiritual renewal, unity experiences, and possible third place experiences. In addition, they are biophilic and contribute to healing gardens and connections to the unknown and things greater than ourselves. Other benefits include increased physical activity, reduced stress, lower heart rate and blood pressure, increased feelings of tranquility, positive emotional responsiveness, and improved concentration, perception, and memory.

Responses to Celestial Phenomena

Observing the *celestial* heavens is an ancient practice and reveals the movement of the Sun, Moon, constellations, comets, and other heavenly bodies. These celestial phenomena were a source of mystery, metaphors, stories, origin and ascension myths (cosmogony), dwelling places of the Gods, and the unexplainable. In ancient times, architectural responses to celestial phenomena were far more important. Stone Age structures were constructed for ceremonial, spiritual, and calendrical reasons – Stonehenge, Newgrange, and Avebury Stone Circle to name a few.

Orientation to both solar and lunar movements was important, and certain dates and times were marked within the structures, especially solstices and equinoxes. For spiritual wellness, celestial phenomena produce a sense of awe and wonder, celestial beauty (sunsets, rainbows, shooting stars, and Northern Lights); they act as windows into the immense size and complexity of space and give us perspective and humility.

There are several spiritual wellness attributes and desired outcomes associated with celestial phenomena. Often they celebrate crepuscular and anticrepuscular skies, occurring at dusk and dawn and during solstices. They include experiences such as the numinous, unity, and transcendence. Further, they include serenity and awe emotions, and spiritual renewal. And they can be elicited by thin places, third places, sanctuary places, labyrinths, and celestial monuments such as Newgrange in Ireland. They are biophilic and can produce connections to architectural experiences and events greater than ourselves. Depending upon the location and specific design of the building, spirit of place can be present and amplified. Contemporary examples of celestial phenomena are less common but often have more subtle connections. For example, many people prefer to have kitchens facing the east for morning light, and some people prefer to have beds oriented to the cardinal directions, with the head of the bed facing north. Since the renewed interest in renewable energy, many dwellings require south orientation for passive solar heating.

Figure 6.10a is a photograph of the light shaft at the winter solstice in Newgrange, Ireland. This light is particularly significant at the winter solstice when the light shaft goes deep into the mound, marking the most sacred time of the year. Figure 6.10b is a photograph of the historic Stonehenge in Wiltshire, United Kingdom, during the summer solstice sunset. Stonehenge was bult in several phases, beginning more than 5,000 years ago. Figure 6.10c shows the interior sundial room in Charles Jencks's home in London. The home, called the Cosmic House, was a postmodern renovation completed in 1983. Several celestial references were featured including the solar stair, moonwell, and the sundial room. Figure 6.10d is a detail of the astrological clock tower on an early Renaissance building facing the Piazza San Marco in Venice. The great clock face in blue and gold, inside a fixed circle of marble, is engraved with the 24 hours of the day in Roman numerals. A golden pointer with an image of the sun moves round this circle and indicates the hour of the day; within the marble circle, beneath the sun pointer, are the signs of the zodiac in gold. Figure 6.10e is the sundial outside of the Galileo Museum in Florence. The shadow cast by the glass polyhedron atop the large bronze gnomon indicates the date and time. These celestial references are strategies that can remind us of the larger world within which we live.

Design for Demateriality

The form and material qualities of a building most often express its function and means of construction. The resulting interior spaces, as previously discussed, can support spiritual wellness either through intimate and more serene scales or through generous and awe-inspiring spaces. The experience of transcendence, however, can be further enhanced through what might be called "dematerialization." This

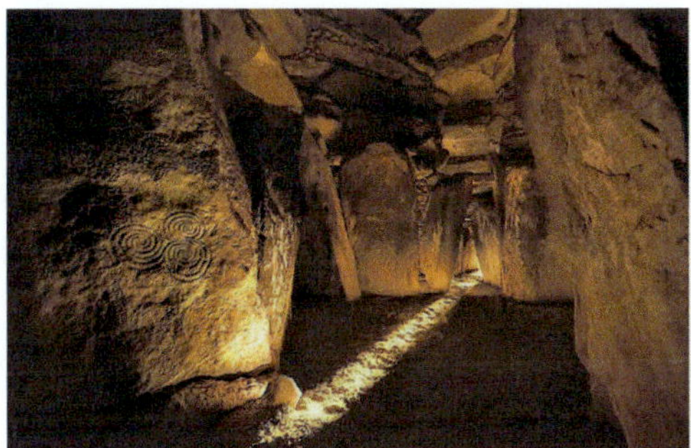

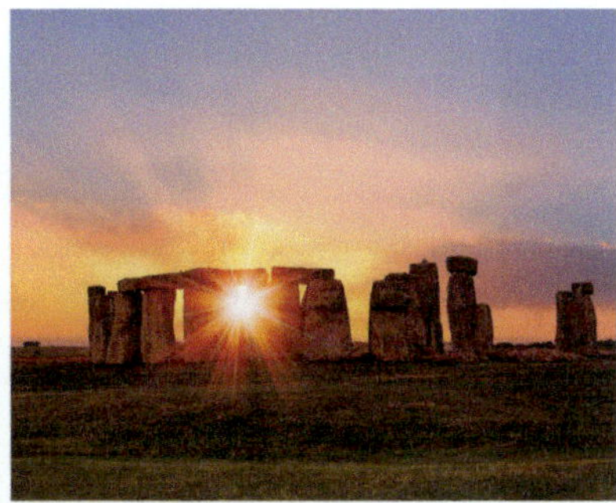

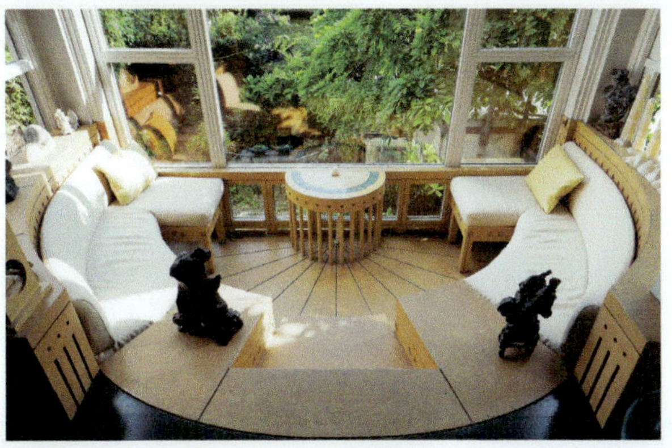

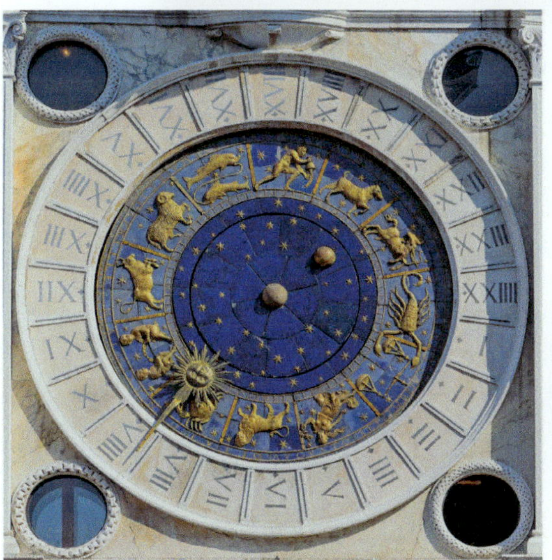

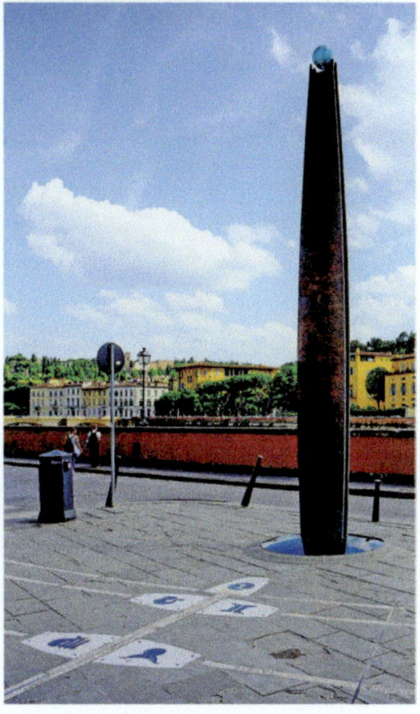

6.10
Celestial Phenomena: (a) Newgrange, Ireland, (b) Stonehenge, Salisbury, UK, (c) Charles Jencks's Sundial Room, London, (d) Piazza San Marco Clock Tower, Venice, (e) Galileo Museum Sundial, Florence

occurs when the physical nature of the material form defining a space begins to disappear through visual optics. Certain Islamic mosques, for example, have beautiful domed spaces defined with incredible sacred Islamic geometry. On the outside, they may employ arabesque patterns resembling wind-blown fields of wheat or desert sand, as in the Sheikh Lotfollah Mosque, Isfahan, Iran, or waves of water that create the visual effect of movement, as in the Royal Mosque in

Isfahan, Iran. On the interior, some mosque spaces have intricate star polygon patterns in which the lines of the geometry direct your eye toward the center or top and then back to the perimeter, and so on. This has the effect of mesmeric movement. Both these examples begin to dematerialize the architectural form and contribute to inner transcendence.

Another method of dematerializing space is through the use of glass, light, and transparency, and these contribute to creating spatial luminosity. This is quite common for religious and spiritual spaces. The translucent nature of glass creates a perceptual shift in the fixed material character of the space, thereby enhancing a more dynamic, transcendent experience. In some examples, the use of color can also create movement, as in St. Gabriel's Passionist Parish Church, Toronto, Canada.[15] According to the architects of St. Gabriel's Parish Church, Roberto Chiotti and Richard Vosko, their design is a meaningful expression of eco-theology, ritual-centeredness, the relevance of religious teachings in the world today, and active participation.[16] There are several strategies for de-materializing architecture for sacred wellness experiences, as follows:

1. **Use of geometry** – geometry expressed in a way that is fluid and interconnected leads the eye, and therefore perception, beyond the static material of the form or space.
2. **Use of transparent materials** – materials that are diaphanous and translucent, such as glass and polycarbonate sheets and fibers, express a lightless and impermanence that seem to defy gravity.
3. **Use of light** – light that glows, streams, and illuminates draws attention away from the physical realm and creates an ineffable effect.

De-materialization of the human body can occur during transformative moments. At the physical level, there are visceral signs, including goose bumps, tingling, chills, shuddering, breathlessness and visible inhalation, momentary freezing of mobility, feeling of suspension, and sense of quiescence. For experiences such as these transformative moments, time typically slows down subjectively. The spiritual wellness outcomes include numinous, serenity, and awe experiences, transcendence and spiritual renewal, and unity experiences. They are geometric and contribute to healing gardens and connections to the unknown and things greater than ourselves.

Biophilic Design for Connections to Nature

Biophilia is an emerging discipline within the confluence of the fields of natural and social sciences, philosophy, anthropology, public health, evolutionary psychology, environmental engineering, planning, urban design, landscape architecture, and architecture. Biophilia has been shown to have both spiritual and wellness effects. Since it is defined as the love of nature and natural processes, in architecture it is important for architects to design for various sensual connections, including physical access to nature.[17] This connection can be a direct experience of nature or ascribed to abstract manifestations, such as the diversity of shapes, forms, patterns, and colors found in the living natural world. According to Kaplan and Kaplan, landscapes today that resemble savannas or are park-like are preferred.[18]

Exposure to nature produces positive effects as experienced by all our senses. Visual, auditory, olfactory, haptic, and gustatory sensations all contribute to this experience. Humans are dominantly visual, but the other senses are important in biophilic design. Natural sounds restore moods, and natural olfactory sensations are important to memory, language, social attraction, and reproduction. Tasting farm-to-table food can be transforming. Haptic sensations – touch – are experienced in gardening and when enjoying horticultural activities. A walk in the rain or snow or playing with domesticated animals creates opportunities for haptic experiences. Moving through varying spaces, either spatially intimate or generous, affects us. The Interface Headquarters in Atlanta is an example of a building that incorporates nature within it.

There are several spiritual wellness attributes and desired outcomes associated with biophilic design and connections to nature. Stephen Kellert, in 2008, expanded on the health and wellness effects of biophilia and presented six dimensions, including environmental features, natural shapes and forms, natural and processed patterns, light and space, place-based relationships, and evolved human–nature relationships, and he identified 72 attributes of biophilic design.[19] These biophilic attributes included the terrestrial elements, views of nature, biomorphy and biomimicry, sensory variability, prospect and refuge, and light in all forms, to name a few. Further, biophilic design includes unity experiences, serenity and awe emotions, and spiritual renewal. Biophilic design and connections to nature are integral to thin places, outdoor third places, sanctuary places, and biophilic architecture. They are wellness-related and spiritual in that they can produce connections to natural and architectural experiences greater than ourselves.

SUMMARY

Spiritual wellness is an ongoing process of self-discovery and active participation shaping the deepest part of us, including our beliefs, values, feelings, behaviors, and lifestyle practices. The wellness benefits are in part achieved through design as the dimensions inform the design opportunities in the built environment. Many of the attributes have a more direct impact upon design opportunities in the built environment, while some attributes have secondary effects on attitudes, convictions, and sensibilities that can influence planning and design decisions.

One of the issues with designing for these spiritual wellness attributes and strategies is the contemporary need to mass build, often hundreds of buildings at a time, where it is difficult and expensive to provide the spiritual wellness amenities discussed in this chapter. Most habitable locations are not near dramatic natural sites. There are many sea-level sites; however, with climate change and rising sea levels, they will be increasing less desirable. While not necessarily an inclusive set of strategies at the architectural scale, there are design guidelines for more spiritually wellness-oriented building designs. Climate change design, appropriate orientation responses, biophilic design, functional as well as uplifting space and

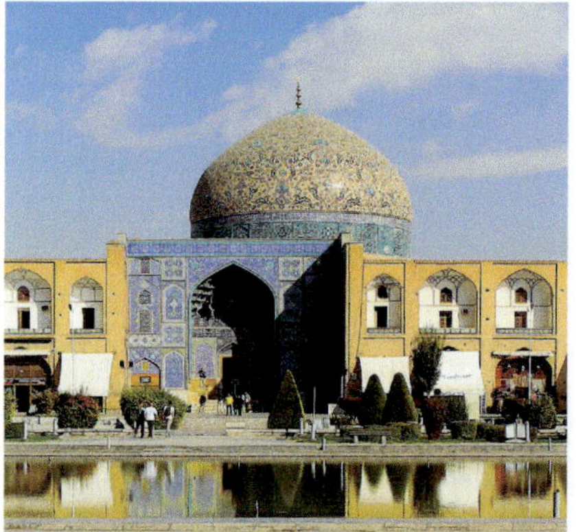
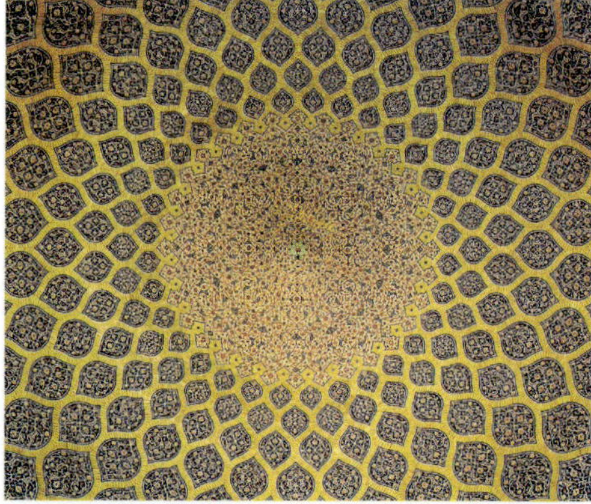
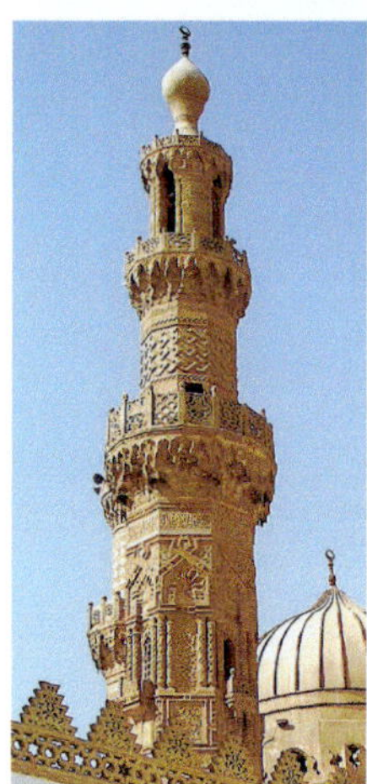
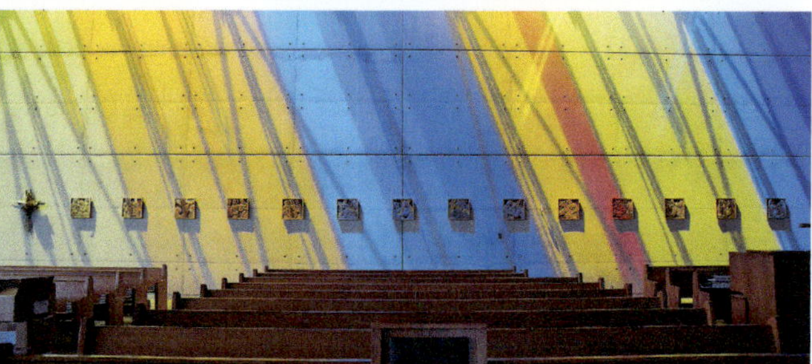

6.11 De-materialization: (a) Sheikh Lotfollah Mosque Exterior, Isfahan, Iran, (b) Sheikh Lotfollah Mosque Interior, (c) Diminishing Perspective of Minaret, (d) St. Gabriel's Passionist Parish Church, Toronto, Canada

light design, among other spiritual wellness strategies, are needed for all building types and scales. Having stated this, there is a distinction between heroic, self-important, and grandiose architecture and more modest, equitable, and soulful examples. The challenge at the architectural scale is to flourish with individual well-being-supporting sustainable lifestyles, connect to nature, and co-exist, cooperate, and participate in planetary stewardship and health.[20] A summary list of spiritual wellness planning and design strategies at the architectural scale follows:

1. Spatial sequencing and passage.
2. Use of sacred geometry.
3. Orientation responses.
4. Design with climate.
5. Creating spatial generosity.
6. Design for luminosity.
7. Incorporating water and blue spaces.
8. Responses to celestial phenomena.
9. Design for de-materiality.
10. Biophilic design for connections to nature.

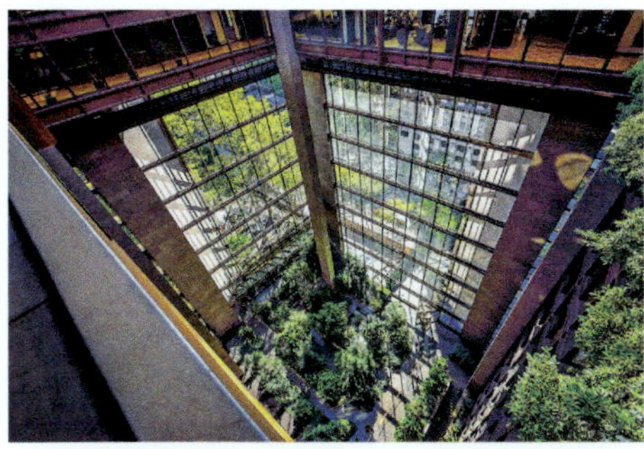

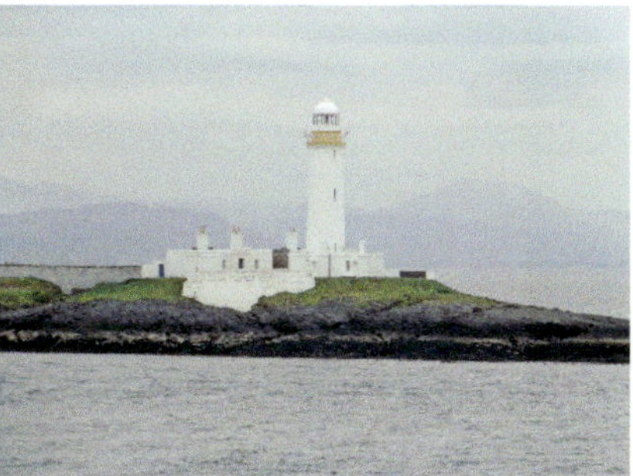

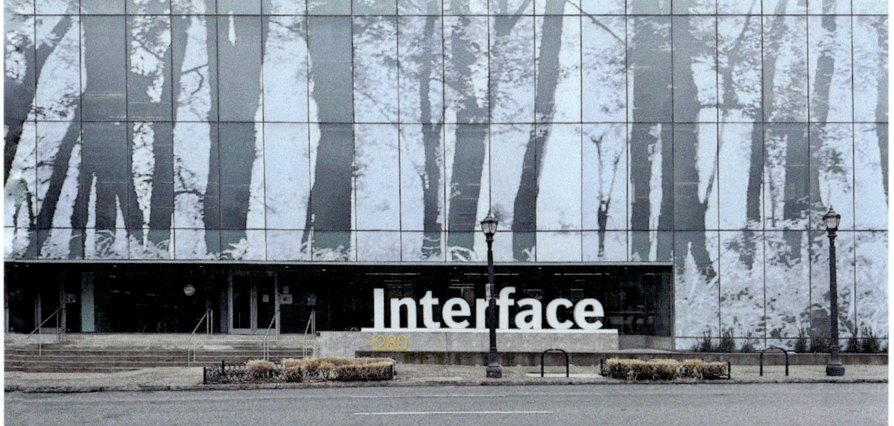

6.12 Connections to Nature: (a) Ford Foundation Headquarters, New York City, (b) Light House in South Haven, Michigan, (c) Abstract Nature on the Interface Headquarters' Façade, Atlanta, Georgia

NOTES

1 Brill, Michael, *Using Place-Creation Myth to Develop Design Guidelines for Scared Space* (Self-published, September 25, 1985), p. 22.
2 Brill, Michael, *The Origin of "Charged" and Mythic Landscapes – A Speculation* (Self-published, November 6, 1991).
3 Lynn, The Vast Immeasurable Dimensions of God's Love (accessed November 10, 2022), https://www.tickledpinklife.com/2014/01/the-vast-immeasurable-dimensions-of-gods-love/.
4 Oliver, Paul, *Dwellings: The House across the World* (Austin, TX: University of Texas Press, 1987), p. 166.
5 Olick, Diana, Zillow Adds Climate Risk Data to Home Listings as Threats Rise (accessed December 1, 2024), https://www.cnbc.com/2024/10/04/zillow-adds-climate-risk-data-to-home-listings.html.
6 Victor Olgyay, *Design with Climate: Bioclimatic Approach to Architectural Regionalism* (Princeton, NJ: Princeton University Press, 1963).
7 Environmental Protection Agency, Improving Your Indoor Environment (accessed April 9, 2025), https://www.epa.gov/indoor-air-quality-iaq/improving-your-indoor-environment#:~:text=Did%20you%20know%20we%20spend,like%20asthma%20and%20heart%20disease.
8 Ott, W.R., Human Activity Patterns: A Review of the Literature for Estimating Time Spent Indoors, Outdoors, and in Transit, in *Proceedings of the Research Planning Conference on Human Activity Patterns* (Las Vegas, NV: EPA National Exposure Research Laboratory, EPA/600/4-89/004, 1989), pp. 3-1–3-38.
9 John Lobell, *Between Silence and Light: Spirit in the Architecture of Louis I. Kahn* (Boulder, CO: Shambala, 1979).

10 Leslie, R.P., Capturing the Daylight Dividend in Buildings: Why and How? *Building and Environment*, February 12, 2024.
11 Ray, Celeste, Ed., *Sacred Waters: A Cross-Cultural Compendium of Hallowed Springs and Holy Wells* (London, UK: Routledge, 2020), pp. 2–3.
12 McAnally, Elizabeth, Buddhism, Bodhisattvas, and the Compassionate Wisdom of Water, in *The Bloomsbury Handbook of Religion and Nature: The Elements*, Laura Hobgood & Whitney Bauman (Eds.) (London, UK: Bloomsbury Academy, 2018), p. 189.
13 Phon, Abby, 10 Reasons Why You Should Drink More Water, March 20, 2012 (accessed November 22, 201), https://www.mindbodygreen.com/0-4287/10-Reasons-Why-You-Should-Drink-More-Water.html.
14 Neil deGrasse Tyson Explains the Tides (accessed August 6, 2024), https://www.bing.com/videos/riverview/relatedvideo?q=what+causes+the+tides&mid=398D73428E78140D3AA7398D73428E78140D3AA7&FORM=VIRE.
15 Tabb, Phillip James, *Thin Place Design: Architecture of the Numinous* (New York, NY: Routledge, 2023).
16 Chiotti, R., & R.S. Vosko, Worship Space Today: Trends in Modern Church Architecture (accessed August 4, 2024), https://www.americamagazine.org/issue/777/article/worship-space-today.
17 Wilson, Edward O. Wilson, *Biophilia* (Cambridge, MA: Harvard University Press, 1984).
18 Kaplan, R., & S. Kaplan, *The Experience of Nature: A Psychological Perspective* (Cambridge, MA: Cambridge University Press, 1989), p. 48.
19 Kellert, Stephen R., Judith H. Heerwagen, & Martin Mador, *Biophilic Design: The Theory, Science, and Practice of Bringing Building to Life* (New York, NY: John Wiley, 2008).
20 Ichioka, Sarah, & Michael Pawlyn, *Flourish: Design Paradigms for Our Planetary Emergency* (Axminster, UK: Triarchy Press, 2021), p. 50.

7 SPIRITUAL WELLNESS AT THE URBAN DESIGN SCALE

INTRODUCTION

Wellness strategies are a mutually supporting set of design approaches that serve as prime actionable elicitors of wellness benefits promoting individual physical health, positive emotional responses, mental clarity, prosocial behaviors, spiritual renewal, and environmental reparation. Most of these strategies have a basis in science, health and wellness, and spirituality informed by the fields of public health, health sciences, religious and spiritual theology, and environmental psychology. The design implications and strategies include an understanding of the basic needs and opportunities at the regional scale. Moreover, they describe design approaches, patterns, elicitors, and several examples that show the effective ways in which spiritual wellness has been responded to and applied in previous works. Health and wellness benefit both human beings and the environments they inhabit, including both natural and built places. The environment-centered benefits have particular importance at the regional scale because they are focused on the natural environment around us and the cities and buildings we occupy.

There are many important planning and design considerations at the urban design scale that involve spatial, functional, and ecological considerations. The spatial implications of spiritual wellness are influenced by responses to ecological flows, natural resource acquisition and management, settlement planning, transportation, and urban form and growth patterns. According to the Global Wellness Institute, wellness real estate was the largest growing market of the 11-sector wellness economy over the years 2019–2023.[1] With this kind of interest and growth in the field, it seems encouraging that, at the urban design scale, many opportunities exist to implement spiritual wellness designs.

While all these are important, a few are directly related to spiritual wellness. From a general wellness viewpoint, sustainability, public health, access to nature, responses to climate change and natural disasters, and inclusion of healthy social spaces are important at this urban design scale. However, the spiritual dimension suggests something beyond these, such as preservation of sacred sites, possible numinous and awe experiences, and connections to the unknown.

DOI: 10.4324/9781003546085-7

URBAN SCALE DESIGN STRATEGIES

Regions are made of geographic characteristics, natural areas, open space and agriculture, and human settlements, whereas the urban design scale deals with the larger scale of groups of buildings, infrastructure, streets, public spaces, entire neighborhoods and districts, and entire cities. The goal is to create urban environments that are equitable, beautiful, performative, and sustainable. The urban design scale involves a blend of disciplines, including planning, landscape architecture, transportation engineering, architecture, and industrial design. The physical planning and design characteristics at the urban design scale generally include zoning, density, typology, land use, movement systems, accessibility, infrastructure, nature, buildings, civil society, growth, and, of course, people.

Another process at the urban design scale is urban expansion, defined as the physical extension of the geographical footprints of towns, cities, and metropolitan areas into the surrounding countryside and agricultural land. Typically, this expansion is initially fragmented and sometimes even leapfrogs vacant open spaces. The piecemeal process of urban expansion does not support sustainable, mixed-use development. This expansion occurs as a result of "growth by addition" through the expansion of more buildings, roads, and infrastructure, often at the expense of agricultural land. Such growth is most often single-use residential development resulting in people being placed further from life support services and functions, and cultural amenities and totally reliant upon the automobile for connectivity.

The urban design scale encompasses a variety of spiritual wellness considerations. Those considerations exist because the urban design scale includes elements that impact well-being; these include city planning, town planning, neighborhoods, rainwater and stormwater management, infrastructure, circulation, zoning, urban parks, urban agriculture, blue spaces, and locations of significant buildings. Fundamental characteristics at this scale include passage and circulation, bounding and identity, spatial hierarchy, more organized urban geometry, placemaking with public spaces, planning for solar access, and interactions with nature. At the urban design scale, the planning and design strategies address spatial organization and urban functional issues that affect the level of well-being. These urban design issues include accessibility, provision of services, safety, cost of living, commuting time, climatic variables and air pollution, and environmental protection. The relationship between urbanized areas or a region and natural areas is critical. Physical planning and design strategies at this scale can have a large impact on comprehensive planning; transportation network engineering, with particular focus on pedestrianization; and the creation and maintenance of urban ecological zones.

Several places located worldwide demonstrate many positive wellness-oriented urban design characteristics (see Figure 7.1). The Metropol Parasol, in Spain, is an urban design intervention in an existing plaza giving it new form and vitality. The Kronsberg district was originally planned to demonstrate sustainable principles for the Expo 2000 World Exposition held in Hanover, Germany. The motto for the fair was "Humankind – Nature – Technology," which guided the exemplary planning approach to Kronsberg.[2] In 2003, Kronsberg had a population of 7,300 residents, making it one of the largest sustainable urban examples at that time.

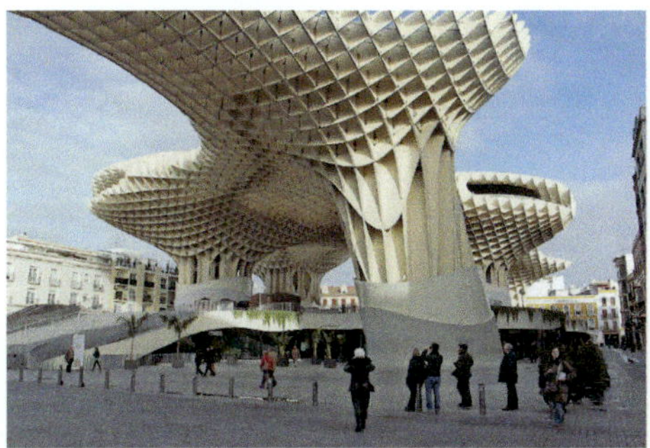
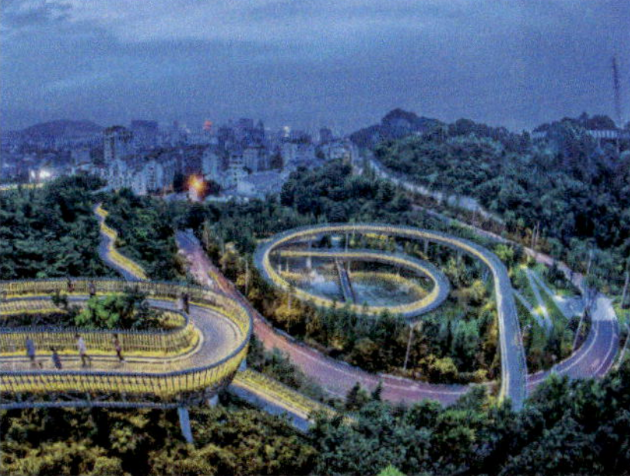
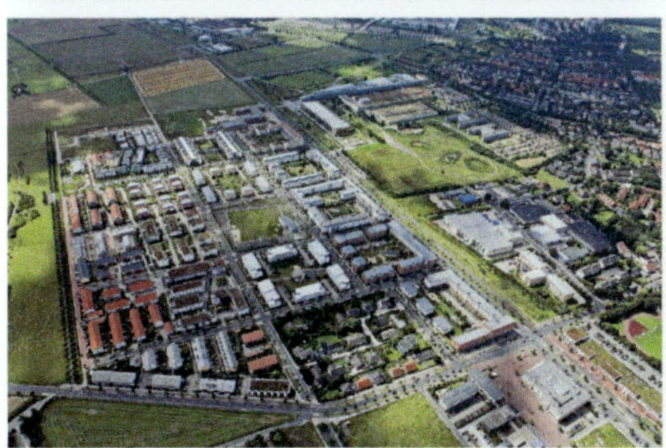
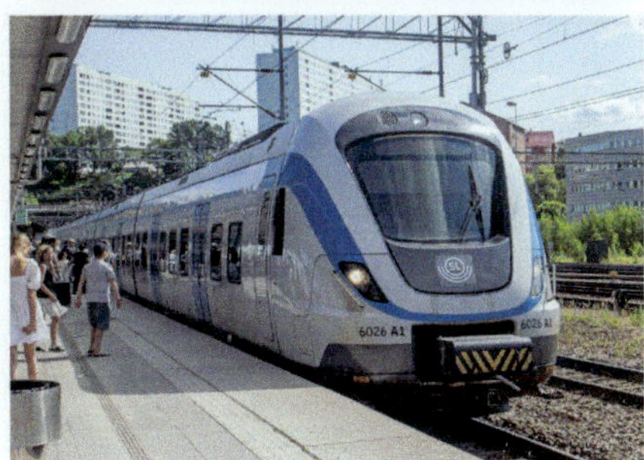

7.1
Urban Design Scale: (a) Metropol Parasol, Spain, (b) Fuzhou Jin Niu Shan Trans-Urban Connector, China, (c) Agriculture Surrounding Kronsberg District, Germany, (d) Stockholm, Sweden, Regional Train

Culoz is a town located in the southeast part of France along the west bank of the River Rhône. It is situated at the base of the foothills of the Alps and the Grand Colombier and is surrounded by the fertile agricultural land along the Rhône. The Stockholm regional train system in Sweden was originally a small, local train service that was expanded in the 1960s. As of 2022, on an ordinary weekday, 342,000 passengers use Stockholm commuter trains.[3] Other examples, not illustrated here, include Michael Sorkin's urban design work in New York City, which promoted urban agriculture and pedestrianization, and the Babcock Ranch, Florida, which has a local renewable energy source of electricity employed within its 440-acre (178-hectare) solar farm.

These examples present issues of urban fabric design and spatial structure design, density, land use, transportation, renewable energy production, and inclusion of nature, all of which affect well-being. At the urban design scale, prioritizing spiritual wellness through accessible green spaces, quiet contemplative areas, and community gathering places fosters a sense of peace, belonging, and connection, contributing to the overall well-being and social cohesion of urban residents. Spiritual wellness is further addressed through the spiritual dimension and its attributes, from the creation of sensitive ecological zones, urban agriculture, and integrated parks and green spaces to renewable infrastructures, integration of civic third places, inspiring streetscapes, and planning for important religious and spiritual ceremonial sites.

Preserving Ecological Zones

Urban ecology is considered the balance between human culture and habitation and any natural process in urban environments, including all living organisms, urban hydrology, and waste amelioration. The ecological systems within and flowing through a given settlement or geographic region should be considered sacred. These systems include waterways, natural areas, biotic living organisms, and air and soil. This is about not only benefitting us now but creating wellness environments for future generations. It seems clear that achieving a balanced urban ecology begins with the recognition that humanity now faces existential crises on multiple fronts: extreme economic disparity; increased competition for resources, including land and water; a severely degraded natural world; and climate change.[4] So what can spiritual wellness bring to address these problems?

Maintaining healthy rivers is key to a balanced ecology. Rivers are an ecological lifeline as they flow through the heart of communities that surround them, providing food, jobs, transportation, energy, and, of course, water. Over 50 percent of the world's population lives within 1.8 miles (3 km) of a surface freshwater body, and only 10 percent of the population lives farther than 6.2 miles (10 km) away.[5] Urban density is not evenly distributed among fresh water-rich locations. Despite this uneven distribution, urban rivers benefit the health of those who live in urban environments, providing access to limited open spaces.

With increasing urban populations, human waste is another central issue within an urban ecology. Scaling waste amelioration is important to public health. Further, creating manageable infrastructures and resilient systems will allow for continued growth while reducing the negative impacts of increasing waste production. From a wellness point of view, this issue relates to disease prevention. Furthermore, from a spiritual point of view, it reinforces the idea that everything is connected in a holistic web and requires our constant care and stewardship.

Natural areas within cities are diverse and usually take the forms of parks, greenways, streetscapes, gardens, urban agriculture, cemeteries, waterways, and residential properties. The public health and wellness effects are well documented with production of oxygen, greenhouse gas sequestering, reduction of the heat island effect, and encouragement of physical activities. Walking or reflecting in a park or garden is a powerful strategy for improved physical and mental health.[6] Although not a medical diagnosis, access to nature helps relieve "nature deficit disorder," coined by Richard Louv in 2005, and can reduce alienation from nature. Ways to make a spiritual connection to nature include urban forest bathing, stargazing, river sitting, wildflower meandering, viewing sunsets, and quiet moments alone.

With the focus on locally grown food, urban agriculture is another important part of urban ecology. Urban agriculture includes animal husbandry, aquaculture, beekeeping, and horticulture. Benefits of urban agriculture include the creation of resilient food systems, reduction of greenhouse gasses, and reduction of the heat island effect. Figures 7.2a and 7.2b are photographs of the Cheonggyecheon Stream in Seoul and Boise River in Idaho, both showing beautiful, tree-lined rivers flowing through urban areas.

The spiritual wellness elements of urban ecology are as follows:

1. **Water and urban hydrology** – are crucial for survival and provide stormwater management, recreation, beauty, habitat for other life forms, preservation of wetlands, and provision of places of spiritual renewal.

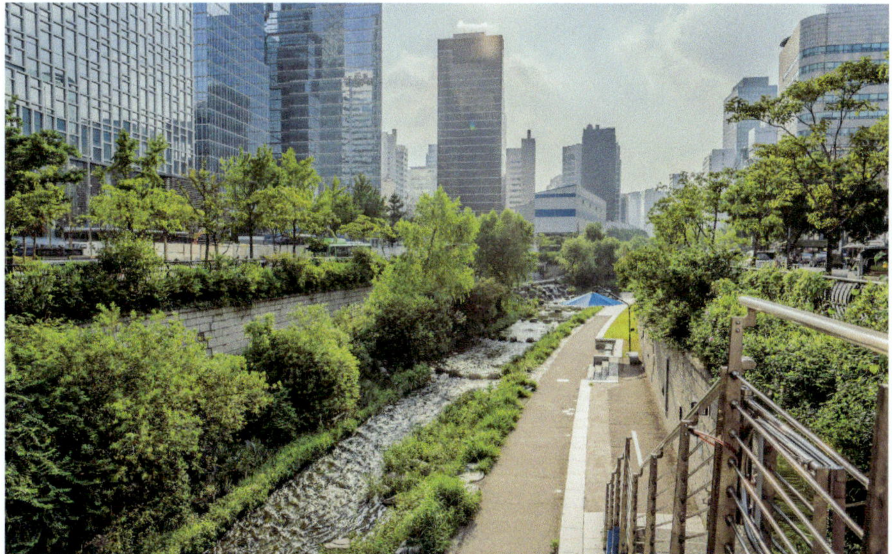

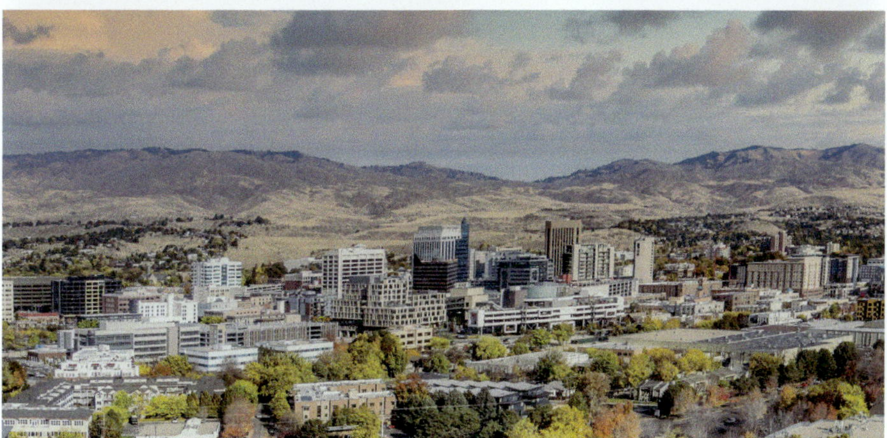

7.2 Ecological Urban Design: (a) Cheonggyecheon Stream, Seoul, (b) Boise River, Idaho

2. **Urban waste** – requires reductions in consumption, increased and improved recycling practices both individually and communally, and improved repurposing of waste.
3. **Urban nature** – provides health, wellness, and spiritual benefits, including boosting physical activity, production of oxygen, greenhouse gas sequestering, and reduction of the heat island effect.
4. **Urban agriculture** – takes the form of community gardens and rooftops and produces local, healthy food that is diverse, resilient, and within easy distribution distance of inhabitants.
5. **Habitat protection** – harbors and promotes urban wildlife as well as migrating species; the richer the animal population, the greater the benefits to human well-being.[7]

There are several spiritual wellness attributes and desired outcomes associated with ecological flows through urban areas. Spiritual wellness can be enhanced together with clean fresh water, intelligent management of waste, inclusion of more natural areas within our cities, increased local agricultural production, and increased habitat protection. Spiritual wellness within urban ecological areas includes numinous, serenity, and awe experiences, transcendence and spiritual renewal, unity experiences, and possible outdoor third place experiences. They are biophilic and contribute to high-level wellness, connectedness, especially to nature, and awareness of the unknown and things greater than ourselves.

Spatial Structure, from Grids to Nucleation

Spatial structure, from grids to nucleation, along with mixed-use zoning and polycultural farming, provides greater opportunities for spiritual wellness. Such structures organize human activities in space. Critical to an urban spatial pattern is the built-in function of growth. A critical question is, "As population and development increase, how does the pattern accommodate growth?" There are several ways this occurs. First is growth by addition, which expands outward. This can occur in variations of linear patterns or in square or rectangular patterns. The second is growth by multiplication: when an optimal size is reached, expansion is achieved by replication into multiple neighborhoods, villages, or suburban enclaves. The multiplication pattern suggests an optimum size based on nucleation and pedestrian access to goods and services, which suggests that populations are in sync with the carrying capacities of our local ecological regions.[8]

Currently, suburb and exurb spatial orders dominate, worldwide. They vary widely, from random orders to serpentine, linear, space-filling orders, and are characterized by single-family dwelling occupancy, homeownership, and automobile commuting.[9] Conversely, single-use zoning and monotonous grids can produce many negative effects. This spatial structure is not without public health consequences. These consequences are wide-ranging and include reduction of physical activity, pedestrian unfriendliness, increased dependence on the automobile and commuting, stormwater issues due to increases in impervious surfaces, and lack of access to nature.

Nucleation has public wellness implications that include the fostering of a sense of community, identity, and social cohesiveness. Further, it can accommodate mixed-use development, density gradients, and pedestrianization. Positive attributes are diversity of land use, proximity to one another and to the center, and sense of place.

The spiritual wellness attributes for urban spatial structure are as follows:

1. **Geometric system** – is a space-filling spatial structure and land-use pattern, from Cartesian grids to radial nucleated patterns.
2. **Growth by addition** – is a growth pattern that expands outward horizontally, typically employing grid patterns, and is usually a function of economic factors. Suburban sprawl is an example of this pattern.
3. **Growth by multiplication** – is a growth pattern that expands by replication where its optimal size is a function of human scale, sense of community, and spiritual wellness creation of place. Neighborhoods, clustered settlements, and nucleated suburbs are examples of this pattern.

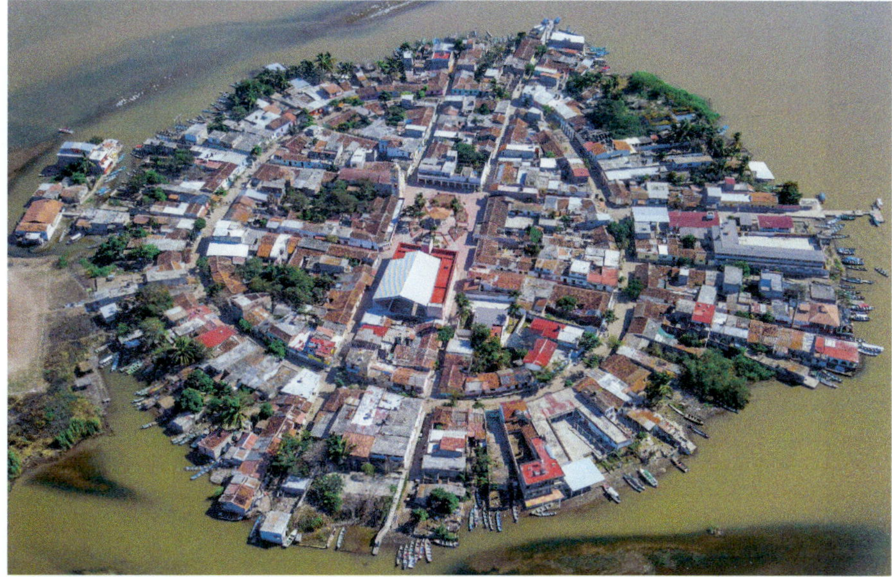

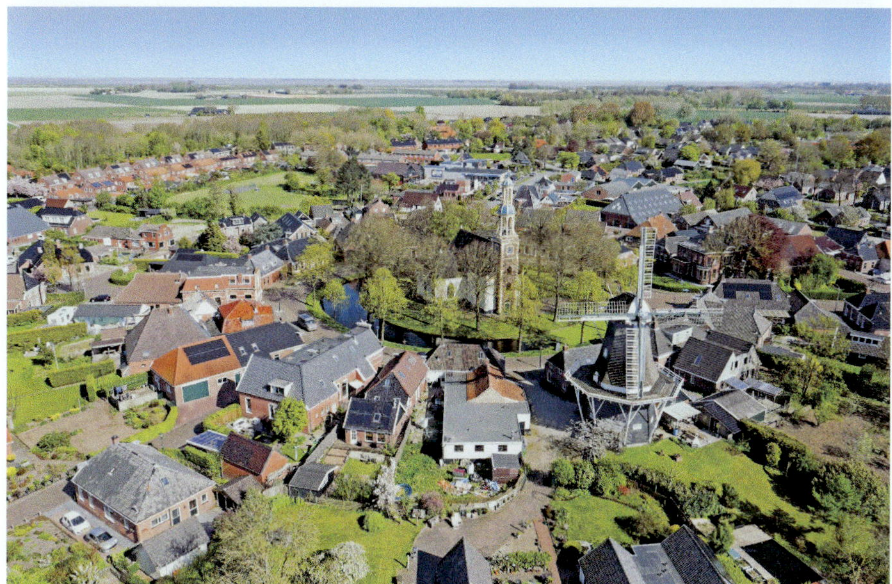

7.3
Nucleated Spatial Structure: (a) Island Village Mexcaltitán, Mexico, (b) Village of Spijk, the Netherlands

Examples of wellness-oriented spatial structures exist globally. Figure 7.3a is an aerial photograph of the island village of Mexcaltitán on the western coast of Mexico. It has a beautiful mandalic plan formed by a double cross and circumferential roads. This island village is nucleated, with a mixed-use plaza in the center. Around the serrated perimeter are residences and boat landings. The spatial order transitions from more random at the perimeter to more organized at the center. Figure 7.3b is an aerial photograph of Spijk, in Groningen, located on the east coast of the Netherlands. It has a radial spatial order dating back to the 7th or 6th century, with a tiny forest and church in the center. Both examples support a strong community focus fostering a strong identity and prosocial behaviors.

There are several wellness attributes and desired outcomes associated with the quality of spatial structures. Social cohesion reinforces relationships and the sense of solidarity among members of a community. Studies have found that people living in or closer to the city center, as in London, United Kingdom, for example, tend to be more satisfied with their lives.[10] Wellness attributes and outcomes include spiritual benefits. These benefits depend upon the spatial structure and include serenity and awe experiences, transcendence and spiritual renewal, unity and possibly third place experiences, and sustainability. For more centralized or nucleated spatial orders, these attributes are more evident. At the urban design scale, a nucleated and well-defined spatial structure fosters a strong sense of place, enhances walkability and social interaction, optimizes infrastructure efficiency, and creates a clear framework for community organization and identity.

Integrating Nature within the Urban Fabric

To best facilitate spiritual wellness, urban planning should carefully consider preserving natural areas and integrating them into the fabric of the design. New natural areas could be created on derelict lands. Strategies for nature in urban areas encompass zoning for parks and natural open spaces, nature-based streetscapes, tree planting and tiny forests, green infrastructure, natural stormwater solutions, and introduction of renewable energy technologies. While isolated islands of natural urban land are good, interconnected ones provide for better pedestrian circulation. Cities developing open-space plans that provide for interconnected systems of green spaces, including parks, gardens, walkways, and stream corridors reap multiple benefits.[11] Furthermore, natural urban areas offer numerous public health and individual spiritual benefits. Some of the spiritual wellness benefits of nature included in urban settings are as follows:

1. **Physical benefits** – engaging in passive and active experiences of outdoor physical activities and opportunities for forest bathing can improve physical health, increase energy, and create pro-individual wellness behaviors.
2. **Social benefits** – participating in shared activities, recreation, and sports improves mood, and, with diverse immersive nature experiences, there is improvement in self-esteem, self-efficacy, resilience, generosity, connectedness, which creates prosocial behaviors.
3. **Environmental benefits** – providing oxygenated air, reduction of urban noise, carbon sequestering, and places for wild animal habitats promotes pro-environmental behaviors and a greater willingness to protect nature.

There are several spiritual wellness attributes and desired outcomes associated with the inclusion of nature within the urban fabric. The wellness benefits of integrating nature in the forms of parks, green spaces, and biophilic environments are well documented. According to the Urban Institute, parks and green spaces intrinsically support healthy and productive lifestyles. In addition, they contribute to resilient and cohesive communities and produce positive health outcomes, such as a reduced risk of cardiovascular disease, diabetes, cancer, and heart disease with averted health expenditures. In addition, they help reduce stress levels and improve mood. Other benefits occur for mental, emotional, social, and environmental wellness, with physical health impacted the most.[12] These benefits include increased energy levels, boosted immune system, reduced stress, and improved mood. Further, the inclusion of parks and green spaces reaps many economic benefits such as increased property values, tax revenues, tourism, and branding potential; improved environmental health; and improved aesthetics. Importantly, urban nature brings abundant environmental, sustainability, and climate action benefits.

Within the urban design context, the principal benefits of natural areas include enhanced biodiversity, improved air and water quality, reduced urban heat island effect, increased opportunities for recreation and well-being, and a greater sense of connection to nature for urban dwellers. The spiritual benefits are numerous and consist of increased serenity experiences, awe experiences, transcendence and spiritual renewal, improved sleep, and, possibly, third place experiences. Additional contributions to spiritual wellness include the biophilic effect, land stewardship, connectedness, experiencing things greater than ourselves, and restoration of optimism and hopeful outlooks on life. Refer to Figure 7.4 for images of Savannah, Georgia, park system, Central Park, New York City, and Rouge Urban National Park in Toronto, Canada. These are just two of many examples worldwide that are preserving and re-naturalizing urban settings.

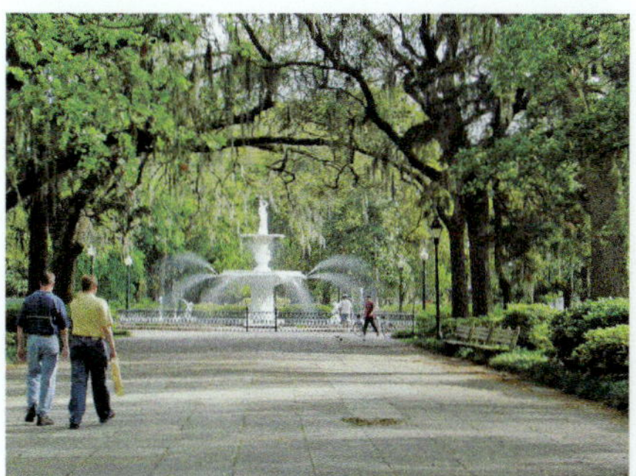

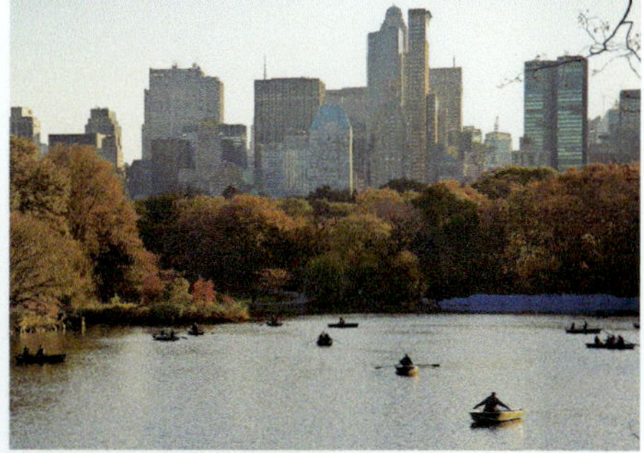

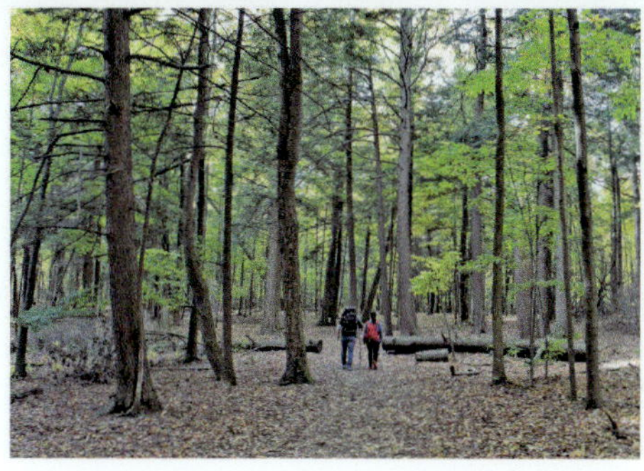

7.4
Nature Within: (a) Savannah, Georgia, Park System, (b) Central Park, New York City, (c) Rouge Urban National Park, Toronto, Canada

Creating Community Agriculture and Gardens

As urban areas expand, farmland is often converted into residential and commercial zones. This expansion reduces agricultural land and pushes it further and further away from end users.

In response, agricultural urbanism is an emerging movement, although not a new one. This movement, bolstered by the belief that local agriculture is healthier, more diverse, and fresher, seeks to integrate a broad range of sustainable food and agricultural systems into city planning.[13] Urban farming, as opposed to farming in rural areas, consists of a local food system growing plants and raising livestock in and around cities. Today, 800 million people around the world rely on urban agriculture for access to fresh, healthy food, which comprises 15–20 percent of the global food supply. Urban agriculture is considered a complement to rural agriculture although it includes different scales, from commercial agricultural facilities to household-level production. It is becoming widely practiced by society in areas of rapid urbanization, cities, suburbs, and towns.

Most grocery stores have food that travels as much as 1,500 miles to reach the shelves. In response, the concept of a 100-mile diet proposes the idea to stop purchasing globally in favor of eating locally by only obtaining food produced within a 100-mile radius of your home.[14] People engaging with the 100-mile diet are considered "locavores." The strategy is simple and emphasizes growing or purchasing locally grown food, including produce, fresh meat, and dairy products. The benefits of urban agriculture include the following:

1. **Provision of healthy nutrition** – locally grown food includes a variety of produce from fruits, vegetables, herbs, and animal husbandry.
2. **Accessibility** – proximity and easy access preserves freshness of food and reduces transport energy costs.
3. **Provides food security** – locally grown food is climate-responsive, responds to residents' needs, and provides security from scarcity.

Edible landscapes double as food-producing gardens, and *foodscapes*, as well as ornamentals full of color and seasonal change, serve a broader function including the entire environment where food is obtained, prepared, discussed, and given meaning. Foodscaping is the practice of integrating edible plants into landscapes.[15] Plants include baby greens, kale, lettuces, tomatoes, beans, peppers, berries (strawberries, cherries, black raspberries), and culinary herbs (rosemary, sage, parsley, dill, and basil). In addition, they should also be pollinator-friendly. Foodscapes encourage interdependence between people, food, and place. Edible streetscapes and verge gardens typically parallel streets, sidewalks, and footpaths.

Many benefits result from organic farming. Organic farming, which eliminates the need for pesticides, is a preferable approach for urban environments and protects public health and well-being. Urban agriculture can contribute to the reduction of rainfall runoff. Further, it assists in climate change mitigation through CO_2 sequestering. It promotes education on sustainability while serving as a platform

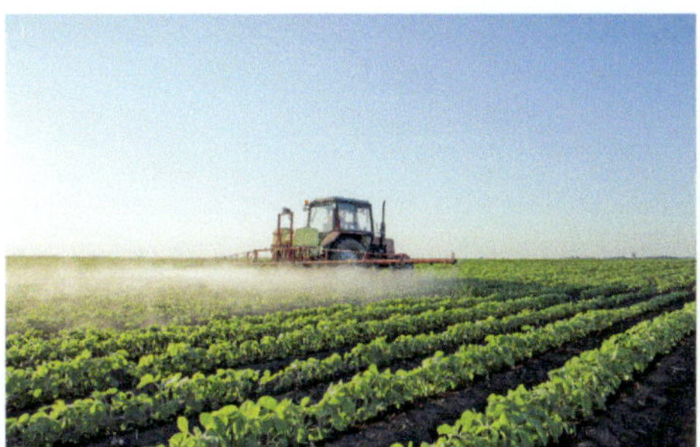

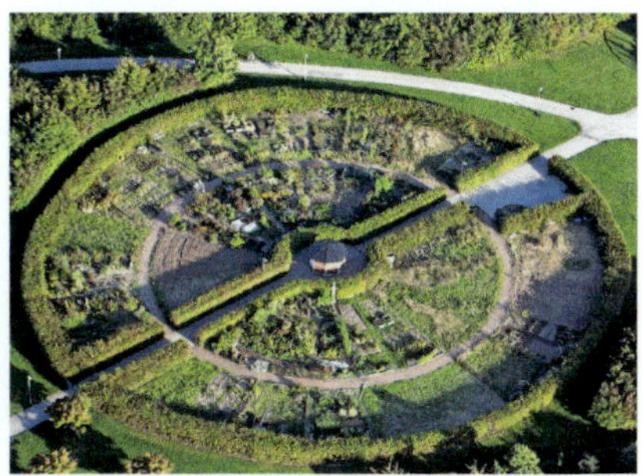

7.5
Urban Agriculture:
(a) Monoculture and Pesticides,
(b) Stinsparken, Swedish Allotment Gardens

for social interaction and it can create local jobs. The wellness benefits include improved response to variable external climatic conditions, improved nutrition and food security, expanded educational opportunities for children, promotion of biodiversity, improved indoor–outdoor access, stress reduction, and promotion of physical activity. In addition, there can be a focus and sense of community, and financial benefits to lower supply chain energy consumption. At the urban design scale, urban agriculture enhances local food security, promotes community engagement, improves green spaces, and fosters a more sustainable and resilient urban ecosystem. The spiritual wellness benefits include numinous, religious, serenity, and awe experiences, transcendence and spiritual renewal, unity experiences, a sense of presence and mindfulness, and connections greater than ourselves. Figure 7.5a is an image of large mono-agriculture far from urban centers. Figure 7.5b is an image of an allotment circle in Stinsparken allotment gardens in Hjarup, Sweden, located between Lund and Malmo.

Circular Regenerative Infrastructure

Urban infrastructure refers to a city's support systems for essential flows, such as streets, energy, water, sanitation, waste management, moving fresh agriculture, and blue/green networks, necessary for urban function and growth. These urban infrastructure systems are among the determining factors for comfort, quality of life, and health and well-being.[16] While urban infrastructure primarily addresses pragmatic, safety, and environmental issues, opportunities exist for spiritual wellness, especially through the development of renewable and regenerative infrastructure. To illustrate, regenerative infrastructure is urban infrastructure that is a place-based and nature-based network connected to wider interconnected ecological, economic, and food-delivery systems.

Renewable infrastructure is a combination of incorporation of renewable energy and power, clean water and waterways, carbon sequestering, pedestrianization, and improved transport modes and networks. Waste includes wastewater, solid municipal waste, and greenhouse gases. Renewable energy extends to solar and wind energy, geothermal heating and cooling, hydroelectricity, biomass, and nuclear fusion. Relatedly, ReGen is a term for "regeneration," where outputs of one system are inputs for another. In biology, it is the process of renewal, restoration, and new growth. ReGen also refers to an integrated and resilient development and an experimental model neighborhood of regenerative homes conceived by James

Ehrlich from Denmark in 2016. Key to the workability of this regenerative system is the on-site integration of electrical energy production, water collection, food production, and distribution to every residence. Benefits of a regenerative infrastructure include the following:

1. **Renewable energy** – includes renewable sources of solar and wind energy, geothermal heating and cooling, hydroelectricity, and biomass.
2. **Water management** – includes preservation of freshwater sources, rainwater collection, efficient flows of water, and stormwater management.
3. **Waste management** – includes municipal and individual waste disposal and management, and recycling and reuse.
4. **Circular systems** – create a local, regenerative infrastructure eco-system that is visible, efficient, and seen as an important part of urban fabric.

There are several spiritual wellness attributes and desired outcomes associated with urban infrastructure. Rivers and streams are natural corridors that transect many urban areas. They provide great opportunities for integrated infrastructure systems that lead to carbon emissions sequestering; recreation enhancements; access to clean air, water, and energy and healthy management of waste; educational opportunities; stress reduction; and increased contact with nature. The spiritual wellness benefits include contemplative and meaningful connections to nature and natural processes, direct experiences of natural resources and our use of them, understanding of connectedness to the system, environmental stewardship, personal mindfulness, and connections greater than ourselves. The circularity is important as it expresses the interconnected nature of energy, water, waste, and human habitation. At the urban design scale, the principal benefits of regenerative infrastructure include enhanced ecological health, improved resource efficiency (water, energy, materials), increased community resilience to environmental changes, and the creation of more livable, biodiverse, and aesthetically pleasing urban environments. Figure 7.6a shows a solar and wind farm in Germany, and Figure 7.6b is Biopolus in Hungary, a closed-loop modular and expandable water, waste, and urban food management system.

Zoning for Mixes of Use and Intergenerational Living

Zoning for mixes of use offers another spiritual wellness contribution at the design scale. Mixed-use zoning allows for greater land-use diversity, increases pedestrianization and socialization, and enhances the character richness of a place. Areas of single-use zoning typically are boring, often dominated by the automobile, and unsustainable in the long term. Cities, towns, villages, and neighborhoods are more sustainable, with abundant mixes of use, than their counterpart single-use zoning. Mixed zoning generally fosters a richer environment with increased casual encounters. Moreover, it promotes a village-style mix of retail, restaurants, offices, civic uses, and multi-family housing. The health and wellness literature reports that people who have contact with family, friends, and community members, both young and old, gain mutual benefits. Planning for such intergenerational living reaps

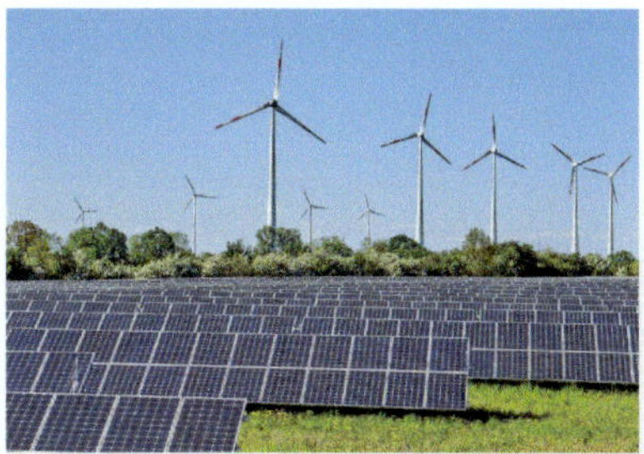
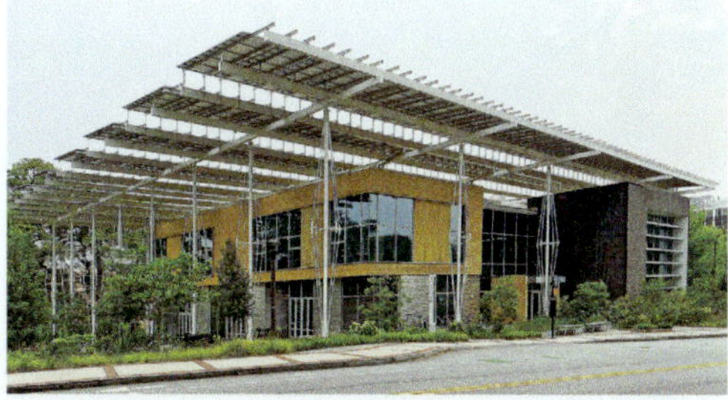
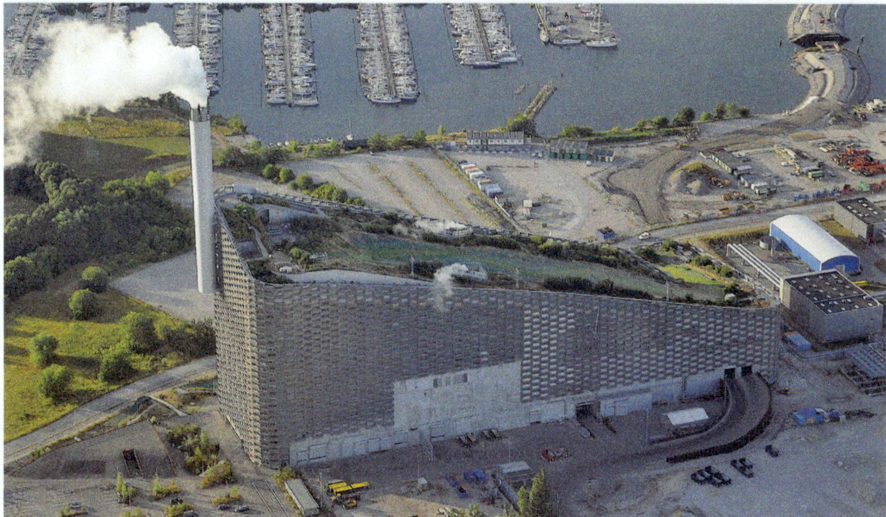

7.6
Regenerative Infrastructure: (a) Solar and Wind Farm, Germany, (b) Kendeda Building, Atlanta, Georgia, (c) Waste-to-Energy Plant, Copenhagen

key benefits. These include reduced loneliness and isolation, increased socialization, legacy building, increased emotional support and sense of purpose, and knowledge transfer. So, planning for intergenerational living is an important mixed-use objective. Benefits of development mixes of use include the following:

1. **Physical well-being** – mixed uses encourage pedestrianization and physical movement.
2. **Social interactions** – mixed uses encourage diversification, social interactions, and casual encounters.
3. **Local economic growth** – mixed uses provide economic opportunities for both national commercial and local businesses, and they often lead to higher property values.
4. **Sustainability** – mixed-use development boosts sustainability by reducing travel distances and increasing pedestrianization and accessibility to critical goods and services.

There are several wellness attributes and desired outcomes associated with appropriate and sustainable mixes of use. They enhance an area's unique identity and development potential. They reduce auto dependency, roadway congestion, and air pollution by co-locating multiple destinations. Mixed-use developments offer

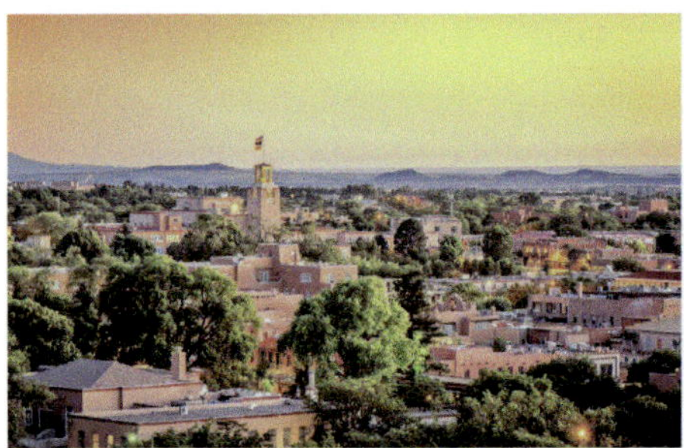

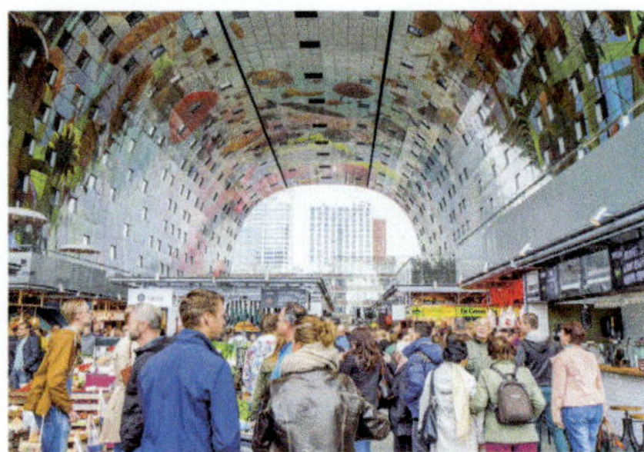

7.7 Mixed-Use Zoning: (a) Old Town, Santa Fe, New Mexico, (b) Rotterdam Market Hall, the Netherlands

residents the convenience of having everything they need within walking distance. This includes restaurants, shopping, entertainment, and public transportation. The synergy created by combining residential, commercial, and leisure spaces makes these areas more desirable, leading to increased demand and, consequently, higher property values.

Numerous spiritual benefits result from mixes of use. These include numinous, religious, serenity, and awe experiences, transcendence and spiritual renewal, and unity experiences. Additionally, mixes of use foster a sense of presence and sense of place, mindfulness, and connections greater than ourselves. Depending upon the actual design, a spirit of place can appear present and be amplified, and this increases a sense of presence and connectedness.

Figure 7.7 shows urban and architectural examples of mixed-use zoning. Santa Fe Plaza is a historical landmark and serves as a gathering place for locals and tourists. Encompassed in the general plaza area are historic monuments, restaurants, businesses and art galleries, the New Mexico Museum of Art, the Cathedral Basilica of Saint Francis of Assisi, and the Loretto Chapel. The Rotterdam Market Hall was designed by MVRDV in 2014. It is a mixed-use residential and office building that houses a large market underneath a large horseshoe-shaped space. The hangar-like structure houses 228 apartments, nearly 50,000 square feet (4,600 square meters) of retail space, and a four-story underground automobile-parking garage. In addition, there are eight restaurants, 15 food shops, and a supermarket. The mixes of use promote social interaction, casual encounters, and support of everyday functions. Implementing mixed-use zoning in communities is crucial for fostering vibrant, walkable neighborhoods, reducing reliance on cars, and promoting a greater sense of community by integrating residential, commercial, and civic spaces. Spiritual wellness occurs because of the spatial generosity, shelter from the elements, diversity of activities, and spirit of place.

Planning for Solar Energy (Access and Denial)

Solar energy can be life-giving but can also be detrimental. In temperate and cold climates, solar energy is welcomed and contributes to creating thermal comfort, especially in extreme conditions. Conversely, in arid and hot climates, solar energy can be overwhelmingly hot and unbearable and can lead to the evaporation of important water reserves. Therefore, solar energy planning needs to be carefully executed and considerate of both the urban context and human needs.

Many pragmatic outcomes are created by responses to solar energy. The sun gives us natural light, relative thermal comfort, and food, and it is life-giving. Further, there are several spiritual wellness attributes and desired outcomes associated with planning for solar energy. They include numinous, religious, serenity, and awe experiences, transcendence and spiritual renewal, and unity experiences and foster a sense of presence and mindfulness, and connections greater than ourselves. Solar delight or celestial beauty is illuminating and transformative and key to sacred architecture. Depending upon the design, a spirit of place can appear present and even amplified, facilitating our ability to cope with existential issues and the unknown. Some of the benefits of planning for solar energy include the following:

1. **Access to natural light** – produces positive health effects, including helping vision, boosting vitamin D, improving sleep, and improving mood.
2. **Energy uses** – include energy for space and hot-water heating, daylighting, and photoelectricity; daylighting reduces the need for conventional lighting sources.
3. **Sunshading and shadowing** – help ameliorate overheating and over-exposure, reduce glare, and increase comfort. They can elicit fractal patterns supporting de-materialization experiences.
4. **Spiritual connections** – the sun is considered the source of life, marks special times during the year (equinoxes and solstices) and day (morning, midday, and evening), signifies positivity and expansion, and is a symbol of divinity.

Solar access is important in areas that need space heating, hot-water heating, and photoelectricity.[17] Typically, both passive and active solar collection requires at least 6 hours of access to the sun throughout the year. In denser urban areas, shading from buildings impinges upon this access. Figure 7.8a is an image of housing in cold climate zones where buildings' southern façades face the southern sun for heat and light. The image in Figure 7.8b is of an off-grid cluster of houses in northern New Mexico, designed by Michael Reynolds.[18] The diagram in Figure 7.8c illustrates the solar window defined by the seasonal extremes of the winter and summer paths of the sun (horizontal curves) and the hourly extents (vertical curves) to which it is efficient to collect solar radiation. Figure 7.8d shows the shadow mask in winter for a single-story structure with morning, noon, and afternoon shadows cast by the house. The shadow mask is a planning tool for planning solar access to adjacent buildings.[19]

Figures 7.8e and 7.8f show hot-arid and hot-humid climate zones where solar energy causes overheating, and, therefore, urban forms and buildings are designed to block the sun, especially during the midday hours. Figure 7.8e is a design by architect Norman Foster in Masdar City, United Arab Emirates, that demonstrates both screening and self-shading. Note how window setbacks and overhanging balconies create shading. Humid climate zones usually have large canopies of trees blocking the sun but have the added problem of high humidity. Therefore, designs are recommended to promote natural air movement through the structures. In these instances, the objective is to block solar energy from entering the interior spaces. Figure 7.8f illustrates the solar shading devices within the Gardens by the

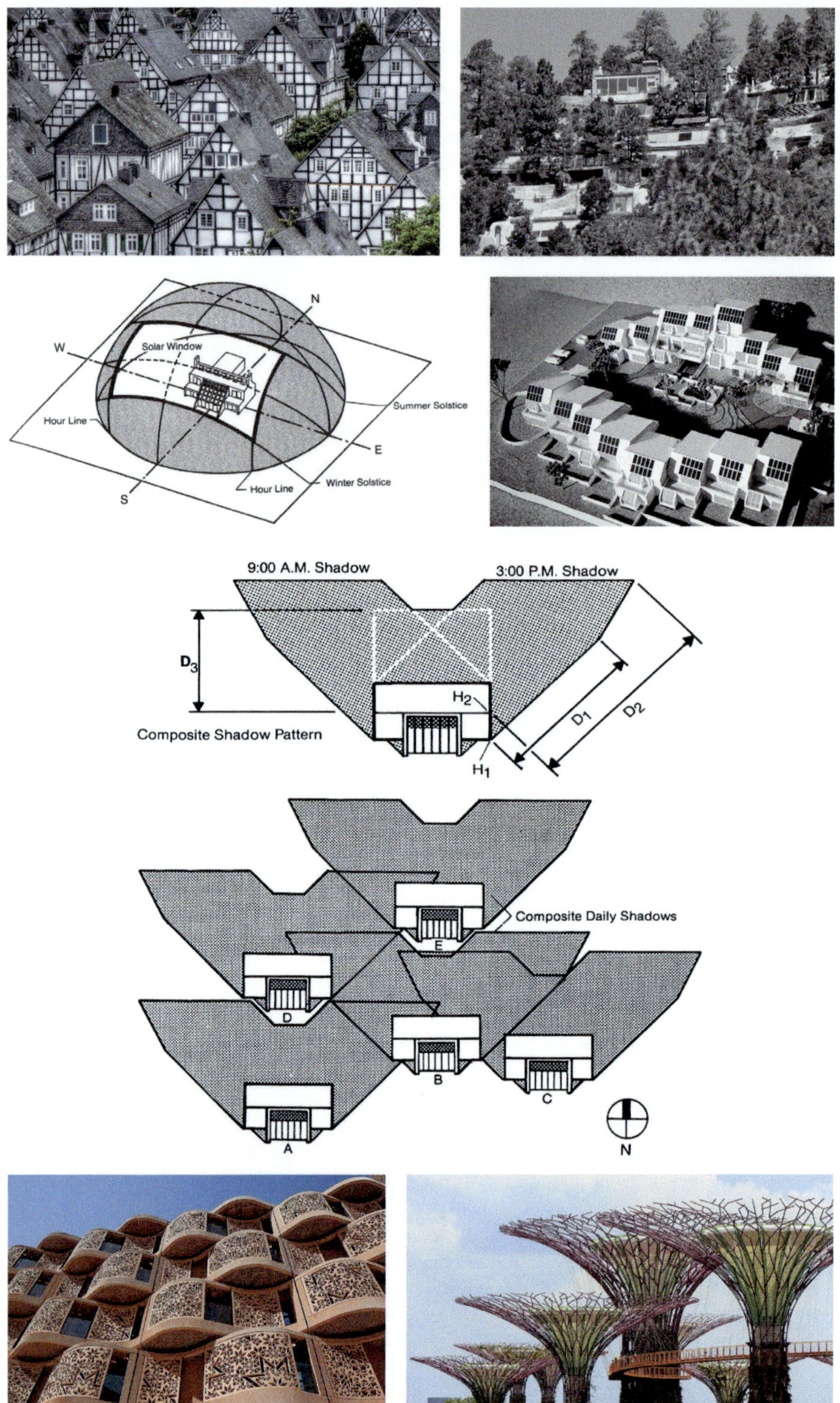

7.8
Solar Energy Responses: (a) Alter Flecken,Freudenberg, (b) Earthship Cluster, New Mexico, (c) Solar Window Diagram, (d) Solar Access to Housing Models, (e) Annual Shadow Mask, (f) Shadow Masks for Multiple Buildings, (g) Self-Shading, Masdar City, UAE, (h) Singapore Gardens by the Bay

Bay in Singapore. It is an urban botanical park consisting of three waterfront gardens, the Flower Dome and Cloud Forest, and sun-shading Supertrees with an elevated walkway.

The wellness benefits include boosting vitamin D, warding off seasonal depression (SAD), improving sleep, reducing eye strain, and generally having positive effects on mood. There are several spiritual wellness attributes and desired outcomes associated with planning for solar energy. They include numinous, religious, serenity, and awe experiences, transcendence and spiritual renewal, and unity experiences. Other attributes include fostering a sense of presence and mindfulness and effecting connections greater than ourselves. Basking in the sunlight can foster a deeper spiritual connection, allowing one to appreciate the life-giving energy. As previously mentioned, the positive attributes of solar energy can help in coping with existential issues and the unknown.

Creating Third Places and Gathering and Ceremonial Places

In the 20th century, city planning was done with automobiles and suburbanization as major design determinants. Since then, many opportunities exist within planned or existing communities to create designs that foster many human social interactions. One type of such designs is third places – that is, places for casual encounters, community gatherings, and ceremonies. The physical manifestations of these third places include, but are not limited to, plazas, parks, blue spaces, indoor and outdoor cafés, restaurants, social clubs, markets, and even bus stops. Third places follow first places (home) and second places (the workplace). Third places are public and most often very familiar and tend to be in socio-economically leveling settings. Their primary function to is foster conversations, exchange of ideas, and having a good time.

Public ceremonial spaces are important for civic, religious, community, and social cohesion. The wellness benefits include stress reduction, improved mood, enhanced cognitive function, boosted physical health, opportunities for greater social connections, and, in the case of spiritual wellness, gratitude and connections to experiences greater than the self. Ceremonial spaces are deeply intertwined with spiritual wellness, offering supportive environments for connection, reflection, and transformation. Participating in rituals and ceremonies within ceremonial spaces helps to connect to deeper and higher powers or universal energies. Further, these spaces can offer support and healing through shared experiences and collective energy.

Benefits of social spaces include the following:

1. **Ceremonial places** – are places of significance and serve a variety of functions, from weddings and funerals to anniversaries and rites of passage. They serve a ritualistic purpose and help elicit spiritual energy.
2. **Social gathering places** – are places of meeting, community, civic engagement, and chance encounters. They support community and sense of place.
3. **Third places** – are special places away from home where one can feel safe, comfortable, playful, and social. They are a home away from home.

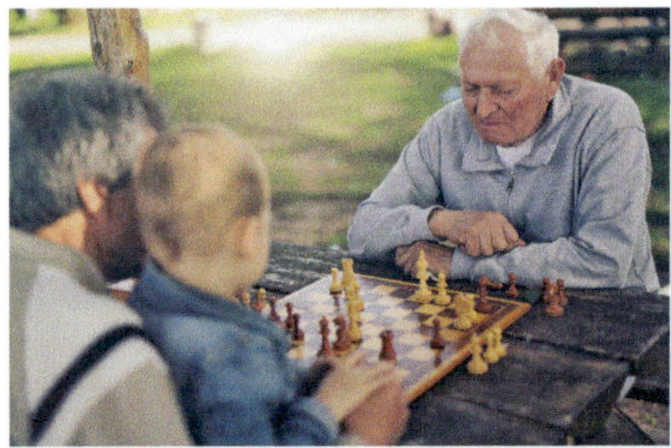

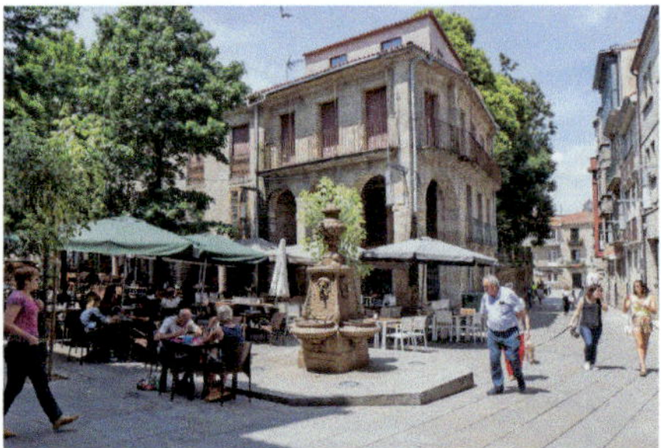

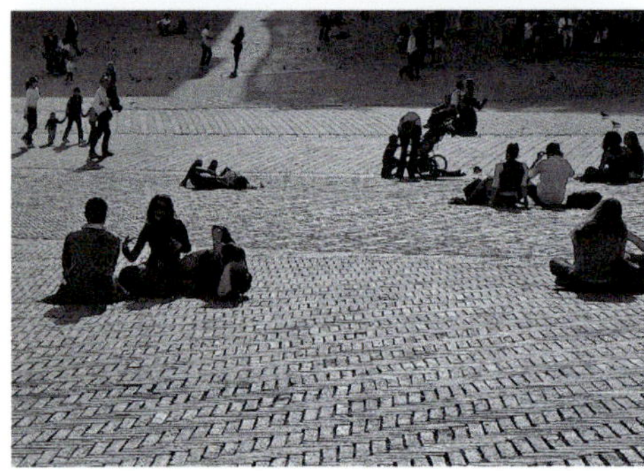

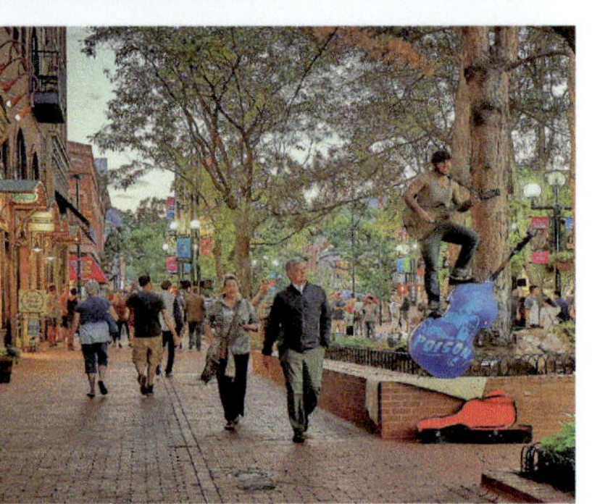

7.9
Mixed Uses and Third Places: (a) Playing Chess in a Park, (b) Pontevedra Square, Spain, (c) Siena Campo, (d) Boulder, Colorado Pedestrian Mall

There are several wellness benefits associated with urban social gathering spaces. They include promoting mental and physical health and reducing morbidity and mortality in urban residents by providing psychological relaxation and stress-alleviating, stimulating social cohesion, supporting physical activity, and reducing exposure to air pollutants, noise, and excessive heat.[20] The spiritual benefits include community building, transcendence above everyday life, unity experiences, fostering a sense of presence and mindfulness, and connecting to things greater than ourselves. Depending upon the actual design, social spaces can foster a sense of presence, amplify prosocial behaviors, and help with stress, the unknown, and existential issues. Certain ceremonial spaces, such as those near water, on mountaintops, or in forests, allow for a deeper connection to the elements and their energies. Figure 7.9 shows several exterior urban spaces supporting social interactions, including playing chess in a park, outdoor dining in a plaza, chatting with friends in Siena's central piazza, and strolling down the Boulder Mall.

Creating Human Streetscapes, Sticky Urbanism, and Walkable Communities

It is no surprise that mobility and the automobile have shaped much of Western planning over the last 75 years, particularly in developing and suburban regions. It is estimated that one-half of a modern American city's land area is dedicated to streets and roads, parking lots, service stations, driveways, signals and traffic signs, automobile-oriented businesses, car dealerships, and more.[21] Strategies now focus on improvements in transportation, convenience, and the experience of movement. Pedestrianization, sticky urbanism, and walkable communities are at the forefront of this change.

According to Brent Toderian, "A street is sticky if as you move along it, you're constantly enticed to slow down, stop and linger to enjoy the public life around you."[22] Sticky urbanism is associated with streetscapes with enticing shop fronts, colorful façades, pedestrian activity, street performers, food carts, cars, bikes, and golf carts creating complexity and constant movement. The character of this kind of streetscape is visually attractive and encourages pedestrianization and social interaction. Visible life on display satisfies innate curiosities. These, in turn, support physical activity, outdoor experiences, and casual encounters. Walkable communities, city centers, and urban enclaves prioritize pedestrians over vehicles and offer easier access to critical necessities. Benefits of streetscapes, sticky urbanism, and walkable communities include the following:

1. **Pedestrianization** – these are urban circulation places that integrate natural, mixed-use, and transportation functions into human scale.
2. **Sticky urbanism** – these are urban streets that are compellingly interesting and active and encourage social interaction.
3. **Walkable communities** – these are settlements, neighborhoods, or urban enclaves that are pedestrian, mixed-use, and user-friendly.

There are several wellness attributes and desired outcomes associated with streetscapes, sticky urbanism, and walkable communities. They include improved physical health and lower risk for diabetes, hypertension, respiratory illnesses, and many cardiovascular and pulmonary diseases. They are strongly associated with social health, which fosters prosocial behaviors. In addition, they support environmental issues such as lower levels of noise and air pollution. Numbers of people along the streets and on sidewalks mean eyes on the street and feelings of safety.

The spiritual benefits of streetscapes, sticky urbanism, and walkable communities can promote a sense of place, identity, and belonging and include numinous, religious, unity, and awe experiences. They also foster a sense of presence, gratitude, and mindfulness and form connections to something greater than ourselves. Figure 7.10a is an aerial photograph of Las Ramblas, located in the heart of Barcelona, which is a tree-lined, pedestrian, cobblestone street stretching three-quarters of a mile (more than 1 kilometer) in length. Along its route are places of art, music, performance, and celebration of Catalan culture. Figure 7.10b depicts Istiklal Avenue in Istanbul, another pedestrian street filled with shops, restaurants, bars, and people.

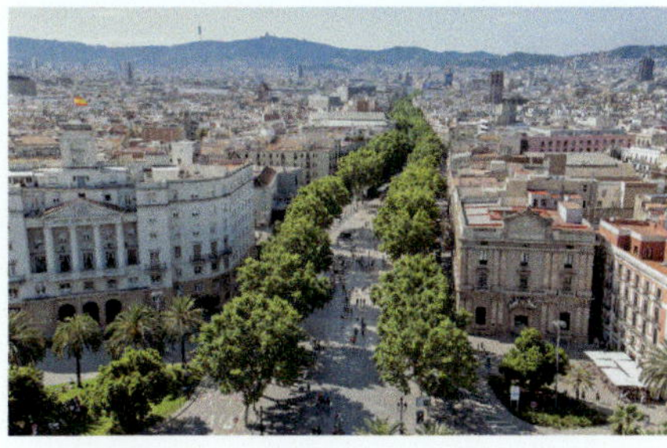

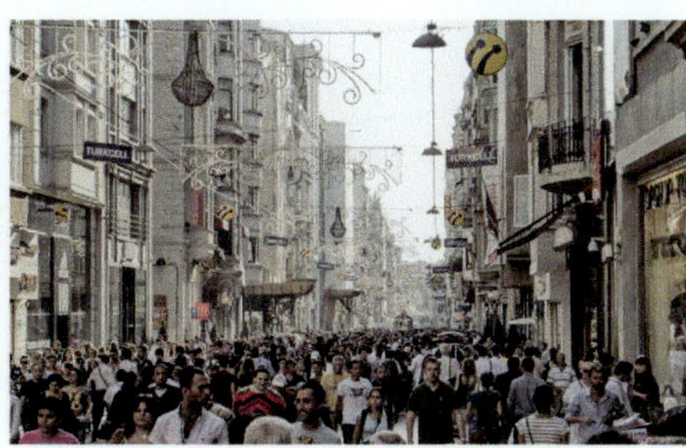

7.10
Streetscapes and Community Well-Being: (a) Las Ramblas, Barcelona, (b) Istiklal Avenue, Istanbul

A tram called Nostalgia connects Taksim Hill to Tunel Square. Both examples serve as incredible social spaces serving a variety of wellness and spiritual purposes.

Providing for Spiritual and Important Civic Spaces and Buildings

Within the fabric of a city, town, village, or neighborhood is the need to preserve or create places that serve higher social and spiritual functions, whether these functions are religious, historic, or civic. Often, these places are prominent, have geometric significance, and are accessible. These sites and buildings can contribute to a sense of place and identity and provide a setting for positive wellness and spiritual experiences. Moreover, these sites often serve as anchors for religious, civic, and community cohesion. Well-known examples include the statue Cristo Redentor in Rio de Janeiro, the Washington Monument in Washington, DC, Trafalgar Square in London, the St. Louis Gateway Park and Arch, the Sacré-Cœur in Paris, Central Park in New York City, and the Cathedral of Santa Maria del Fiore in Florence. Figure 7.11 shows two examples, one a spiritual place, the Sagrada Família in Barcelona, and the other a monument to the French Revolution and Napoleonic Wars in Paris. The significance of the siting and the power of geometry and form are apparent. Benefits of providing spiritual and important civic spaces and buildings include the following:

1. **Geometric significance** – special places in significant locations, such as in centers, on axes, or on geographically or historically important sites.
2. **Creating significant places** – special civic, spiritual, community, or natural places that contribute to identity, branding, and community cohesion.
3. **Featuring significant buildings or monuments** – located on significant sites, near important public spaces, encouraging extraordinary architecture and public art installations.

There are several wellness attributes and desired outcomes associated with important sacred, social, and civic spaces. They contribute to community cohesion; improve neighborhood safety; offer opportunities for reflection, renewal, and revitalization; reduce mental distress; and promote physical and emotional well-being. Further desired outcomes include fostering a sense of optimism, hope for

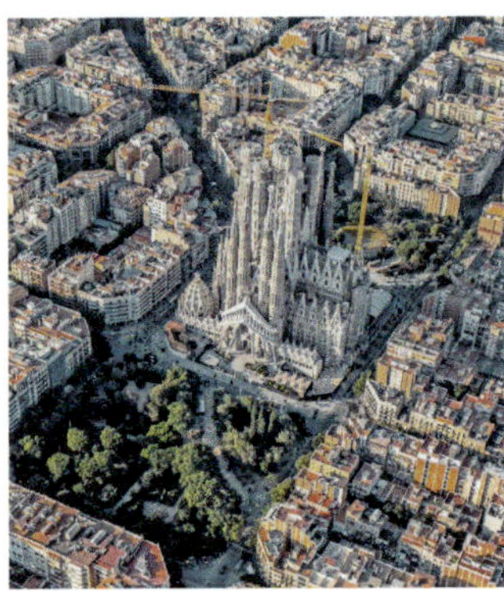

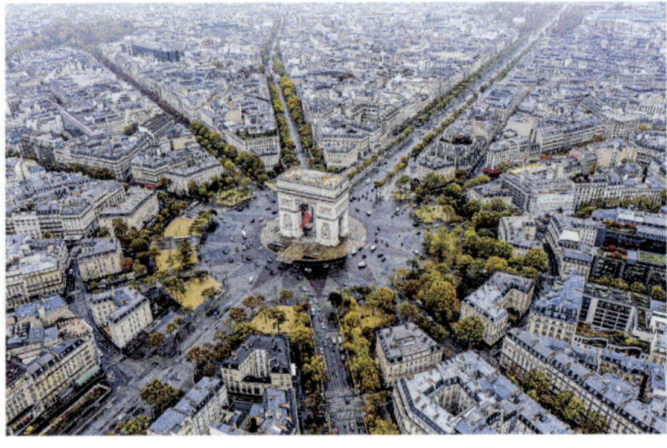

7.11
Special Land-Use Designations: (a) Sagrada Família Cathedral, Barcelona, Spain, (b) the Arc de Triomphe, Paris, France

the future, connectedness, and collective well-being. The spiritual benefits include spirit of place, numinous and religious experiences, transcendence and spiritual renewal, unity experiences, fostering a sense of presence and mindfulness, and connections to places greater than ourselves. Depending upon the actual design and location, these sites and buildings can elicit and amplify numinous and awe emotional responses. They help to cope with existential issues and unknown experiences. Special places like these can also occur in everyday locations, as in Figure 7.12, where the site plan and photographs show natural and planned sacred sites located within the Serenbe community in Georgia. As seen in Figure 7.12a, 35 different sacred and land art sites exist throughout the community. Two of these are shown in Figures 7.12b and 7.12c, with the waterfalls identified on the plan as number 30, and a land art sculpture as number 24. While the subjective benefits of special civic, religious, and spiritual places within communities are difficult to measure, they do contribute to the social and spiritual wellness capital of these places in positive ways.

Summary

Spiritual wellness is an ongoing process of self-discovery and active participation shaping the deepest part of us, including our beliefs, values, feelings, behaviors, and lifestyle practices. The wellness benefits in part are achieved through design, as the wellness dimensions inform the design opportunities in the built environment. Many of the attributes have a more direct impact upon design opportunities in the built environment. Others have secondary effects on attitudes, convictions, and sensibilities, which can influence planning and design decisions. The challenge at the urban design scale is to flourish with collective well-being toward the development of climax communities that are equitable, and to co-exist, cooperate, and participate in planetary stewardship and health.[23] A summary list of the planning and design strategies for the urban design scale follows:

1. Preserving ecological zones.
2. Urban spatial structures.
3. Integrating nature within the urban fabric.
4. Creating community agriculture and gardens.
5. Circular regenerative infrastructure.
6. Zoning for mixes of use and intergenerational living.
7. Planning for solar energy (access and denial).
8. Creating third places and gathering and ceremonial places.
9. Creating human streetscapes and walkable communities.
10. Providing for significant spiritual and civic sites and buildings.

The urban design scale offers opportunities for specific design strategies to incorporate spiritual, health, and wellness benefits. These benefits include positive responses to ecological and hydrological cycles, climate change mitigation, reduction of greenhouse gas emissions, clean air and water, and encouragement of physical activity through greater pedestrian connections and networks. This scale

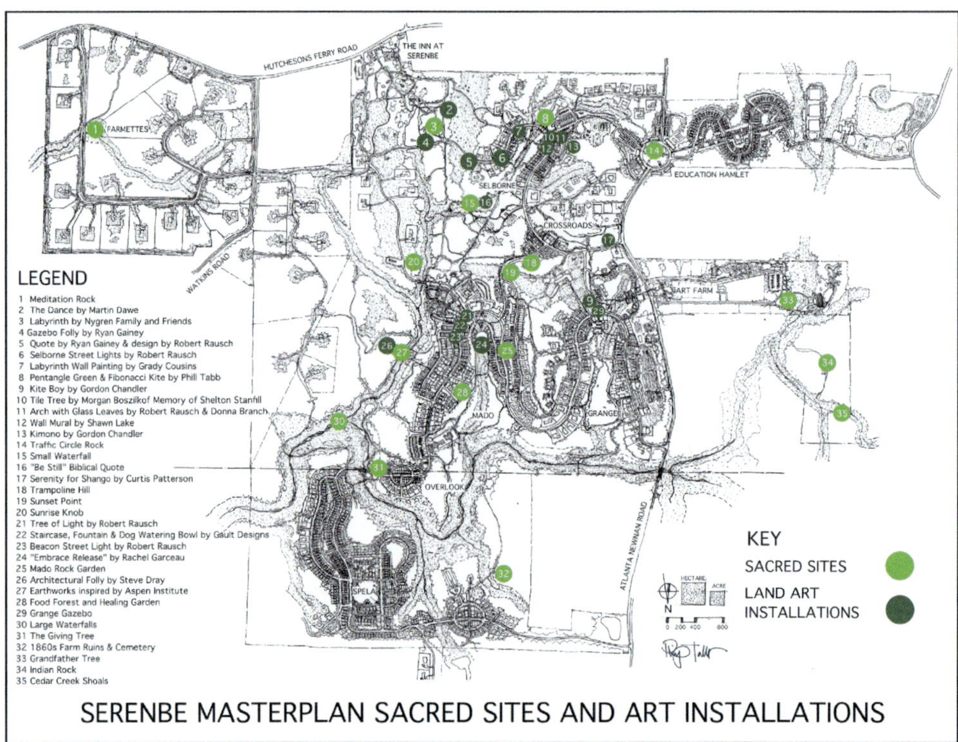

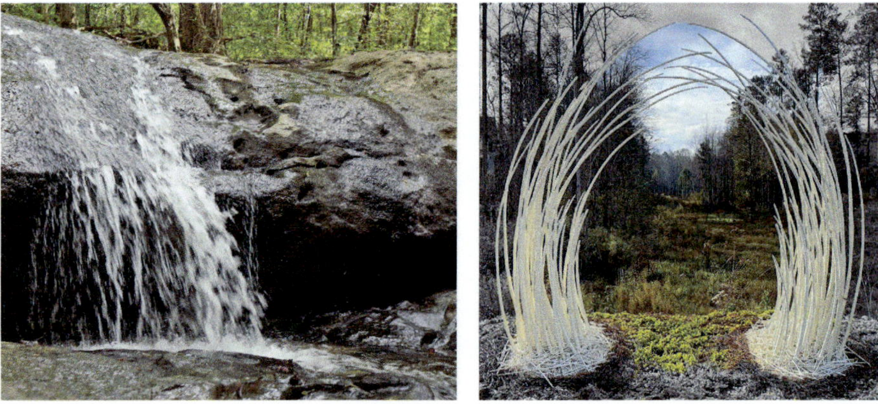

7.12

Streetscapes and Significant Sites: (a) Serenbe Sacred Sites and Land Art Installations, Georgia, (b) Large Waterfalls #30, (c) Embrace-Release Land Art #24

offers the opportunity to create a more seamless connection between urban areas (climatic forms, renewable infrastructure, mixes of use, and the positive effects of densification) and nature (parks, green streetscapes, and urban agriculture). This scale also sets the scene and physical context within which the other scales are placed (such as personal space, architecture, interiors, and landscapes). Owing to the larger impact of the urban design scale, wellness design strategies and opportunities can quite easily be addressed with both existing and new construction. Providing mixes of use and the many wellness design strategies within the suburban, single-use context is a challenge, yet very important for wellness, social, and sustainability outcomes. In addition, the outcomes at this scale contribute to pro-individual benefits through intimate and everyday wellness strategies and to prosocial benefits by fostering community and family and friend gatherings in public settings. They can also lead to pro-environmental benefits through protection from negative climatic effects and providing positive interactions with urban nature. It must be noted here that implementation of these wellness design strategies does not guarantee positive health outcomes but can provide greater opportunities for them to occur. Finally, this scale can also promote pro-spiritual benefits through careful integration of ecological, green, and blue spaces and provision of special spiritual and civic sites which support wellness activities.

The following Chapters 8–11 focus the spiritual wellness attributes and design strategies into specific themes that help elucidate spiritual wellness in the built environment. These themes are defined with certain guiding principles, illustrated with specific examples, and described with explanatory stories. These stories or narrative vignettes are intended to give voice to firsthand, insightful, and accessible connections to the experience of spiritual wellness. They are lived experiences and portraits of personal experiences that reveal real events with encounters with the transformative power of spiritually charged well-places. These narrative vignettes include the significance of solar energy, the role of sacred geometry, the value of mythic landscapes, and the importance of pilgrimages.

NOTES

1 Global Wellness Institute, 2024 Wellness Real Estate Market Growth (2019–1013) and Future Development, (accessed August 12, 2024), https://globalwellnessinstitute.org/industry-research/wellness-real-estate-market-growth-2019-2023-and-future-developments/?utm_campaign=Industry%20Research%20%26%20Trends&utm_medium=email&_hsenc=p2ANqtz-9JnDUR1J8kDMblrOrd33vNp5DRC9I22Zo80_7XWPa9sqV9Wdfxf9U7_pc8SNcJwFvBw_HXdKy-uMMUwtQwCdGz9Qd0-Q&_hsmi=319484537&utm_content=319484537&utm_source=hs_email.

2 Hootz, Eva, & Karl Johaentges, *Living on Kronsberg* (Hanover, Germany: City of Hanover, 2000).

3 SJ kör pendeltågstrafiken i Stockholmsregionen från den 3 mars 2024. *Mynewsdesk* (in Swedish) (accessed November 1, 2023), https://sl.se/aktuellt/nyheter/sj-tar-over-pendeltagstrafiken.

4 Amster, Randall, & Linda Bell Grdina, Individual Well-Being with Environmental Systems (accessed August 9, 2024), https://ssir.org/articles/entry/integrating_individual_well_being_with_environmental_systemsInegrating.

5 Kummu, Matti, Hans de Moel, Philip Ward, & Olli Varis, How Close Do We Live to Water? A Global Analysis of Population Distance to Freshwater Bodies (accessed September 9, 2024), https://www.ncbi.nlm.nih.gov/pmc/articles/PMC3110782/.

6 Frumkin, Howard, The Health Superpowers of Parks (accessed September 9, 2024), https://www.tpl.org/parks-promote-health-report.

7 Mastrorosa, Erika, Urban Wildlife: Threats and Benefits of Humans–Animals Interactions (accessed September 9, 2024), https://greentumble.com/urban-wildlife-threats-and-benefits.

8 Krier, Leon, *Houses, Palaces, Cities* (London, UK: Architectural Design Editions, 1984), pp. 32–38.
9 Moos, Markus, & Pablo Mendez, Suburban Ways of Living and the Geography of Income: How Homeownership, Single-Family Dwellings and Automobile Use Define the Metropolitan Social Space. *Urban Studies*, 52(10), 2015, 1864–1882.
10 Ala-Mantila, S., J. Heinonen, S. Junnila, & P. Saarsalmi, Spatial Nature of Urban Well-Being (accessed September 12, 2024), https://www.tandfonline.com/doi/full/10.1080/00343404.2017.1360485#d1e275.
11 Arvanitis, Agni Vlanianos, "BIOPOLIS": Biopolicy for Greener and More Livable Cities (accessed August 12, 2024), http://www.cadmusjournal.org/node/350.
12 Cohen, Mychal, Kimberly Burrowes, and Peace Gwam, The Health Benefits of Parks and their Economic Impacts (accessed December 12, 2024), https://www.urban.org/sites/default/files/2022-03/the-health-benefits-of-parks-and-their-economic-impacts_0.pdf.
13 de la Salle, Janine, & Mark Holland, *Agricultural Urbanism: Handbook for Building Sustainable Food & Agriculture Systems in 21st Century* (Green Frigate Books, 2010).
14 Belsey-Priebe, An Overview of the 100-Mile Diet (accessed September 10, 2024), https://ecolife.com/food/eating-local/100-mile-diet/.
15 A Landscaping Just as Good as Beautiful (accessed September 10, 2024), https://gardenculturemagazine.com/foodscaping-a-new-way-to-create-a-garden/.
16 Hassan Bazazzadeh, Behnam Pourahmadi, Peiman Pilehchi ha, Seyedeh Sara, Hashemi Safaei, & Umberto Berardi, Chapter 12: Urban Scale Climate Change Adaptation through Smart Technologies (accessed August 10, 2024), https://www.sciencedirect.com/topics/social-sciences/urban-infrastructure.
17 Tabb, Phillip, *Solar Energy Planning* (New York, NY: McGraw-Hill, 1984).
18 Michael Reynolds designs Earthships as autonomous, off-grid homes constructed with natural and recycled materials such as earth-packed automobile tires, aiming for self-sufficiency in energy, water, and waste management. These innovative structures utilize passive solar heating and cooling, thermal mass, and rainwater harvesting to create sustainable and comfortable living spaces.
19 The solar window and shadow patterns were taken from Tabb, Phillip, *Solar Energy Planning* (New York, NY: McGraw-Hill, 1984).
20 WHO, Urban Green Spaces and Health (accessed September 12, 2024), https://iris.who.int/bitstream/handle/10665/345751/WHO-EURO-2016-3352-43111-60341-eng.pdf?sequence=3&isAllowed=y.
21 Melosi, Martin, The Reshaping of City Cores That Were Designed for Cars (accessed September 12, 2024), https://www.forbes.com/sites/johnfrazer1/2019/08/06/the-reshaping-of-city-cores-that-were-designed-for-cars/.
22 IBI Group, Creating Sticky Streets (accessed September 12, 2924), https://www.ibigroup.com/ibi-insights/creating-sticky-streets/.
23 Ichioka, Sarah & Michael Pawlyn, *Flourish: Design Paradigms for Our Planetary Emergency*, (Axminster, UK: Triarchy Press, 2021), p. 50.

8 NARRATIVE VIGNETTE 1

The Significance of Solar Energy

INTRODUCTION

The narrative vignettes are first-person descriptive examples of my experiences with several attribute clusters of spiritual dimensions of wellness. They are intended to give voice to firsthand, insightful, and accessible connections to the experience of spiritual wellness. They are portraits of personal stories that reveal real events with encounters with the transformative power of spiritually charged well-places. Included are focuses on the function of sacred geometry and the role of myths in the physical and cultural landscapes of placemaking, the influence of solar energy in planning and design, and the importance of pilgrimages as well as everyday experiences of spiritual wellness. Finally, I discuss the intentions and design of my own home in Georgia as representing spiritual wellness. The purpose of the narrative vignettes is to discover the spiritual dimensions of wellness and their attributes in very specific and more anecdotal ways. While, generally, vignettes evoke poignant moments in time, they too can be a weaving, capturing plots or processes over time.

NARRATIVE VIGNETTES

The narrative vignettes that follow are written by several differing voices depending upon the nature of the story and subject. Those that are more informational and descriptive in content are written in a more academic and professional language, while others are written with a more experiential, personal, and, in some instances, esoteric language. The four narrative vignettes present personal stories that reveal specific spiritual wellness concepts and insights. They occur over the next four chapters. The vignettes present experiences that cover time from the early 1970s through to the present. While they do not necessarily address all the dimensions or attributes of spiritual wellness, they do contain and communicate some important strategies, insights, and benefits. Taken together, they represent an accumulation of interests, practices, and life experiences. The narrative vignettes that occur in the following chapters are listed below:

1. The Significance of Solar Energy (Chapter 8).
2. The Role of Sacred Geometry (Chapter 9).
3. The Value of Mythic Landscapes (Chapter 10).
4. The Importance of Pilgrimages (Chapter 11).

DOI: 10.4324/9781003546085-8

THE SIGNIFICANCE OF SOLAR ENERGY

The sun has been a focus of worship in many cultures, and its symbolism has been used in various spiritual practices. The sun has been a symbol of immense power, life, divinity, and rebirth. It, too, is a source of health, wellness, and spiritual renewal and rebirth. The sun is a source of immense energy. In a religious context, the sun is often seen as a symbol of divine power and enlightenment, representing the light of truth and wisdom that illuminates the darkness of ignorance and confusion.[1] Its spiritual meaning derives from its ability to emanate light, its enduring power, its transformative ability, and its ability to provide a connection to our inner selves, and its scale is certainly larger than ourselves. The sun facilitates circadian lighting following the 24-hour internal clock. The area of the brain called the hypothalamus controls each person's circadian rhythm by receiving signals from the eyes that report when it is daytime and nighttime. The hypothalamus, in turn, controls the amount of melatonin released to correlate sleepiness with darkness and alertness with light.[2]

The solstices identify the two times in the year when the sun reaches its highest or lowest position in the sky at noon, resulting in the longest and shortest days of the year. The sun also creates what is called the "golden hour." This is the hour after the sun rises in the morning and the hour before the sun sets in the evening. It is golden because, as the sun approaches the horizon, it becomes more golden in color and radiance. These transitions during the day and the solstices during the year are considered the most sacred times. They mark profound transitions and transformations.

It is the midwinter sunrise (northern hemisphere) that is considered the most sacred time of the year. The twilight or golden hour before sunrise transforms in three phases, with the black or indigo night sky changing into blue, red, and finally golden colors, creating the primary colors and a natural ethereal display. This time signifies the moment that the day is at its shortest, and thereafter, there is a daily increase in daylight and the promise of new beginnings. The darkness of the winter solstice represents introspection, reflection, and the fertile void from which new beginnings emerge. In contrast, light symbolizes hope, illumination, and the promise of renewal. The summer solstice is a symbol of vitality, illumination, and abundance.[3] During both the summer and winter solstices, the sun appears to stand still, not gaining or loosing daylight for several days; hence, it is a time of reflection. Refer to Figure 8.1 showing a golden sunset.

The spiritual meaning of the sun is deeply rooted in various cultures and religions throughout history. In Egypt, the sun was worshiped as the god Ra; in Greece, it was the god Helios; in Geek mythology, it was associated with Apollo; in Hinduism, it is the god Surya; in China, the sun was associated with yang energy or the creative; and, in Native American culture, it is often associated with the eagle. Knowing the healing effects of sunlight throughout history is important to understanding why it is still essential today. To name a couple, it helped cure the "disease of darkness," or vitamin D deficiency, and Florence Nightingale observed that patients in east-facing sunlit rooms recovered faster. With the phenomenon of people spending most of their time indoors – more than 90 percent – it is no

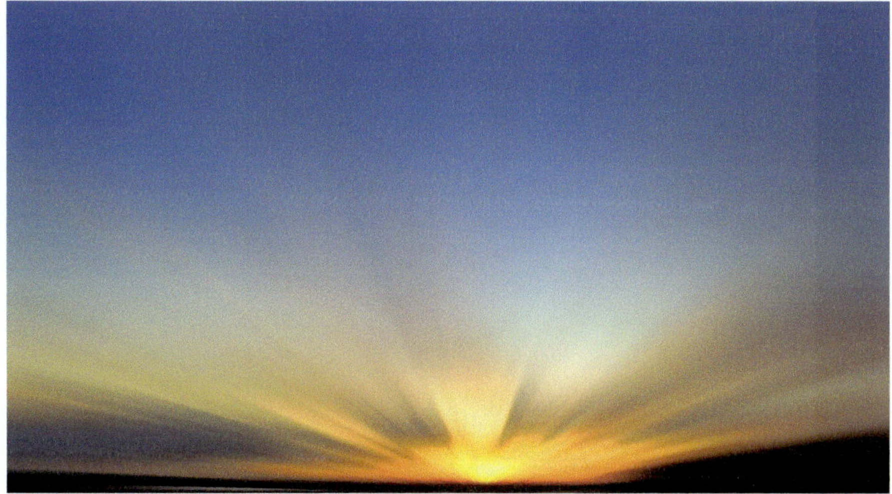

8.1
Solar
Energy: Sunset over the Horizon

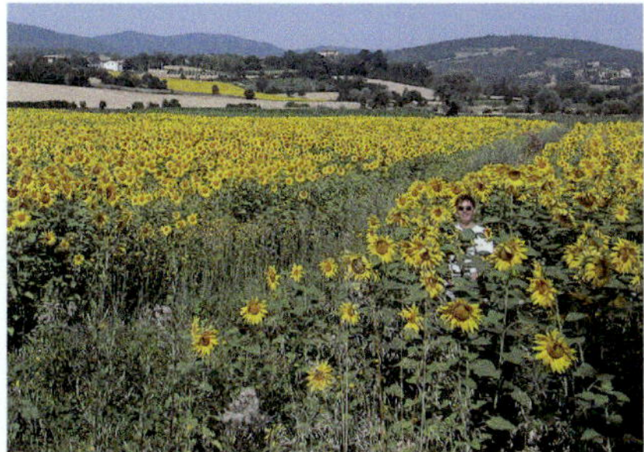

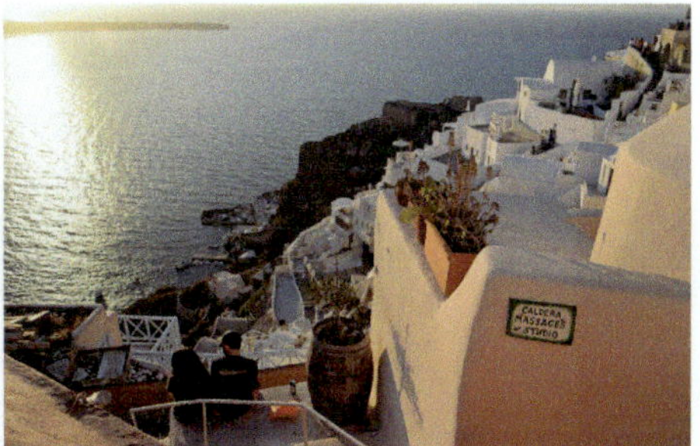

8.2
Solar Energy: (a) Tuscany Sunflower Field, (b) Oia, Santorini, Sunset

wonder that more outdoor experiences and safe exposure to the sun have both spiritual and wellness outcomes.

The sun emits infrared, visible, and ultraviolet waves that reach Earth. Almost all life on Earth relies on solar energy for light, food, and warmth. Daylight affects both our eye functions and our inherent circadian rhythms. Light expresses in many forms and is related to luminosity, the ethereal, inspiration, and the numinous. Solar delight in the places we occupy has long been of interest to architects and planners. For me, positive sun experiences have occurred when sunbathing on the San Jean beach in St. Barts, viewing a sunset in midsummer in Santorini, the anticipation of the midwinter sunrise, watching the sparkling reflections off the Buffalo River in Idaho, or stopping by a Tuscany sunflower field (see Figure 8.2). Most of us have delightful experiences not too unlike these in everyday life, no matter where we live.

The 1973 oil crisis started in October 1973, when the members of the Organization of Arab Petroleum Exporting Countries, or OAPEC, consisting of the Arab members of OPEC plus Egypt, Syria, and Tunisia, proclaimed an oil embargo. This occurred as a response to the US decision to re-supply the Israeli military during the Yom Kippur War. Daniel Yergin explained, "The embargo and its consequences sent shock radiating through the social fabric of the industrial nations."[4] Long lines occurred routinely at gas stations, and often they were closed. There was a fourfold increase in the price of oil, from $3 a barrel to $12. By January of 1974, Secretary of State Henry Kissinger had negotiated an Israeli troop withdrawal from parts of the Sinai Peninsula. The promise of a negotiated settlement between Israel and Syria was sufficient to convince Arab oil producers to lift the embargo in March 1974. The National Maximum Speed Law in the United States was a provision of the 1974 Emergency Highway Energy Conservation Act and prohibited speed limits higher than 55 miles per hour (88.5 kilometers per hour). Following the embargo, there was an increase in domestic oil production and a greater emphasis on efficiency and renewable sources of energy.

In 1974, the first of several solar energy bills became law, and federal research jumped substantially. Congress responded by enacting the Solar Energy Research, Development and Demonstration Act of 1974. The Act stated that it was henceforth the policy of the federal government to "pursue a vigorous and viable program of research and resource assessment of solar energy as a major source of energy for our national needs." The Act's scope embraced all energy sources that were renewable by the sun – including solar thermal energy and photovoltaic energy – and energy derived from wind, sea thermal gradients, and photosynthesis. The Solar Heating and Cooling Demonstration Act of 1974 followed. The AIA Research Corporation, directed by John Eberhard, participated in solar energy research to help fulfill the charge of the solar demonstration programs. They were given the task of identifying the available types of solar energy systems and components and the ways in which they could be integrated into varying housing typologies in different climatic contexts as part of the Department of Housing and Urban Development Solar Demonstration projects.

The first examples of active solar architecture simply applied the emergent technologies unceremoniously to buildings, usually rooftops. Solar collector arrays faced cardinal directions for optimal efficiency and often did not match building orientations, resulting in an awkward massing. Eventually, building forms assimilated the blossoming technologies, where solar collector orientation, tilt angle, and area intensiveness became more integrative. The early demonstrations of active solar architecture, especially in temperate and cold climates, revealed competition for sunlight between the area requirements of the opaque solar collector arrays and daylight needs of the users inside. From a spiritual wellness point of view, natural light should favor human use first over the technology.

Other examples involved the dramatic integration of solar technologies into the building form, such as the Odeillo solar furnace in the southwest of France, which I visited in 1978 (see Figure 8.3a). There is a field of mirrors that track the sun and reflect its energy onto a large parabolic mirror in the belly of a ten-story research building. The mirror then focuses the energy onto a small boiler that produces extremely high temperatures. The ten-story building and enormous parabolic collector array are fully integrated.

On my visit to Taos, New Mexico, to visit my friend and former classmate Michael Reynolds, I stayed in one of his Earthships for a couple days. The experience was wonderful, and the location, especially during sunrise and sunset, was spectacular. We drove around the 650-acre (243-hectare) Greater World Earthship

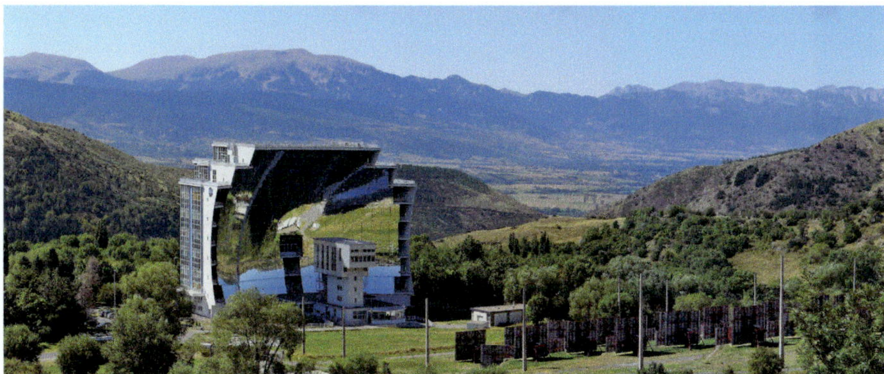

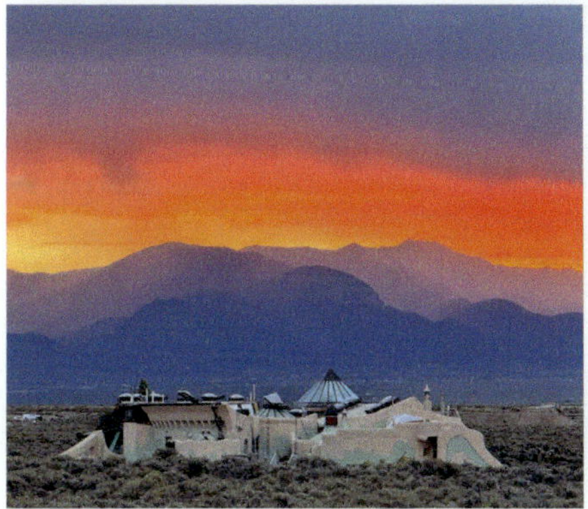

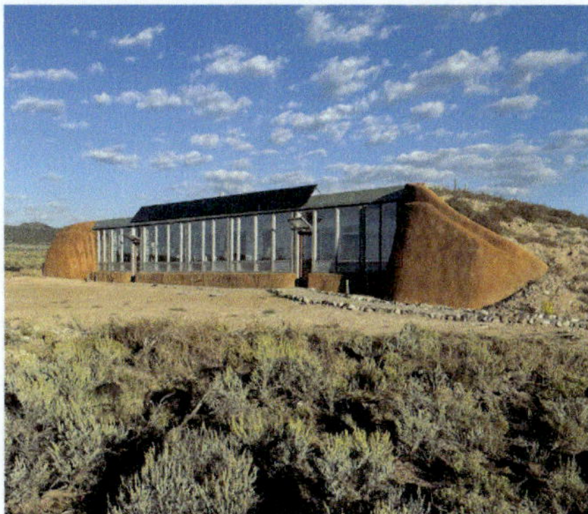

8.3
Solar Energy Architectural Examples: (a) Odeillo Solar Furnace, France, (b) Atlantis Earthship, New Mexico, (c) Refuge Earthship, New Mexico

Community discussing his ideas. It is amazing hanging out in a completely off-grid residence where shelter is provided by the Earth, heat comes from the sun, water is captured from rain and recycled four times, and electricity is generated by a photovoltaic array. Inside is a long, south-facing garden full of plants – flowers and herbs. Figures 8.3b and 8.3c show the Atlantis and Refuge Earthships.

Full passive solar systems consisted of three major types. They were the direct-gain distributed-mass system, the concentrated-mass system, and the sunspace system. There were two types of concentrated-mass systems, which used either water or masonry for storage. And there were two types of sunspaces, isolated gain and integrated sunrooms. The effectiveness of a passive solar system depended upon ways in which the architecture responded to the entire solar system's functions, including accommodating the area intensiveness of collection, adequately matching solar glazing to internal thermal mass for overnight storage, efficiently coupling solar-charged spaces with other internal spaces, and responding to potential overheating conditions. The wellness benefits might include decreases in greenhouse emissions and lower electric bills, energy independence, and low maintenance, and health benefits such as reductions in respiratory and cardiovascular issues.

The oil embargo brought a revived interest in the sun and its utilization as an energy source. As an architect working on the world's largest solar building at that time, I was fascinated by its emerging technology, but also intrigued by the larger cultural and spiritual implications of moving away from centralized nuclear power to decentralized solar energy. Interest in solar energy also expanded awareness of even greater celestial phenomena. The photovoltaic effect was discovered in 1839 by Edmund Becquerel. By 2016, the United States was obtaining 1 percent of its power from 1 million installations. The principal benefit is that solar energy is a local, on-site, free resource, available everywhere but most effective in sunny climate regions. I dedicated the rest of my professional career to its function in planning and design and grew more involved with its spiritual healing power. Part of what I learned is that technology is mutable and always changing, while the solar source is unchangeable.

The sunflower field image in Figure 8.2a is a wonderful demonstration of phototropic design and a natural process for solar access. Each sunflower and its petals function as its own solar collector, responding to the changing movement of the sun. Within the context of the entire field, they find the space for sunlight access and freedom from obstruction. Phototropism is most often observed in plants and in other organisms such as fungi, but also can occur within the built environment. This natural biological response is a good model for low-density solar energy access in planning and urban design.

SOLAR GEOMETRY

It is important to understand solar geometry as it reflects the changing dynamic of the sun's relationship to Earth. After the 1973 oil embargo, solar geometry became an important area of study, applied to the design of both solar technology and solar buildings. The annual orbit around the sun, the daily rotation around our own axis, and the fixed position of the axis are all causes of the varying seasons, climatic phenomena, and weather. In winter in the northern hemisphere, the Earth's axial tilt is cause for the land to receive less direct solar radiation as there are greater reflections of the surface. This is what is known as an increased incident angle.[5] In summer, the sun angles are higher in the sky and generate more heat and absorption. The reverse occurs in the southern hemisphere.

Sun angles are critical to the functioning of solar systems and need to be considered in building design. This is true for both overheating and under-heating climatic zones. The solar window is a good construct that aids in designing for solar access or solar shading. The window geometry is defined by the latitude of a given site, the midwinter and midsummer sun paths across the south sky, and the sunlit hours of the day, usually between 9:00 am and 3:00 pm. This polygonal shape is the space within which the sun shines throughout the year and day. For solar heating, it is important to keep this space free of any obstructions, and, for cooling, it is important to shade this space. Refer to the solar window diagram in Chapter 7, Figure 7.8c.[6]

SIGNIFICANCE OF SOLAR ENERGY IN PROJECTS

This vignette recalls and explores this interest in solar energy, its wellness qualities, and its prominence in several of my architectural projects. In the late 1970s, my firm was architect for the Celestial Seasonings Herb Teas headquarters building (1978), Stonebraker Student Housing (1975), Bramwell House (1982), the Tresemer, Dubose, Goldman, and Overmeyer off-grid residences (1990s), and my own solar home in Serenbe (2016). While solar techniques have been used for millennia, the term *passive*, meaning not relying on mechanical or electrical components, was popularized during the 1970s by a friend, Richard Crowther of Denver, Colorado. Passive solar architecture was attractive to architects at this time because it was less about "attaching" solar technology to a building and more about designing the building "as solar technology." Our architectural practice worked on a great number of passive and active solar projects, and we received several national solar demonstration awards from the American Institute of Architects Research Corporation, the Department of Housing and Urban Development, and the Department of Energy. In the mid-1970s, I added a passive sunspace to my house in Boulder and I had long dreamed of designing my own fully off-grid home.

Figure 8.4 shows three early projects incorporating hydronic solar energy technologies. The first project is a model of the initial design for the Community College of Denver West Campus, now called Front Range Community College. It was designed in 1973 in the Denver architectural offices of Anderson, Barker, Rinker, Seacat. The design featured a quarter-mile-long (403-meter) linear building with an interior undulating spine connecting all of the college's academic programs. One could walk along the spine and see into each of the programmatic areas, getting a wholistic sense of the college. On top of the sawtooth roof were placed the solar collector arrays. Figure 8.4a is a photograph of the model with the roof off, showing the interior circulation, classrooms, and studios. The heart-shaped form housed the counseling and administrative functions for the college. While this specific design was not realized, the eventual building was constructed utilizing a linear, but far simpler, design. This design incorporated the contrast between the formal technological constrains of the building systems and the informal and serendipitous people places.

The second project was research for the American Institute of Architects Research Corporation in 1974. This was an outgrowth of the Solar Heating and Cooling Act of 1974, and our newly formed architectural practice, along with Dr. Jan Kreider, PE, won one of the research projects, which focused on the integration of various solar energy technologies with multiple housing schemes. The model photograph in Figure 8.4b is one of the schemes developed from this research. It shows an east–west linear design with a slightly curving or zigzag south façade. The highly efficient solar collector arrays were positioned away from the corners of the zigzag in order to avoid self-shadowing. This design strategy was used on the Boulder Student Housing project described later in this chapter. The work was published in 1976 in *Solar Dwelling Design Concepts*, by Michael Holtz and the AIA/RC.[7]

The third project is a model of the Celestial Seasonings Herb Teas headquarters. It was an interesting project in that the client was young, progressive, and interested in pursuing solar energy applications in the design. The design featured the tea production process occurring beneath a large solar collector array, while the administrative offices form a courtyard with abundant natural daylighting. We applied for and won a Passive Solar Demonstration Award from the Department of

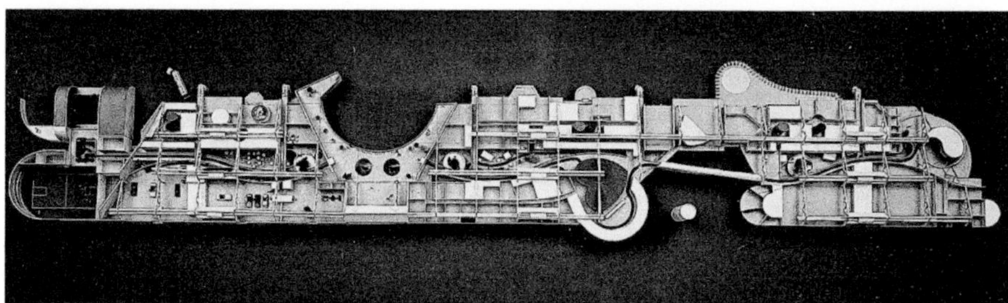

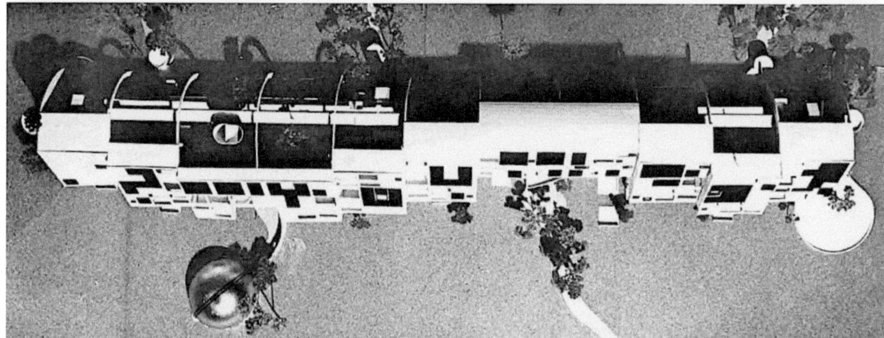

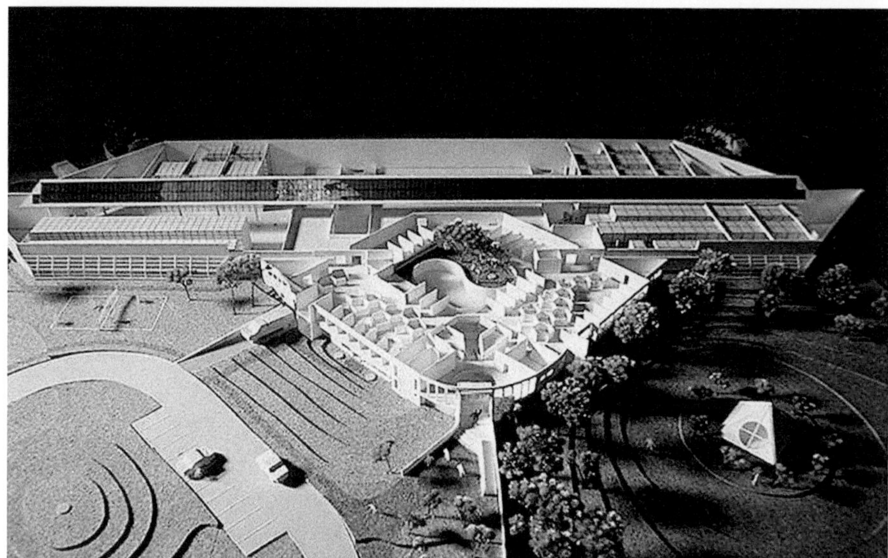

8.4
Solar Energy Projects: (a) Model of Community College of Denver West Campus, Colorado (1973), (b) AIA Research Corporation Study Model (1974), (c) Celestial Seasonings Headquarters Building Model, Boulder (1978)

Energy for the active solar system and a passive greenhouse pre-heating system.[8] However, in 1978, the client chose to stop the project. The model with the roofs off, in Figure 8.4c, shows the tea production, administration, courtyard, and an employee meditation pavilion. These three projects provided an initial understanding of solar applications that informed later work.

Figure 8.5 shows a number of solar-oriented buildings my firm designed over the years from 1976 to 1997. Figure 8.5a is a photograph of the Boulder Flatirons, which served as inspiration for the active solar energy student housing project completed in Boulder, Colorado, in 1975. Figure 8.5b is a photograph of the completed Boulder

Student Housing building designed by my firm, Joint Venture Architects (architects Alan Brown, Roland Hower, and myself). The Boulder Student Housing project addressed the issue of active solar technology integration into architectural form. The project was based on the American Institute of Architects Research Corporation work that we previously completed in 1974 where we investigated the integration of four different active solar system types into multi-family housing. This building was designed with approximately 70 percent of the space-heating and domestic-hot-water-heating requirements provided by an active solar system. The building responded to the systems' orientation constraints, collector area requirements, and optimal tilt angle with sloping south façades.

The Boulder Student Housing building was oriented along an east–west axis with about a 2:1 aspect ratio. It was designed with five solar collector arrays having a combined solar collector area of 700 square feet (65 square meters). The south façade was shifted into four distinct, yet attached, parts by a "pushing and pulling" of the sloping secondary forms. This allowed the in-between spaces to accommodate stairs and balconies and facilitated daylight penetration deep into the interior spaces.[9] The living, dining, and kitchen spaces faced south, while all the bedrooms and bathrooms faced north. The plan was organized with four attached four-bedroom units stacked on top of one another, accommodating a total of 32 units. I lived a block away from the project and was able to observe construction, which was completed in 1976. Important to me with this project was the integrative qualities of the solar technologies and the overall building form. The solar collectors were extant and present, having a large visual impact. But, because they were so fully integrated into the overall form, they were not obtrusive.

In the early 1980s, I was commissioned to design the Bramwell House located in Florissant, Colorado. For me, this was an important project because it incorporated hybrid passive and active solar systems (Figure 8.5c). All the primary rooms of the house face south and employ direct-gain passive solar collection. In the center of the house is a two-story sunspace utilizing high-performance heat mirror glazing. At the top of the sunspace are three active domestic-hot-water solar collectors with a heat recovery subsystem delivering captured heat to rockbed storage. At the top of the house is a clerestory, bringing natural light into the circulation corridor beneath it.

In the early 1990s, I designed a community-oriented sacred building in the foothills of the Rocky Mountains, three miles outside of Boulder, Colorado. I have written about this project in previous books and later in Chapter 9, but here will focus on the spiritual wellness aspects and the use of solar energy. The StarHouse was a building based upon sacred and astronomical geometrical principles, including solar energy. A careful process was conducted on site using a surveying transit and pole tracing shadow patterns to determine true south. Once we felt we had determined the north–south line, we double-checked at night by finding the pole star. Another line we created was to the southeast, toward the midwinter solstice sunrise. The winter solstice sunrise, occurring during the shortest day of the year, is one of the most sacred moments of the year as it represents the slow increase in sunlit hours of the day until the summer solstice. This increase of sunlight is seen as a sign of

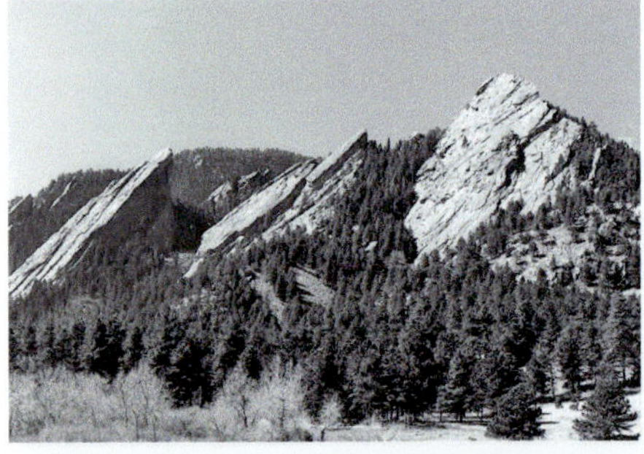
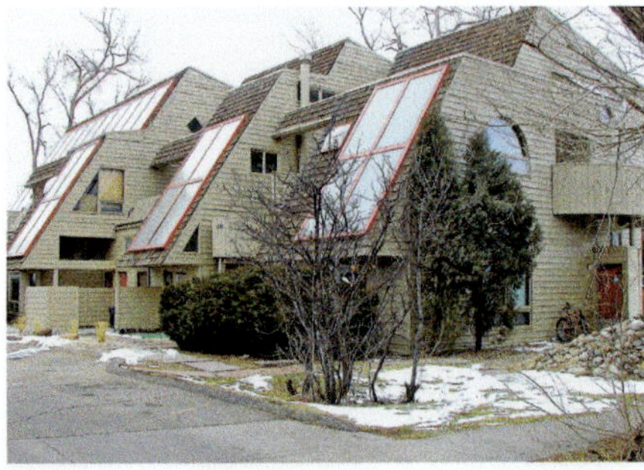
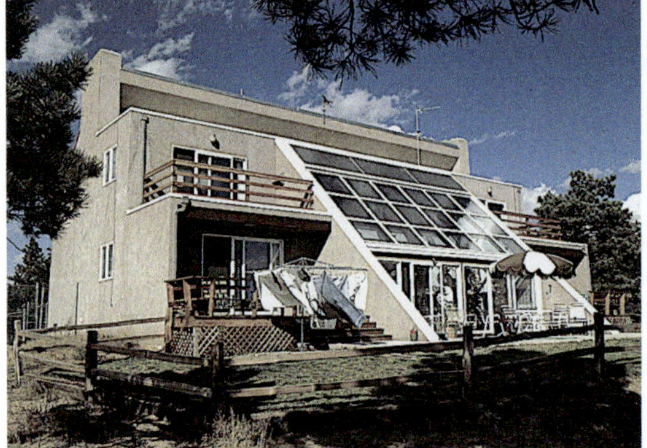
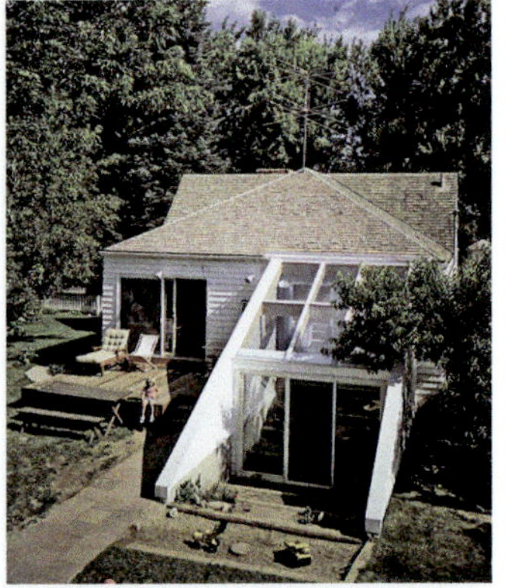
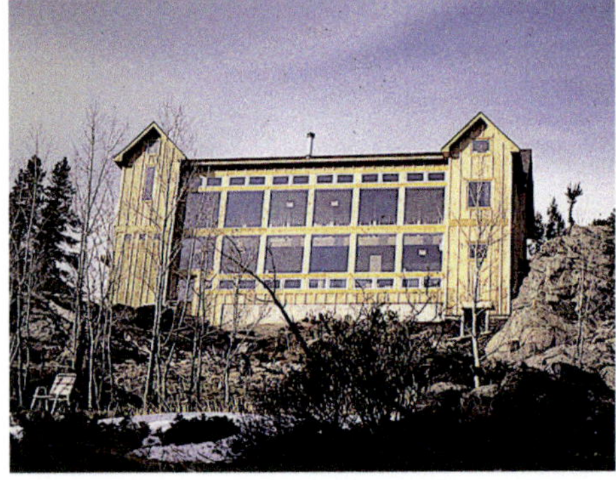
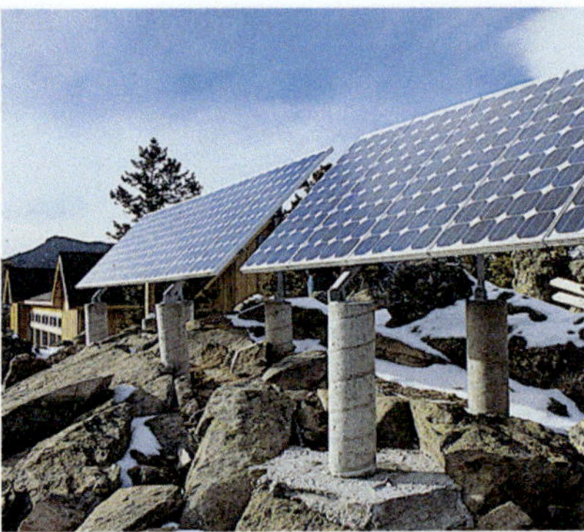

8.5
Solar Architectural Projects: (a) Boulder Flatirons, (b) Boulder Student Housing (1976), (c) Bramwell Residence (1982), (d) Tabb Boulder Sunspace (1983), (e) Overmeyer Off-Grid Residence (1997), (f) Detached Overmeyer Photovoltaic Arrays

rebirth and inner growth and as a triumph of hope over despair. In order to keep the building energetically clean, we decided to have no electricity running through the building. Since Boulder can get quite cold in winter, this meant that the building had to heat itself. This we did through the use of lots of insulation, heat mirror glazing, and passive solar heating. In addition, we included a highly efficient wood-burning stove in the north corner of the building.

Figure 8.5 shows a number of solar-oriented buildings I designed over the years, from 1976 to 1997. Figure 8.5a shows a photograph of the Boulder Flatirons that were inspiration for an active solar energy student housing project completed in Boulder in 1975 (Figure 8.5b). Designed in 1975 by my firm, Joint Venture Architects, the Student Housing project in Boulder, Colorado, addressed this issue with 70 percent of the space-heating and domestic-hot-water-heating requirements provided by the active solar system. The building responded to the systems' orientation constraints with a collector area of 700 square feet (65 square meters) and optimal tilt angle with sloping south façades. The south façade was broken up by a "pushing and pulling" of secondary forms allowing in-between spaces for stairs and balconies and allowing daylight to penetrate deep into usable spaces.

Figure 8.5c is a passive solar house completed in Florissant, Colorado, in 1982. It features a sunspace glazed with heat mirror glass and sidewalls of insulated concrete block for thermal storage. Two heat-recovery ducts collect stratified hot air and deliver it to two remote rockbeds located on the north side of the house. All of the primary living spaces have south access and, therefore, are passively solar heated. Located in south-central Colorado, the architectural language is reflective of Northern New Mexico. While teaching a course on solar energy technologies at the University of Colorado, I decided to add a sunspace to my home in Boulder. The two-story sunspace was positioned over cascading planter beds (Figure 8.5d). Within the sunspace is a heat-stratifying duct and fan delivering solar-heated air to the room below. The Overmeyer Residence has a large isolated-gain sunspace with vertical glass. The project employs a remote photovoltaic array that serves to provide electricity for the home.

In the mid- to late 1990s, the photovoltaic industry created panels that were more cost-effective and so facilitated off-grid designs. The Overmeyer Residence was my first fully off-grid design, completed in 1997. It featured a vertical, south-facing, double-glazed isolated gain sunspace and rockbed storage system (Figure 8.5e). Operable awning windows were placed at the top and bottom of the passive solar wall for natural summer ventilation. The photovoltaic array was positioned separate from the house for easy access for maintenance (Figure 8.5f).

In the early 1980s through to the sunsetting of the Windfall Profit Tax Act in 1985, credits were given to projects, and I was involved in a number of solar renovations and additions throughout Colorado. This included my own house in Boulder. Built in 1991, the Moss Residence is located high in the foothills of the Rocky Mountains, near Estes Park, Colorado. This three-bedroom home was designed for nearly 100 percent passive solar heating. This was accomplished with a super-insulated envelope, full vertical glazing on the south side with insulated shutters, and a rockbed thermal storage system. The highly insulated roof was sloped to direct the cold winter wind up and over the house. Figure 8.6a shows the south façade, with both fixed and operable windows, and Figure 8.6b shows the owner, Larry Moss, discussing the interior of that same glazing wall and the functioning of the insulating shutters. It was important to see if passive solar projects, especially in cold climates, could provide all or most of the required space heating. The Zimmerman isolated-gain sunspace addition and rockbed storage below it are shown in Figures 8.6c and 8.6d. The sunspace glass wall was positioned at the optimum tilt angle for winter solar gain. Two small passive solar greenhouse projects were also completed in the early 1980s, which included active domestic-hot-water collectors (Figures 8.6e and 8.6f). The costs for small projects like these were offset by state and federal energy tax credits, amounting to 70 percent of expenditures up to $10,000.

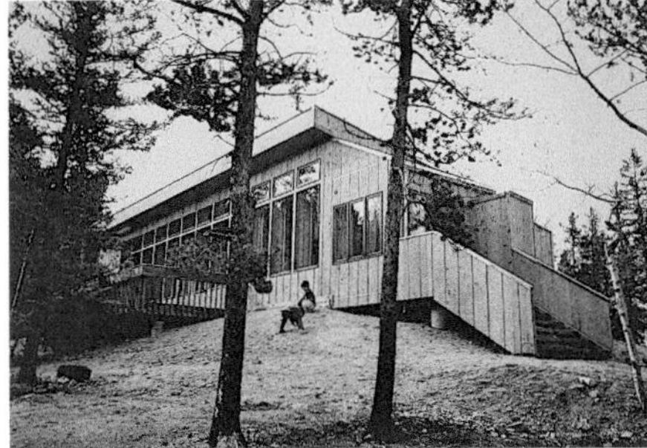

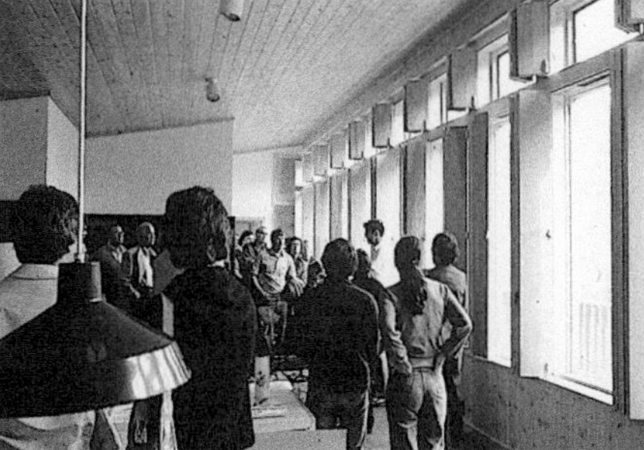

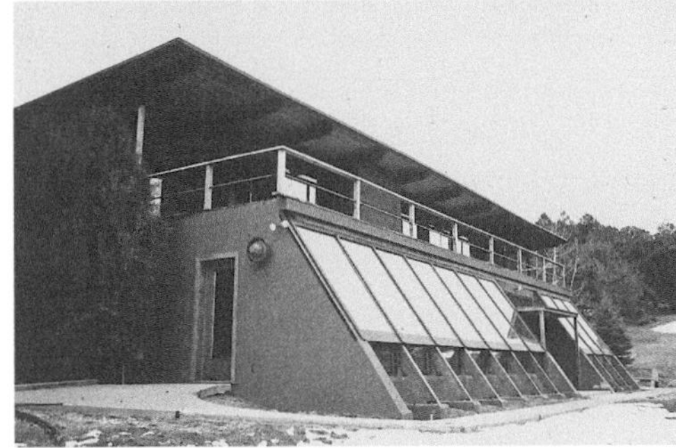

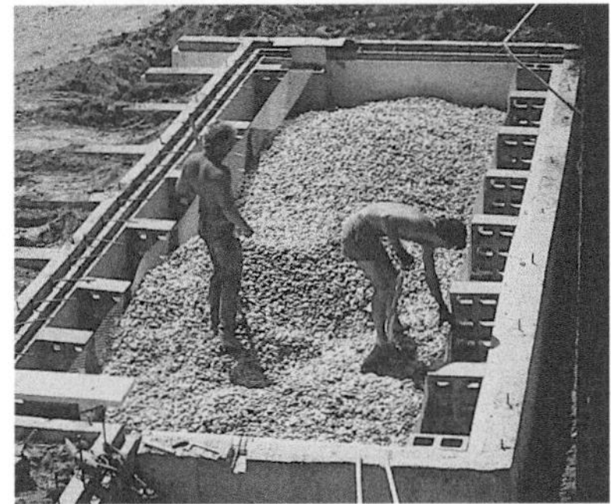

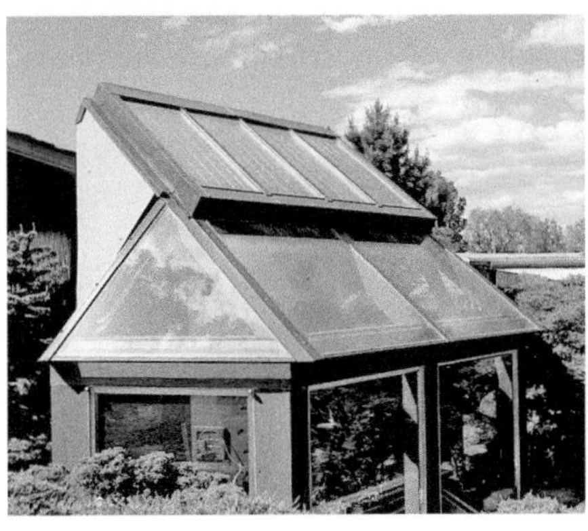

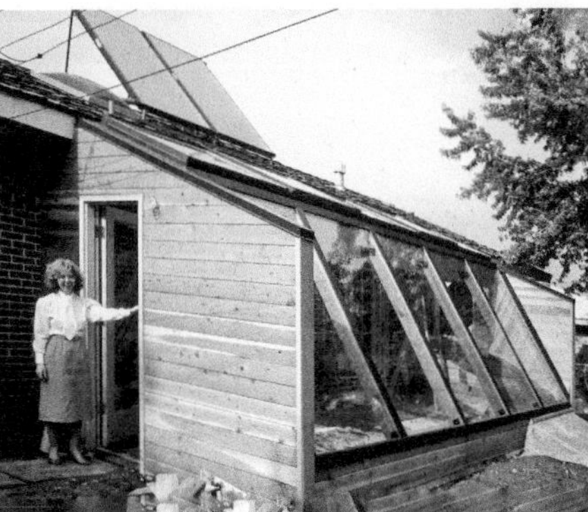

8.6
Solar Additions and Retrofits: (a) Moss Residence Exterior (1991), (b) Moss Residence Interior, (c) Zimmerman Sunspace Addition, (d) Zimmerman Rockbed Storage, (e) Johnson Detached Greenhouse (1980), (f) Attached Greenhouse Addition (1982)

The Goldman Residence is located in the foothills of the Rocky Mountains, west of Boulder, Colorado (Figures 8.7a–8.7c). It was constructed in the early 1990s. The initial analysis of the 35-acre site included a geomantic study of the Hartmann grid and positive energy paths through the land.[10] The exact site location was selected by the client. A courtyard form was preferred for the design. The building courtyard was considered the center and was surrounded by more public spaces on the south and west sides and more privates spaces on the north side. The square dwelling form is placed within a circle comprised of decks and retaining walls. The three photovoltaic collector arrays, with 40 panels, are located to the northwest of the main building, seen in the upper left of Figure 8.7b. In the center of the courtyard is a garden and flow-form water purification fountain.

In the late 1970s, our firm, Joint Venture Architects, designed for Boulder Springs a mixed-use hot-tub facility with a series of hot tubs facing an interior garden. As can be seen in the architectural model, Figure 8.7a, there are two solar

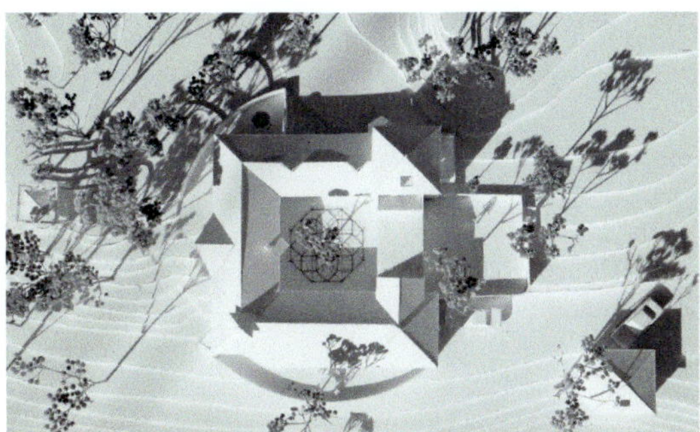

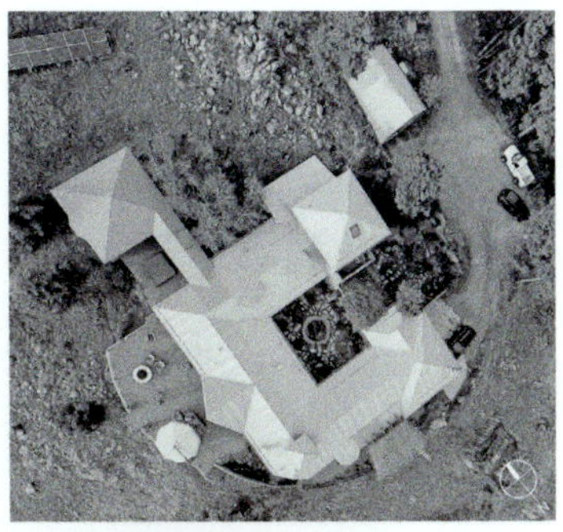

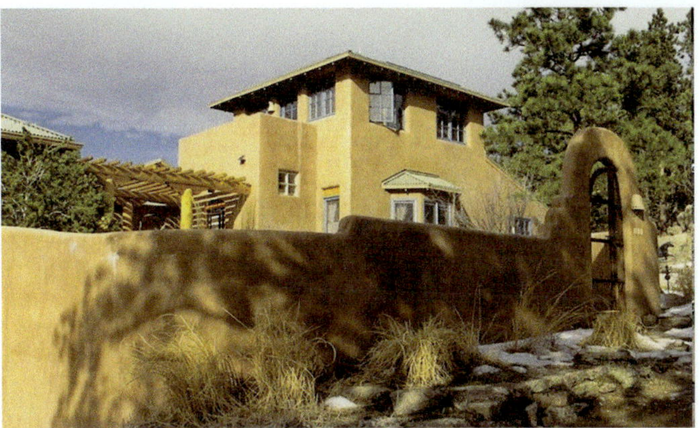

8.7 Courtyard Residence: (a) Goldman Residence Model, (b) Goldman Residence Aerial Photograph (1992), (c) Goldman Residence Ground-View Photograph

collector arrays for heating the hot-tub water. In addition, the facility has a cold plunge and men and women changing rooms. Facing south and southeast are two-story reflective bronze glass block walls. This allows natural light in while offering protection from being viewed from the outside (Figure 8.8c). The City of Boulder at that time required on-site parking, and so we included a small garage with office space above it. Boulder Springs became a "third place" for many Boulder residents during the 1980s.

Finally, in 2015, I designed my Georgia home with passive solar heating and included a large photovoltaic array on the vaulted roof and a Tesla Powerwall. Two years after the first 30 panels were installed, I added five more to make a total of 35 panels. The eight large south-facing windows and French patio doors provide passive solar heating and connect the main living spaces with the walled-in garden. As much as I wanted a solar residence, it is the play of natural sunlight throughout the seasons and day that are the most healing and spiritual. My home is further described in detail in Chapter 12.

I was aware that solar energy was effective with single buildings, especially those with what were called "skin-dominated" thermal energy interactions, mainly residential building types.[11] These are buildings that lose or gain solar energy around the envelope. In the early 1980s, I became interested in solar applications to multiple buildings and issues of solar access. In order that solar energy be utilized in a broader context, access to the sun during critical hours of the day and density were necessary for multiple buildings. I, therefore, was influenced by Ralph Knowles's work with the relationship between energy and form.[12] Knowles's work was inspiring, and he and his students at the University of Southern California were able to design city blocks with densities of up to 50 units per acre (120 units per hectare), with solar access to all the dwelling units. Solar access was primarily targeted at roofs, south walls, and south lots. Providing adequate solar access, while responding to flexible site designs for difficult and varying site conditions, was challenging while achieving higher-density developments.

In most instances, elemental architecture is phototropic, meaning that there is a formal relationship to the presence of light. The Greek *photo* means "light," and *tropos* means "a turning." Phototropic derives from the botanical world and the chemical and biological processes plants possess; it is the tendency to respond to the external stimulus of solar radiation by rearranging plant chloroplasts in order to enhance the process of photosynthesis and facilitate growth. This principle is important at the urban design scale, especially in temperate and cold climates, to ensure every building within a development or neighborhood has solar access.

With the help of my students at the University of Colorado, I focused on planning scale issues and later published my first book with McGraw-Hill, *Solar Energy Planning*.[13] We studied the limitations of solar energy utilization, which were location, diffused nature of the source, technology efficiency and design requirements, cost, and scale or density. We then looked at four different scales of application, including the single building, cluster, neighborhood, and, finally, settlements. The application of solar technologies is very achievable with single buildings and within lower densities. However, in higher densities and with larger, more complicated mixed-use buildings, such as hospitals or high-rises, achieving high solar fractions (percentage of solar utilization) is difficult. Figure 7.8d is a model showing the solar access to active and passive solar systems of two rows of apartment buildings. Figure 7.8e shows an annual shadow mask site plan positioning dwellings outside of shadows. Decoupling buildings from solar technology, as in solar farms, is gaining popularity. However, individual control of the system is lost with this approach. Remember that the source of solar energy is generally accessible, is not owned by anyone, and is healthy.

With the threat of climate change, production of greenhouse gas emissions resulting from human activity, and a growing world population, renewable energy sources are seen as one strategy to meet these problems. However, our modern, technology-driven lifestyles require vast amounts of global energy that are difficult for renewable energy sources to meet. Typically, we place faith in new innovations and technologies, such as fusion energy, to solve these problems. It seems clear that the sources of energy we use in the future will have wellness consequences. I am not convinced about the spiritual qualities of fusion energy, but I am sure about the spiritual qualities of solar energy.

Sunlight has several benefits, including photosynthesis, boosting mood, enabling better sleep, helping with vitamin D production, killing bacteria, reducing high blood pressure, increasing energy, improving melatonin production and regulating the body's circadian rhythms, reducing stress, and extending life expectancy.[14] The sun initiates both spiritual and aesthetic experiences. Overexposure to the sun,

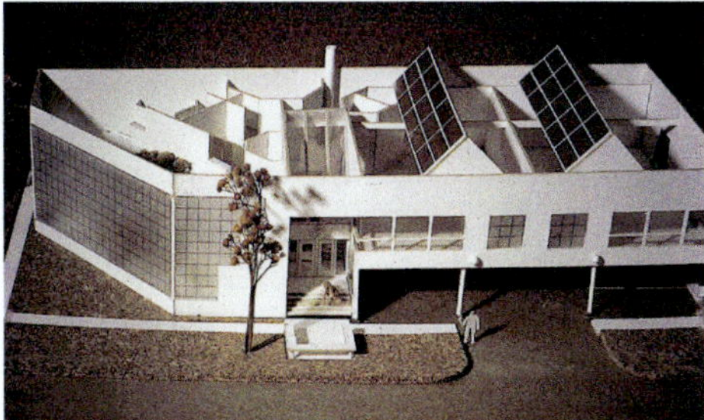

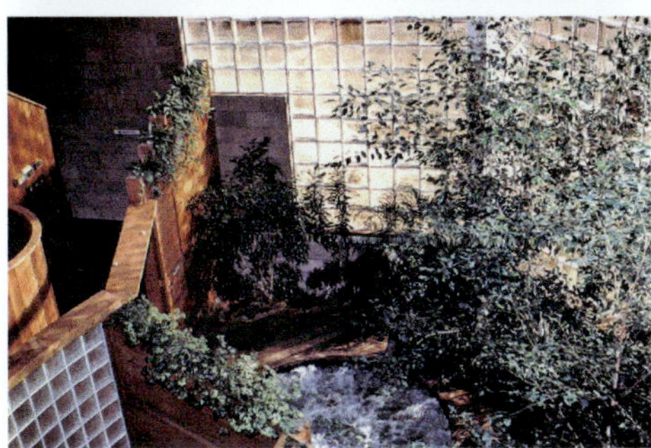

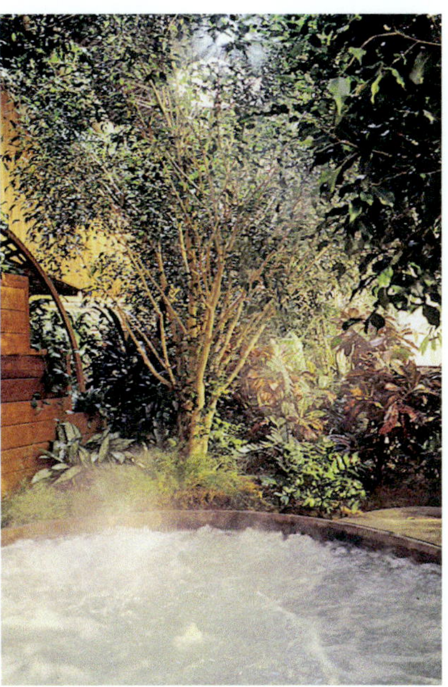

8.8
Solar Hot-Tub Garden Facility: (a) Model of Boulder Springs, Boulder, Colorado (1980), (b) HotTub, (c) Interior of Boulder Springs

conversely, can cause health problems, including too much exposure to ultraviolet radiation. A Yale University study, The Nature of Americans National Report, found that more than half of adults reported spending five hours or less in nature each week.[15] This is not good for wellness, let alone spiritual wellness. The sun and its energy have been revered as spiritual throughout our human history. Beyond the physical benefits of its light, vitamin D, energy, and warmth, the spiritual dimension offers a profound connection to nature, a sense of vitality and endurance, and radiance.

SUMMARY

Throughout the 1970s and 1980s, in my early solar energy days, I loved learning about the nature of this energy, its geometry, its thermal dynamic qualities, and the ways in which we could harness it as a source of energy that is decentralized, free, accessible to most people, and renewable. As an architect, I enjoyed the challenge of integrating the technology in functional and aesthetic ways. Despite the skepticism surrounding its use and effectiveness, I felt it was a healthy pursuit with potential spiritual benefits. Solar energy is seen as life-giving, illuminating, and transformative. Since the beginning of this century, there has been less attention given to solar energy, although, more recently, there has been renewed interest in renewable energy usage. However, I have noticed that most development projects do not incorporate solar energy technologies into their building designs. Let us not forget Apollo's fiery chariot making its way across the sky, bringing life-giving light and warmth to the planet. The significance of solar energy cannot be overstated especially as we move into climate change and post-fossil fuel eras.

■ NARRATIVE VIGNETTE 1: THE SIGNIFICANCE OF SOLAR ENERGY

Energy is produced by electricity, earth's gravity, the attraction of things to one another, the power of wind and water, or the emotional influence of solar energy. It is a kind of numinous emotion, coming from the Latin word *emotere*, meaning energy in motion and the power to sustain continuous activity. Originally from the Greek *aitherios* plus *-al*, ethereality pertains to the divine or an agency of the supernatural, considered otherworldly, pure, and perfect. In nature, ethereal experiences occur with sunrises and sunsets, night skies, rainbows, unspoiled beaches, mountaintops, waterfalls, geothermal features, and other beautiful and unusual landscapes. In buildings and urban forms, solar energy is not only essential but also functional, life-giving, healing, and beautiful. Its wellness benefits derive from its abundant light, its contribution to our food supply, its warmth, and its life-giving energy. It marks our time and seasonal cycles. The spiritual benefits are numerous. Apart from the physical, emotional, and environmental benefits, solar energy has been a symbol of great power, hope, and spiritual renewal from time immemorial. This includes its wonderful changing light qualities that occur at special times of the day and throughout the year. For me, it still has this power and meaning and is an important part of my daily life. Where the early1970s sparked a renewed interest in solar energy and its applications to buildings, it seems, unfortunately, to have lost a bit of its luster. Having said that, while it might seem like solar applications to buildings have lost momentum, the data suggest a more nuanced picture. While some sectors and regions have experienced a slowdown, the overall trend indicates continued growth in solar energy adoption for buildings.[16] With the emergence of biophilic, wellness, and spiritual trends, these interconnected concepts contribute to a growing underlying motivation for adopting solar energy in buildings.

In the future, energy is likely to come from a mix of sources, whether renewable energy, hydroelectricity, fossil fuels, hydrogen, or nuclear energy. A key issue is the centralization versus decentralization of these energy sources. These will impact future directions in the built environment. New, contemporary architectural forms, including parametric and AI-generated designs, will affect integrated building approaches. Many young architectural designers are at the forefront of the sustainable movement that will include urban designers and land and city planners. Hopefully, not only will the pragmatic and sustainable functions of solar energy be considered, but also the spiritual wellness dimension will be rekindled.

NOTES

1 Telxelra, Pedro, Spiritual Meanings of the Sun (accessed September 6, 2024), https://www.askthesoul.com/spiritual-meanings-of-the-sun/#:~:text=The%20sun%20is%20the%20most%20powerful%20source%20of,is%20also%20associated%20with%20spiritual%20awakening%20and%20enlightenment.

2 What Is Circadian Lighting? (accessed September 22, 2024), https://www.thelightingpractice.com/what-is-circadian-lighting/#:~:text=Known%20as%20circadian%20lighting%2C%20these,a%2024%2Dhour%20internal%20clock.

3 Luke, Understanding the Spiritual Meaning of Winter Solstice (accessed September 22, 2024), https://spiritualityshepherd.com/spiritual-meaning-of-winter-solstice/.

4 Yergin, Daniel, The Prize: The Epic Quest for Oil, Money & Power (accessed April 10, 2025), https://www.iwp.edu/wp-content/uploads/2020/06/The-Prize-The-Epic-Quest-for-Oil-Money-and-Power-by-Daniel-Yergin.pdf p. 615.

5 The incident angle is the angle between the incident ray (the ray of light or other wave striking the surface) and the normal. If the incident ray is itself perpendicular to the surface, it lies along the normal line. Therefore, the angle between the incident ray and the normal is zero.
6 Tabb, Phillip, *Solar Energy Planning: A Guide to Residential Development* (New York, NY: McGraw-Hill, 1984).
7 Holtz, Michael, *Solar Dwelling Design Concepts* (Washington, DC: U.S. Department of Housing and Urban Development, 1976), pp. 128–133.
8 In the late 1970s, the US Department of Housing and Urban Development and the US Department of Energy, in cooperation with the Solar Energy Research Institute, held the "First Residential Passive Solar Design Competition and Demonstration." This program recognized innovative applications of passive solar design in residential buildings. A publication detailing the award-winning projects was released in January 1979. This indicates a historical precedent for government-led initiatives in this area.
9 Tabb, Phillip, *Solar Energy Planning: A Guide to Residential Development* (New York, NY: McGraw Hill, 1984), pp. 76–77.
10 The Hartmann grid was observed by the German physician Ernest Hartmann. The invisible energetic grid has not been scientifically proven; however, there is a magnetosphere, or magnetic field, around the Earth that is measurable.
11 A skin-dominated building, also known as a skin-load-dominated building or envelope-dominated building, is a building where the energy usage for heating and cooling is primarily influenced by the transfer of heat through its external surfaces – the roof, walls, windows, and floors – owing to the impact of the outside climate.
12 Knowles, Ralph, *Sun Rhythm Form* (Cambridge, MA: MIT Press, 1981).
13 Tabb, Phillip, *Solar Energy Planning: A Guide to Residential Development* (New York, NY: McGraw-Hill, 1984).
14 Kerslake, Risa, 10 Benefits of Sunlight for Your Health (accessed July 28, 2024), https://www.singlecare.com/blog/benefits-of-sunlight/.
15 Yale School of the Environment, U.S. Study Shows Widening Disconnect with Nature, and Potential Solution (accessed July 28, 2024), https://e360.yale.edu/digest/u-s-study-shows-widening-disconnect-with-nature-and-potential-solutions?source=post_page.
16 Solar Industry Research Data (accessed April 10, 2025), https://seia.org/research-resources/solar-industry-research-data/.

9 NARRATIVE VIGNETTE 2

The Role of Sacred Geometry

INTRODUCTION

Sacred geometry is seen as one way to connect to spiritual wellness. According to dictionary definitions, sacred geometry ascribes symbolic and sacred meanings to certain geometric shapes, symmetries, and proportions. Sacred geometry organizes material, space, and nature, enabling transcendent experiences. These include awe and serene experiences, love of nature, healing, and spiritual renewal. In planning, sacred geometry is the organization of the urban fabric. It is constituted of elements according to cardinal directions, procession of streets, transects and placement of significant buildings, designs for health and wellness, and respect for and adoration of on-site natural features and processes. While, traditionally, sacred geometry has been characterized by powerful symmetries and star polygonal forms, such as castles, cathedrals, airports, sports stadiums, and even prisons, sacred geometry also can be expressed through more organic and modest nature-driven designs found in villages, cottages, healing gardens, and interior spaces. Cities, such as Paris and Washington, DC, villages such as Bourtange, in the Netherlands, hill forts, monasteries, and religious monuments such as Chartres Cathedral and Stonehenge employ sacred geometry. Historically, sacred geometry expresses through quite formal and monumental geometries, but also informs more modest, informal, organic, and domestic forms as well.

While traveling, I found a more intimate quality of sacred experience in smaller domestic buildings in Europe. While traveling in Great Britain, I often photographed rural cottages and was fascinated by the simple geometry, which I found was both beautiful and functional. Shapes and proportions were harmonious, and the design elements were highly functional, such as chimneys, dormers, window locations, cornices, string courses, and roof overhangs (Figure 9.1a). My appreciation for smaller structures was magnified when Dr. Keith Critchlow introduced me to a book titled *Buildings of the Scottish Countryside*, by Robert Naismith. In this book was a study of proportional cottage systems and cottage façades. I found interesting the fact that the builders incorporated a "self-dimensioning" system of growing the design using the square and its diagonal.[1] The overall width of the cottage was determined by identifying the desired height and then duplicating it on the ground. Then, using this self-dimensioning method, the cottage could be expanded horizontally (Figure 9.1c, adapted from Naismith). The overall shape of the cottage and the relationship between all the elements were determined by

DOI: 10.4324/9781003546085-9

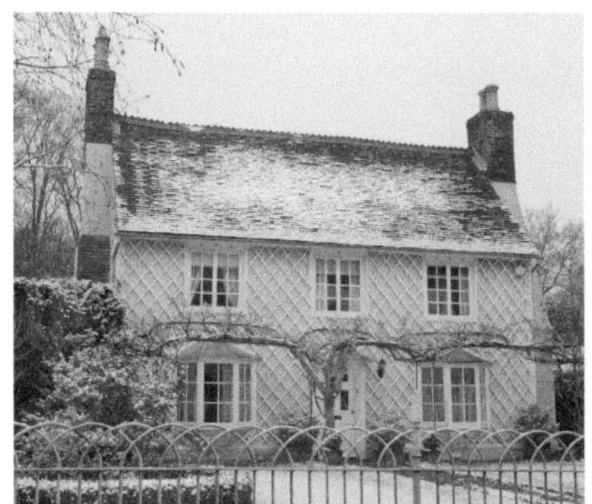

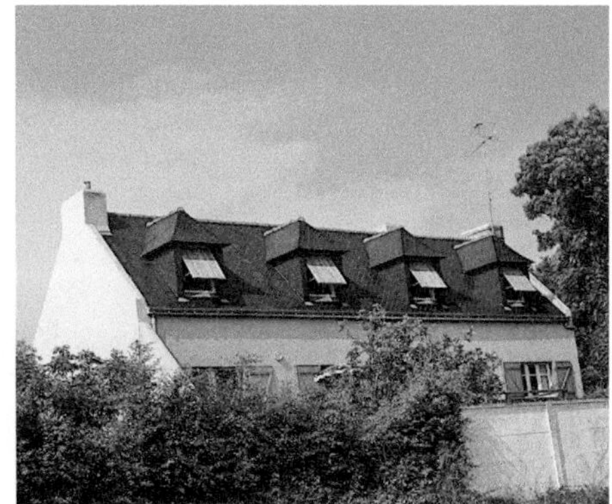

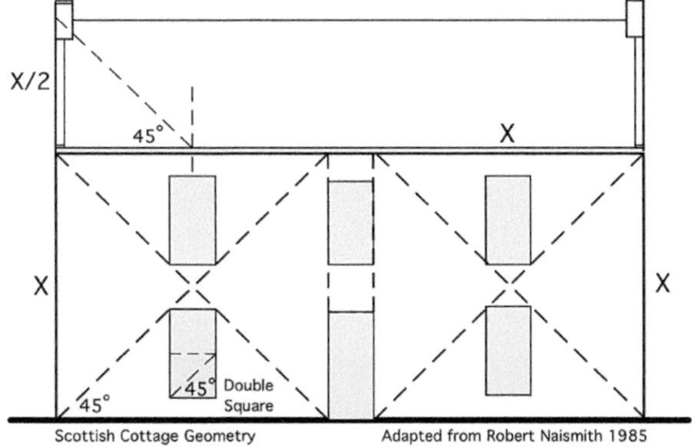

9.1 Everyday Applications: (a) Scottish Cottage, (b) Normandy Cottage, France, (c) Cottage Geometry

geometric and measurable means. Through analysis of some 1,000 photographs of Scottish cottages, Naismith was able to confirm that nearly 60 percent of the cottages conformed to this proportionality. What I loved about this example was that what we call "sacred geometry" was used in a beautiful and secular way, meaning that sacred geometry need not be overly formal and controllingly powerful. It can be domestic, soulful, and charming. I found Naismith's study interesting and, following my understanding of it, I saw rural cottages in a new way – a way in which the sacred geometry was less obvious, yet still present. Typical cottages found in Normandy and Brittany, in France, possess similar geometric principles and proportions (Figure 9.1b).

THE ROLE OF SACRED GEOMETRY

Use of sacred geometry in contemporary settings is rare, but does occur with significant and religious buildings and in small applications, such as in garden planning, meditation spaces, and even table settings. Figure 9.2a is a plan view of the space-filling street grid in the old city of Barcelona, Spain, designed by Ildefons Cerdà, showing an octagon-square grid system. The overall street system is guided by the square Cartesian grid, while the corners are organized by the octagon, creating more of a sense of place at the intersections. The perimeters of the blocks were built up and limited in height in order to preserve natural light reaching the interior courtyard of each block. This design certainly reflects the concern for public wellness and social equity. The intersection nodes create social spaces, and the grid is applied uniformly.

Designs of Islamic structures and spaces provide another interesting example of sacred geometry. In the early 1990s, my best friend, the architect Bob Armon, and I taught a series of workshops in Abiquiu, New Mexico. The workshops were in a beautiful setting within the Dar al Islam Madrassa designed by Hassan Fathy. In our research on Islamic geometry, we discovered what was called the "Foundation Orders of Islamic Patterns of Design." These "Orders" included complex star polygons, tessellations, linear repeat patterns, and arabesques. Of interest to us was the fact that these foundation orders were applied to all scales of design, from large mosques to book covers. These foundation orders could also be applied to cities, with nucleated center (complex star polygon), street and infrastructure systems (tessellations), and agriculture and natural boundaries (linear repeat pattern). Another Islamic design element was crenelation, where the tops of walls and buildings have a repeating stair-stepping or zigzag form with positive shapes echoed with negative spaces. This is a play with the earthly realm (solid) and the sacred realm (space). I experienced many crenelations with my visits to Istanbul and Cairo and felt they were a visually interesting sacred design strategy,

Also in the 1990s, I took workshops on feng shui because of the concept's relationship to building orientation and siting, spatial arrangements, and other formal characteristics. Feng shui was born out of the Chinese philosophical system and had practical applications to architecture and planning. Historically, feng shui was used to site and situate buildings in the most auspicious ways. Of importance was the orientation of rooms, the placement of furniture, and the circulation into and through the spaces. Thus, the design for a building was a terrestrial response to the context and the energetic qualities of the internal spaces and circulation through them. The purpose was to design or place the formal aspects of a building such that *chi*, or the life energy, and the health of the occupants were most achievable. To that end, in many of my architectural projects in the 1990s, clients requested a professional geomancer to identify the Hartman electromagnetic cells and grid and to locate both positive and negative fissures in the ground. A site plan documenting this information then initiated the design process. I found spending a morning pacing the site and documenting the grid a wonderful process. In fact, for me, the concept of *chi* energy within a site and designing for the most auspicious relationship to it seemed part of a spiritual wellness process.

More broadly, geometry has other uses and functions in design. It has long been used as a survival tool in defensive planning against inclement weather, predatory creatures, and military attacks. As an example, prehistoric hill forts emerged around 1100 BC and were a kind of refuge located on elevated land, giving residents a defensive advantage. Geometry was also useful in organizing religious monastic compounds, providing a safe haven, isolation, and self-sufficiency. Many cities were fortified, and even the Great Wall of China is a form of fortification. Place types that are fortified include nuclear plants, military bases, quarantine sites, central banks, prisons and jails, and gated communities. Central to fortification is the use of polygonal shapes that offer multiple defensive angles, height for perspective and prospect, and powerful gating or entry controls. In addition, geometry has been used in the adoration of special, spiritual, and religious places to enhance their transformative abilities. Geometry has been used to communicate or project a certain "form language" about the function, branding, importance, control, or status of a place or building.

Geometry is intrinsic to form language. Courtrooms, libraries, churches, and corporate headquarters are good examples where geometry helps shape images, establish hierarchies, suggest movement patterns, and encourage certain behaviors. High-rise towers fight for supremacy, identity, and national pride. If created distinctly, form languages can project a powerful brand and the values for which they stand, such as with corporate or public building types. Courtrooms in the United States generally follow form languages of colonial times, featuring an adversarial prosecutor or plaintiff versus defendants, attorneys, presiding judge, a jury of peers, court personnel, and a spectator gallery. As in these examples, the geometry follows historic forms.

Corporate headquarters, on the other hand, such as those of Apple and Google, create new forms projecting different values (Figures 9.2c and 9.2d). Apple headquarters, located in Cupertino, California, and designed by Foster + Partners, features a singular circular ringed form with plantings, including fruit trees, inside the circular form. According to Paul Goldberger, the Apple headquarters has geometric rigidity but has a serene and safe interior. It projects the values of innovation, simplicity, and sustainability with a pro-environmental emphasis. The Google

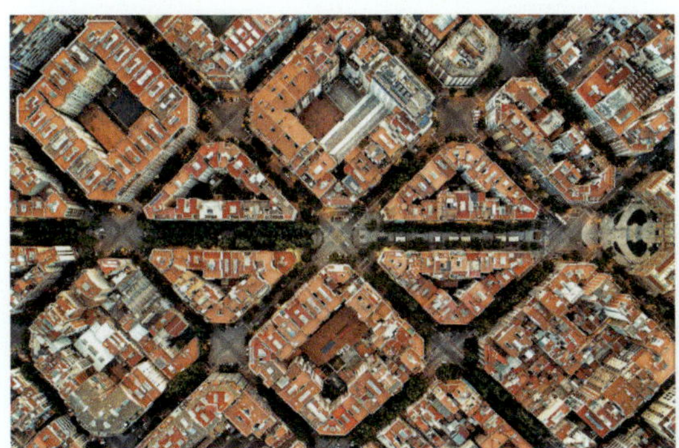
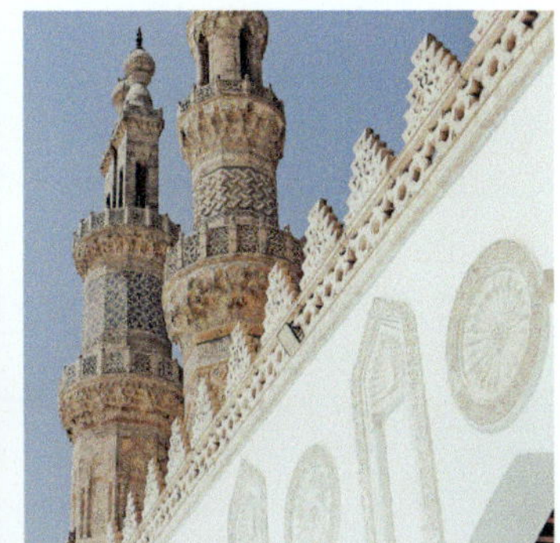
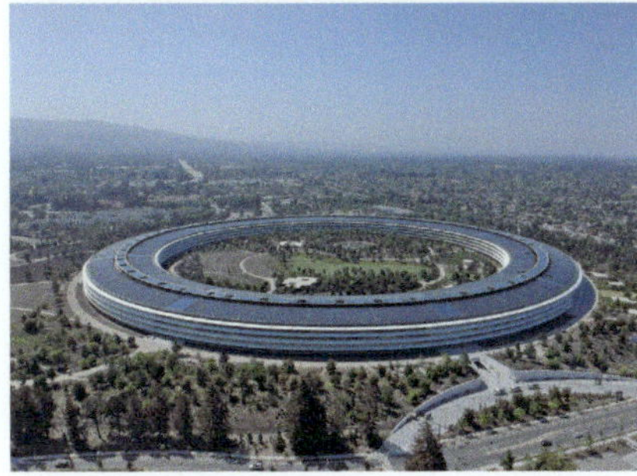
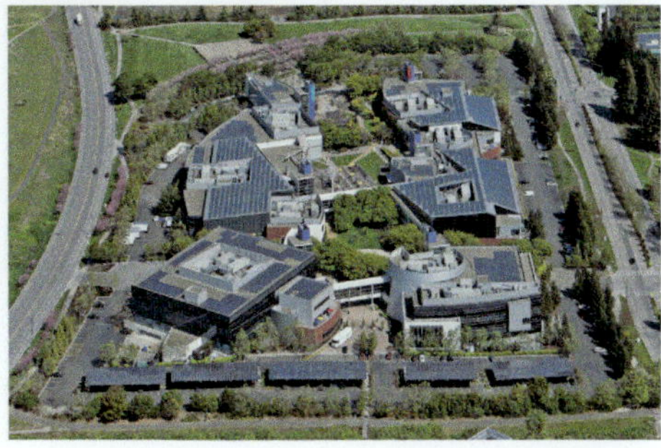

9.2 Sacred Geometry and Form Language: (a) Barcelona Streets, (b) Islamic Crenelation, (c) Apple Headquarters, California, (d) Google Headquarters, California

headquarters, located in Mountainview, California, was designed by architect Clive Wilkinson for Silicon Graphics and later acquired by Google. In Wilkinson's design, the form language is drastically different: complex, random, and colorful, with whimsical elements. It projects the values of creativity, innovation, and the priority of individuals within a vibrant company culture and with a prosocial emphasis. Both headquarter designs project a sense of unity, the former through a singular form and the latter through a connection of parts.

I became interested in geometry in my sophomore year of high school and in sacred geometry in the summer of 1984. My family and I attended the first of what later would come to be a number of workshops on sacred geometry led by Dr. Keith Critchlow, Robert Lawlor, and Rachel Fetcher. The first several workshops were conducted over a two-week period in Crestone, Colorado, located in south central Colorado. The location for the workshop was at the edge of the San Louis Valley and Sangre de Cristo Mountain Range, a powerful and incredibly beautiful site. The workshop took place at the Lindisfarne facilities on a large, wooded site. The building was designed by Californian architect Sim Van der Ryn. The workshop faculty stayed in the main house while students, including my family and me, camped nearby in teepees.

The attendees functioned as a small learning community where we shared meals, classes, walks, and evening discussions. Until the first workshop, I thought spiritual and symbolic ideas such as these were personal. After a day or so, I was blown away with the feelings that emerged and the sense that scholars and theologians have been interested, for millennia, in understanding the higher meanings and functions of something as simple as the concepts of geometry. Occurring in two parts, the workshop was organized along the classical liberal arts principles of the quadrivium.[2] The quadrivium, according to Keith Critchlow, was a curriculum focusing on number (*pure number*), geometry (*number in space*), music (*number in time*), and astronomy (*number in space and time*).[3] Mornings were filled with lectures and presentations, while afternoons were for hands-on drawing exercises. According to Robert Lawlor, one of the instructors, a diagram as simple as the *vesica pisces*, Figure 9.3a, contains profound meaning with the overlap of the solar (universal truths) and lunar (mutable or changeable) principles.[4] The vesica pisces is created by the overlap of these two circles (mediation principle). Nigel Pennick identifies proportion and commensurability as two fundamental factors that create sacred architecture.[5] The vesica, or vessel, in the center of the diagram mediates between these differences. Born from the vesica pisces were philosophical principles, the construction of what was called transcendental geometric proportions with pi, $\sqrt{2}$, $\sqrt{3}$, and golden mean geometry $(\sqrt{5}+1)/2$, and the unfolding of the first primary polygons (Figures 9.3b and 9.3c). These root numbers generate non-repeating decimals and were considered windows into the immeasurable or unknown realms. In addition, they create geometries that inform sacred proportional designs.

The first numbers – 1, 2, 3, 4, and 5 – represent distinct qualities, principles, and symbolic meanings. Relatedly, numbers can inform the dimensions of geometry, from a point to a volume, and the first principles.[6] Sacred numbers can help

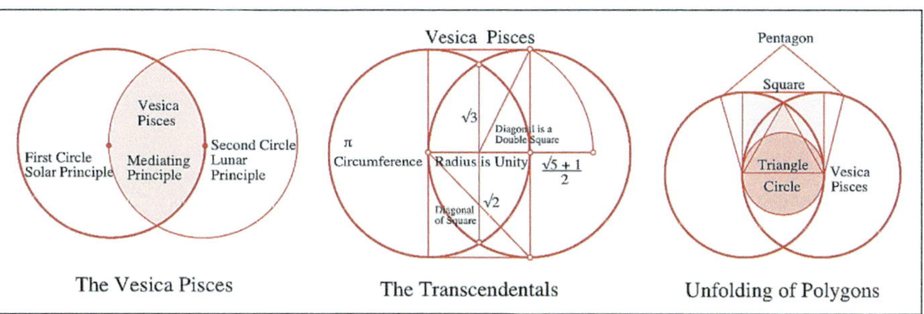

9.3 Sacred Geometry: (a) Vesica Pisces, (b) the Transcendentals, (c) Unfolding Polygons

deepen your spiritual connections, they can enhance self-awareness, contribute to higher levels of inclusiveness, and promote healing. According to Robert Lawlor, the goal of sacred geometry is to lead the mind back to a sense of "oneness" through a succession of proportional relationships.[7] The significant numbers and first principles are further explained as follows:

- **One** – unity principle, onefold-ness, unity, monad, the point/circle, and pi.
- **Two** – generative principle, twofold-ness, duality, dyad, the line, and √2.
- **Three** – formative principle, threefold-ness, triad and the plane, and √3.
- **Four** – corporeal principle, fourfold-ness, tetrad, and the volumetric world.
- **Five** – regenerative principle, fivefold-ness, pentad, sustenance and enhancement, and phi ((√5+1)/2).

First principles, according to Plato, were manifestations of goodness (*commodity*), truth (*firmness*), and beauty (*delight*).[8] According to Robert Lawlor, in architecture, the first principles are realized through the unity, generative, formative, corporeal, and regenerative principles or processes.[9] Robin Waterfield, in *The Theology of Arithmetic*, explained that numbers are divine principles and, by extension, are allegorical, with inspirational powers.[10] Numbers can be viewed as rather static quantitative measures, but they can be seen as the dynamic embodiment of certain principles and processes. For example, the number one represents oneness (unity), two is duality (dark/light), three is stability and prudence (spirit, form, and matter), four is physical materiality and the four corners of the Earth (east, south, west, and north), and five is transformative (human proportion and DNA). These numbers, geometries, and forms are not intended exclusively for religious applications because they can be employed for any building or use. The proportional systems have been used over millennia and embodied in such works of architecture as the Great Pyramids, the Parthenon, as well as the United Nations Building by Le Corbusier and Farnsworth House by Mies van der Rohe. Sacred geometry, with its inherent mathematical harmony and recurring patterns found in nature, can create a subtle resonance within our bodies, mirroring the underlying order fostering a sense of well-being and connection.

Sacred geometry is commonly found in nature, from atoms and cells to planets and galaxies, as seen in Figure 9.4. The recurring appearance of significant numbers and geometric shapes such as spirals, fractals, and Platonic solids suggests a

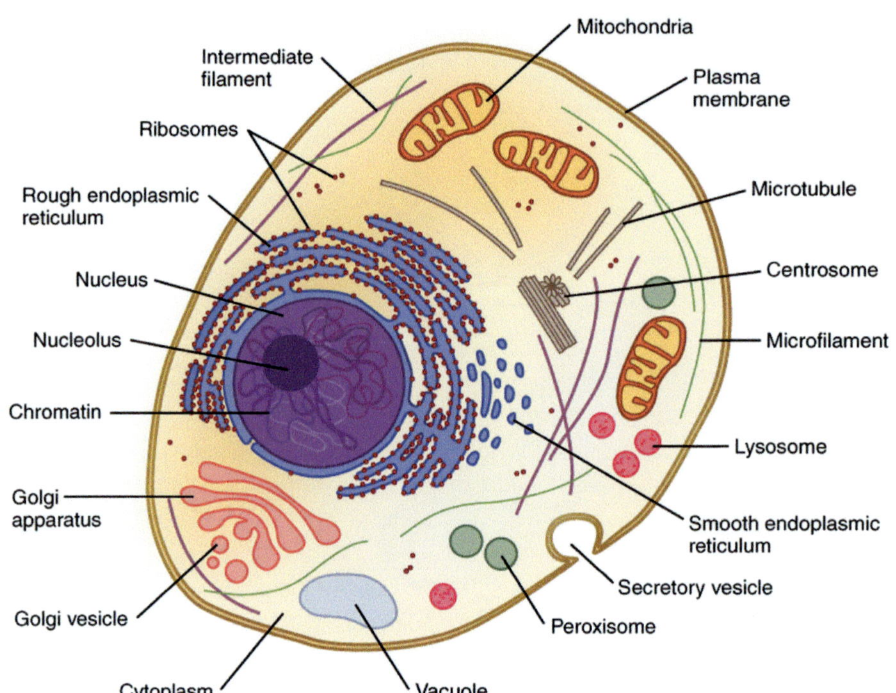

9.4
Sacred Geometry in Nature: (a) Animal Cell, (b) Snowflake, (c) Tree Branching, (d) Flower/Spider Geometry, (e) Moon Spherical Geometry, (f) Galaxy Spiral Geometry

fundamental, underlying order to the universe. This can be seen as evidence of a deeper, universal set of principles, perhaps even divine designs. The inherent beauty and complexity of these patterns in nature are undeniable. The magnitude of scale is clearly explained in Charles and Ray Eames's film *Power of Ten* (1977 version).[11] This journey beyond ourselves into the expanse of our world inspires awe and wonder, and what is remarkable is the interconnectedness that occurs at every scale. It is no wonder that biomimicry is an emerging and compelling design strategy.

After moving to London in 1986, I had the rare opportunity to be working with Dr. Critchlow in his Kairos School of Sacred Architecture and with the Krishnamurti Study Centre in Brockwood Park, Hampshire (Figures 9.5a and 9.5c). Critchlow was the architect for the new building. Jiddu Krishnamurti was an Indian philosopher, author, and spiritual figure.[12] He emphasized continuous inquiry, awareness of the present, and freedom from religious and spiritual authorities (including himself). From my readings of his work, I recall that each of us is responsible for our own spiritual development and life. According to Critchlow, the initial goals for the center were to create an atmosphere, quality, and permanence, and, for Krishnamurti, there was a desire for a space dedicated to quiet contemplation and continuous movement of learning.[13] Opened in 1987, the center is a quiet retreat designed for adults to explore the work of Krishnamurti and its relevance to their lives. The center's accommodation consists of 20 en-suite rooms and two flats, with a library, sitting room, conservatory, video rooms, dining room, courtyard, and unique quiet room. As a spiritual wellness facility, it has many characteristics that contribute to its

9.4
(Continued)

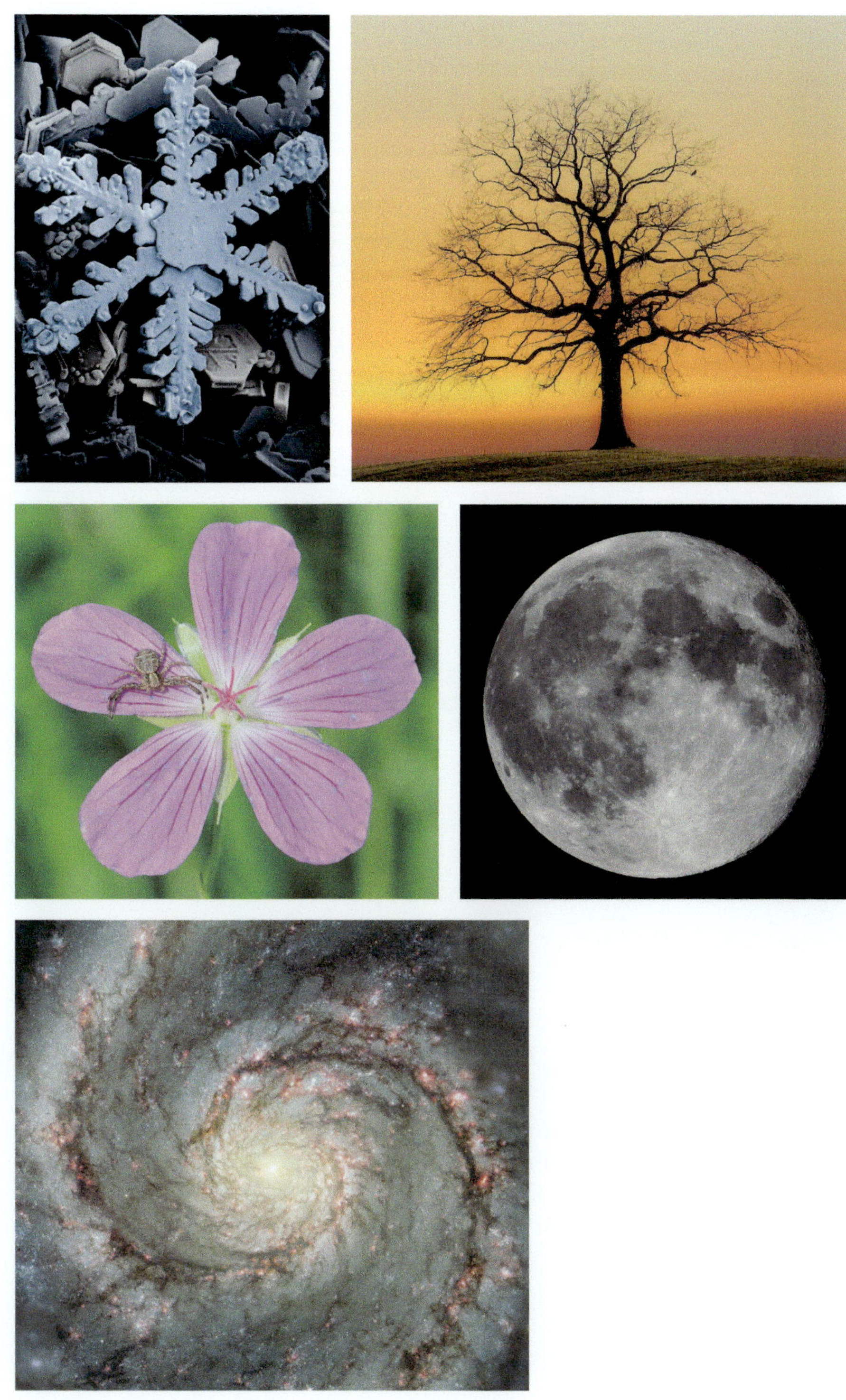

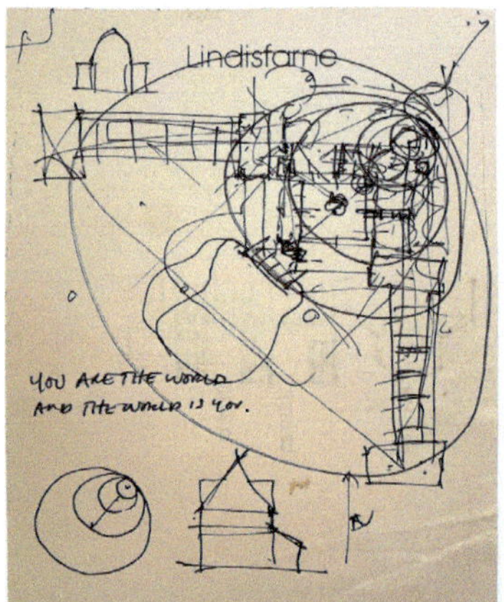

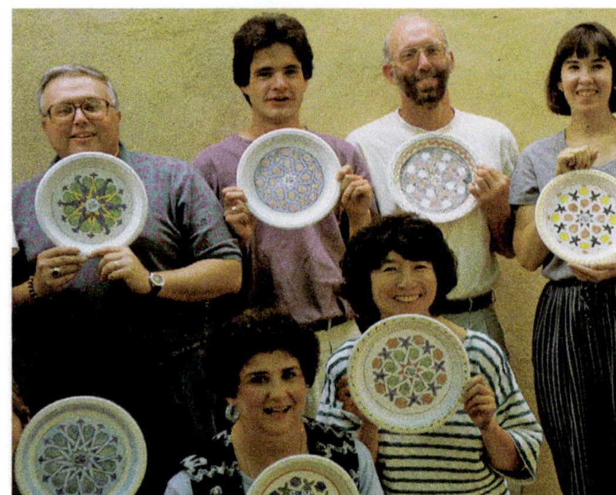

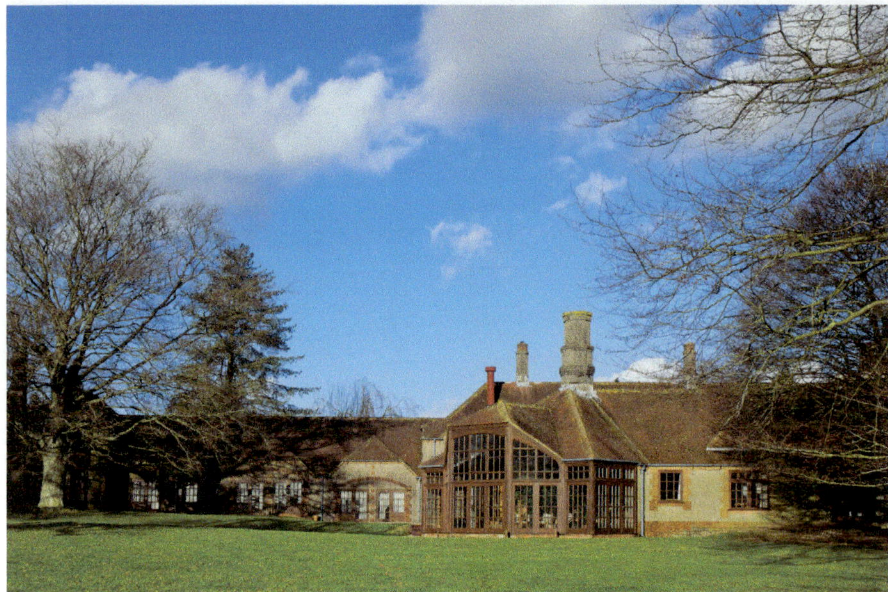

9.5
Sacred Geometry: (a) Sketch by Dr. Keith Critchlow, (b) Dar al Islam Workshop, (c) Krishnamurti Study Centre Exterior, Brockwood Park, United Kingdom

spiritual wellness, including significant geometry, connection to nature, and a contemplative and meditative space (Figure 9.5b). The design "unfolds" from the quiet meditation room at the head, expanding into the other adjacent spaces that form a central courtyard and then outward into the landscape with bedrooms. There was the design intention to create a sense of harmony with a connection to the human form (the plan). For me, it was an extraordinary experience to work on this very special project with Dr. Critchlow in an office a block away from Westminster Abbey.

My personal interest in sacred geometry became a professional interest. Following the work with Dr. Critchlow, architect Robert Armon and I facilitated a series of workshops in the mid-1990s on Islamic sacred geometry at the Dar al Islam mosque and madrassa in Abiquiu, New Mexico. The two-day workshops were directed at American high school teachers of social studies, history, and fine art and focused on the foundations of Islamic geometry. The students were taught the underlying principles of sacred geometry and then were given drawing exercises.

My first opportunity to apply sacred geometry to an architectural project occurred in the late 1980s in Boulder, Colorado. It was the design of a small art therapy studio and one-bedroom apartment. The owner envisioned something more than a studio. She also wanted a place for working with music, painting, and engaging in healing activities. The site was located along the very western border of Boulder, next to the open space at the base of the Rocky Mountain foothills. The original inspiration was given by a friend of the client, Roger Burrows, in the form of an old eight-sided stone building in England. Since the buildable area of the site was very small (25 by 40 feet), it required a two-story structure. I placed the studio on the upper floor and the apartment on the lower. A sunspace stairway connected the two floors. While the plan was organized as an octagon, I proportioned the section and elevations with golden mean geometry. The studio was capped by a curved, eight-sided dome on the interior and a copper roof on the exterior (Figure 9.6b).

My second opportunity to apply sacred geometry occurred in the early 1990s for a client who wanted a special community-oriented structure located on a 105-acre (6-hectare) mountain site north of Boulder, Colorado. In Chapter 8, I wrote about the StarHouse and its solar energy implications. It is a non-toxic, sustainable building based upon sacred and astronomical geometrical principles. It was intended as a multicultural setting for ceremonial practices, especially celestial moments related to the changing of the seasons. The design for the StarHouse was based on the Native American Drum Dance Lodge, an open ceremonial structure widely used across the Great Plains.[14] The circular or 12-sided geometric perimeter signified the universe; in its center was a large drum placed in the earthen floor, representing the underworld, and above, in the ceiling, was a four-sided cupola for the sky world. The geometry for the StarHouse derives from a 12-sided circle and the vesica pisces (the overlapping of two identical circles), as seen in Figure 9.7. A double square crosses through the 12-sided geometry, defining eight of the 12 sides and the cupola above and kiva-like storage space below. The diagonals of the crossing complete the geometry with 12 equal sides. Two circles define the perimeter of the space. The first circle defines the exterior wall, while the inner circle defines the post locations. The owner requested that he be able to sit and experience the geometry rather than it be locked within the walls, hence the double-circumferential geometry.

To this day, the building is used for meditation, dance, music, theater, weddings, lectures, courses, workshops, seasonal ceremonies, and celebrations. In addition, the site has other sacred amenities surrounding it, including a standing stone, a labyrinth, an outdoor meditation grove, a meditation dodecahedron, a year-around well, and a land-art tetractys. The combination of the Native American symbolism and celestial orientation of the theosophical teachings led to the design for the StarHouse and use of the building as a sanctuary and All Seasons Chalice. Overall, the plan is an overlap of four-sided geometry (representing Earth) and 12-sided geometry (representing Heaven).

The third project was completed in 1995 for the Tashi Gomang Stupa in Crestone, Colorado. I was given an elevation of the stupa on graph paper by a Buddhist bhante. I was commissioned to determine the exact height of the stupa, oversee structural engineering, and prepare the construction drawings. Because the soil was so sandy (near the Sand Dunes National Park), the stupa was constructed upon a reinforced concrete table foundation. At 40-feet tall, the stupa was too small for humans to enter; however, within it were placed special objects and offerings. The stupa commemorates the 16th Karmapa, Rangjung Dorje. The stupa is known as "Stupa of Many Auspicious Doors" (Figure 9.6a). For me, it was a special project and serves as a beacon overlooking the beautiful San Louis Valley.

While integrating sacred geometry was interesting, more importantly I discovered the usefulness of the concept of "maintaining the golden thread," taught by Dr. Critchlow. The *golden thread* is a continuous guiding, remembering, and reinforcing of the intentions and purpose for which a building is constructed.[15] Throughout the initial conception, design process, construction, consecration, and use, the sacred intentions are remembered. With the StarHouse, the concept of a sacred meeting place, celestial orientation, use of non-toxic materials, and conscious building practices were maintained throughout the entire process. The intentional thread was reinforced with celebrations at the site ceremony midway in the erection of the structure; with what we called the "beam walk," where the owner,

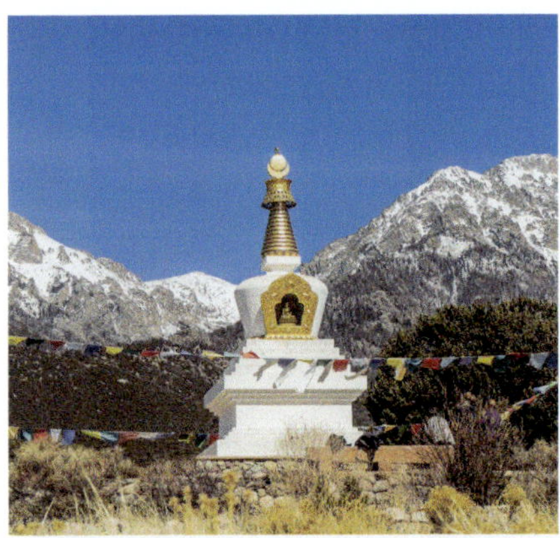

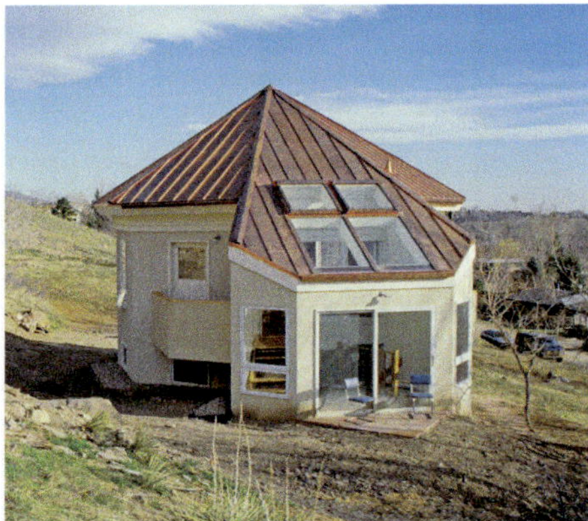

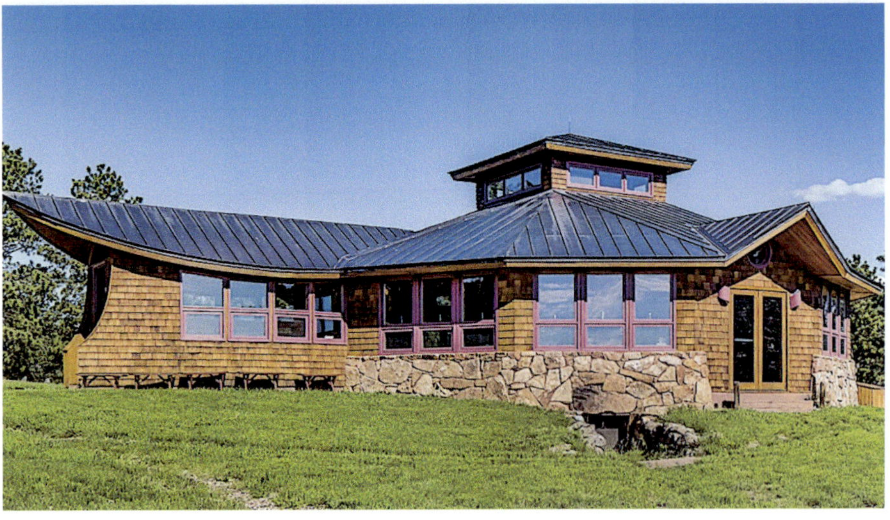

9.6
Sacred Architecture Projects: (a) Tashi Gomang Stupa (1995), (b) Stetson Art Therapy Studio, Boulder, Colorado (1988), (c) the StarHouse Exterior, Boulder, Colorado (1991)

designers, and builders all climbed on top of the beams and walked the full circle; and, finally, at the consecration of the completed project. The logs for the structural posts were selected from trees growing on the site and were chosen for their position around the 12-sided plan. Each morning, before work began, there was a brief, quiet meditation. The owners insisted on a clean construction site throughout the building process. For them, the cleaning of the site each late afternoon was one way of honoring and remembering of the sacred intentions of the project.

Figure 9.6c is a view of the StarHouse from the southwest showing the entrance vesica, cupola, and copper roof. Surrounding the building are standing stones marking certain sun angles throughout the year. The StarHouse is a good example of a thin place because of its intention, design, construction process, and function. According to the StarHouse website, "It is a space that is both incredibly alive and yet peacefully still."[16] The building was designed with non-toxic materials, typically wood from the site, stone, and a copper roof. And it is considered off-grid except for one duplex outlet connected to a nearby generator. The StarHouse is seen as an energetic field for refuge and appreciation of the changing seasons. The interior can accommodate 179 occupants.

The geometry for the StarHouse derived from the vesica pisces (the overlapping of two identical circles). Within the almond-shaped vesica pisces is a double circle that is divided into 12 segments and defined by 12 posts. The southern entrance and passage space are also defined by a vesica shape. The outer circle, with a 40-foot (12-meter) diameter, defines the exterior façade or skin of the building, while the inner circle defines the exposed structural posts and surrounding benches (Figure 9.7). Its axis is aligned with the North Star, and it is perfectly oriented to the four directions. The winter solstice sunrise occurs southeast of the center. The lack of electrical currents running throughout the structure allows it to be less artificially charged and more "energetically clean."

In the workshops I attended and taught on sacred geometry, I found it interesting to see some students gravitate to certain golden mean geometry and biomimicry-like geometric forms. For example, they would design a residence using the nautilus shell form. I found this to be an appropriation, rather than a naturally occurring process, and an inappropriate use of sacred geometry. The nautilus shell is the result of a naturally occurring internal chamber growth over time. The nautilus is born with four chambers in the shell which can grow to as many as 30. Although an interesting design phenomenon, the nautilus shell does not necessarily relate to the functional and spatial requirements of a human home. Another common appropriation of sacred geometry is the star polygonal or circular geometry for many secular situations. The powerful quality of focus on the center renders this form useful in certain circumstances, as in religious, performance, ceremonial, and centrally focused building types. Since this form of growth is natural for the nautilus, it is a difficult form to appropriate in domestic buildings, multiple buildings, and with urban fabrics. Therefore, care should be taken when considering specific sacred geometries and biomimicking approaches.

In the early 2000s, I was commissioned to design a masterplan for the Serenbe Community located in Georgia. The client was interested in an environmentally oriented design that incorporated a strong sense of community, connections to the

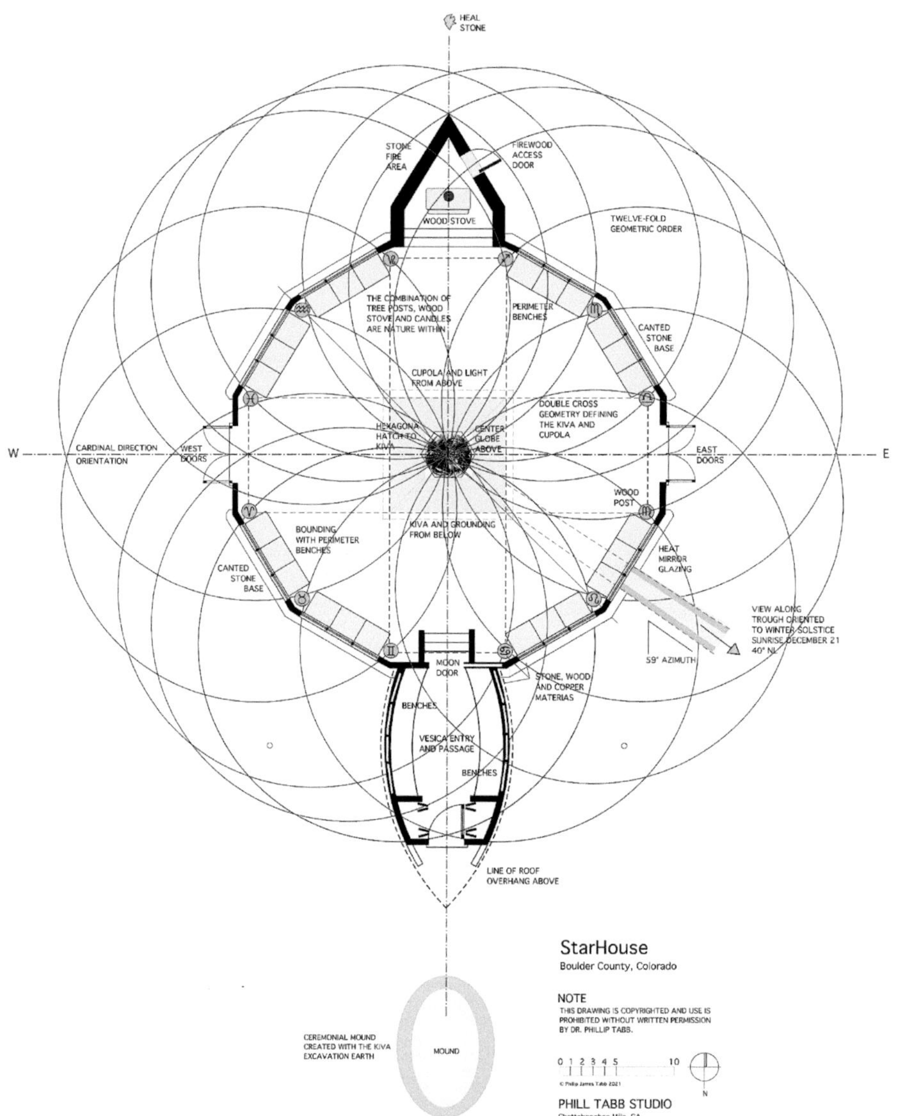

9.7
The StarHouse Geometry and Plan

land, and sacred geometry. This gave me the opportunity to come up with a land-based concept that achieved both connections to nature and to creating community. The solution was a network or constellation of omega-shaped neighborhoods. Selborne, pictured in Figures 9.8a and 9.8b, was the first to be constructed utilizing the omega form. Planned for the center of the omega was an open-ended part, and at the apex was a public "outdoor room" that served as a weekly artists' and farmers' market for the community. The conceptual geometry and shape grammar of the omega form are described in Figure 9.8c with its concentration at the apex and openness at the southern end. The omega form is not a circle or a U-shape but rather an open shape, "Ω." While the omega symbolizes the end of things or events from alpha to omega, it also is considered as a positive through its evolving rebirth.[17]

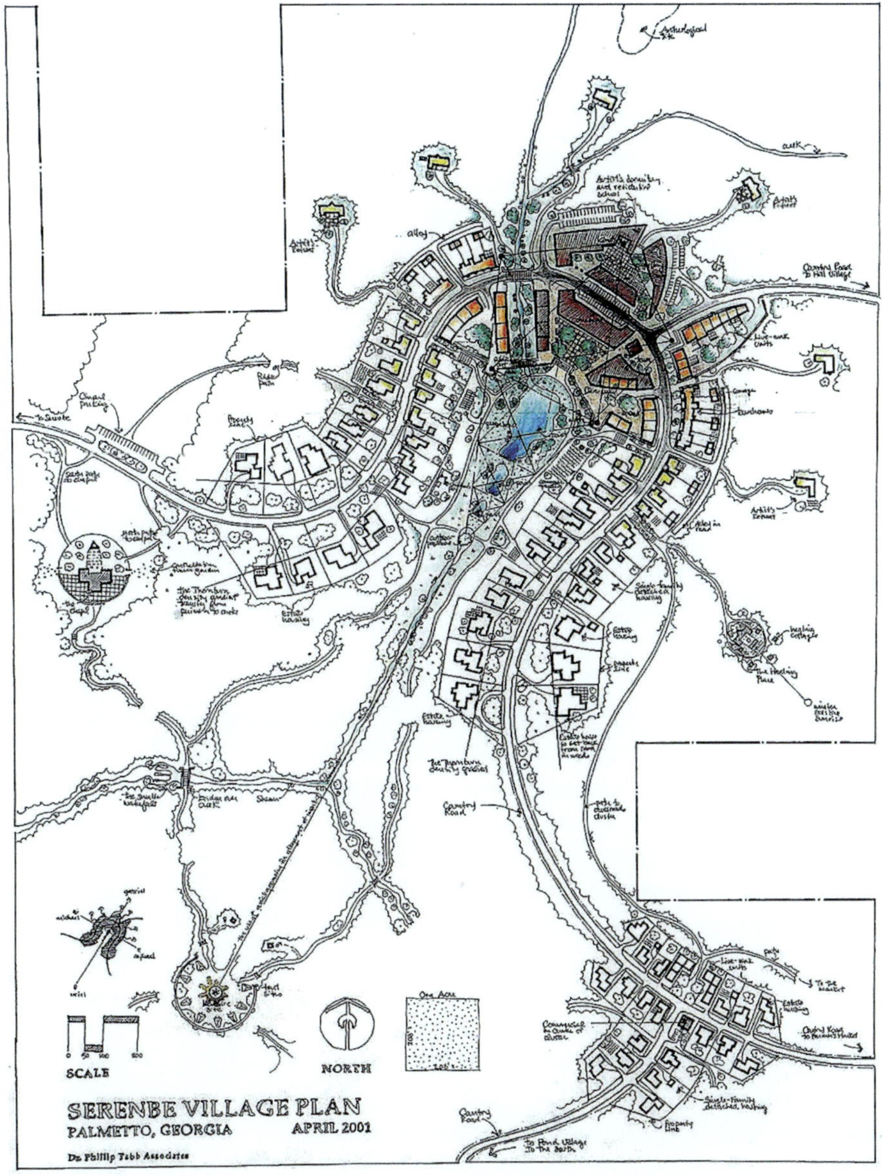

9.8
Planning Scale Geometry: (a) Selborne Concept Plan (2001), (b) Selborne Neighborhood, (c) Shape Grammar, (d) Grange Neighborhood, (e) Mado Neighborhood, (f) Site Plan, Powder Mountain, Utah (2012), (g) Site Plan, Powder Mountain, Utah

As illustrated in Figures 9.8b, 9.8d, and 9.8e, the centers of the omegas are a tributary in Selborne, a tributary and lake in Grange, and a stormwater catchment in Mado. The sacred wellness geometric strategies are more subtle, organic, site-responsive, and place-bound. The shape grammar of the omega form, with its inherent open-endedness and potential for iterative development, offers a valuable framework in planning by allowing for flexible adaptation to the site, exploration of diverse spatial configurations, and the generation of innovative programming that can evolve through time. The omegas also occur through the neighborhood land-use programming and planning, and through the different communities' amenities

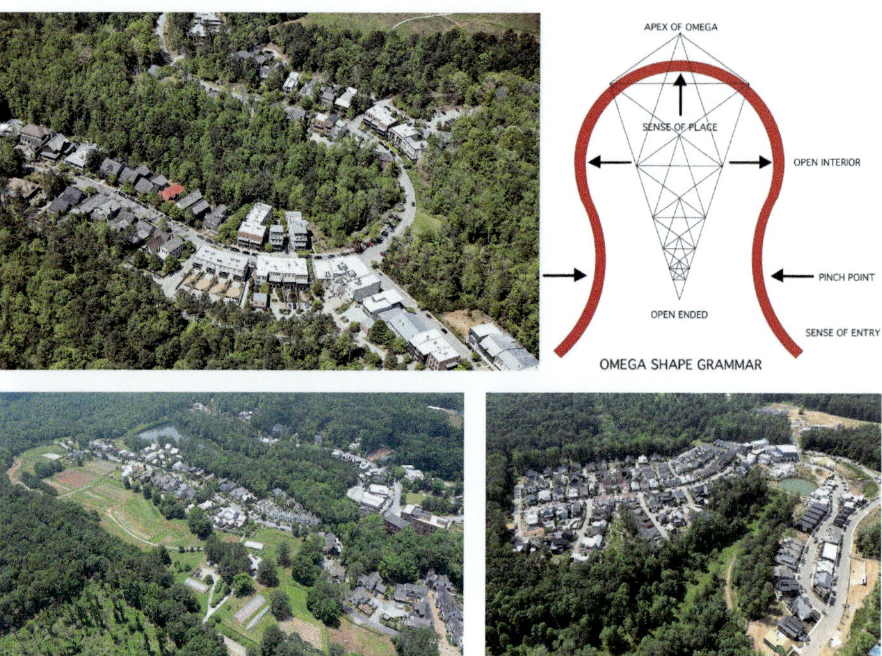

9.8 (Continued)

provided in each neighborhood. The role of sacred geometry embodied in the omega shape gives form to a powerful and identifiable shape that organizes building plots with continuously varying perspectives as you move through the community. Because of the strength of this geometry, it allows for a variety of building forms, types, and architectural languages and contributes to an overall unity of place. There is a play between the formal geometry of the omega and the informal quality of the varied architectural responses.

Another example of the use of sacred geometry at the planning scale is the village plan for the Summit Series Powder Mountain in Utah. The design was the result of a charrette organized in Summit Series Saddle Village, led by Summit Series and with invited professionals nationwide. The charrette was conducted in Eden, Utah, adjacent to the mountain site, on May 12–16, 2012. The result is a dynamic plan that features the Summit Series activities at the center and is supported by seasonal residents. A ski line runs down the center of the village form providing opportunities for residents to ski down to the lift that delivers them to the village center. The purpose of Summit Series is to bring together a community of diverse planetary thought leaders and global makers in a place of beauty to share ideas and experiences. Further, it was intended to create a world-class ski resort. Spiritual wellness is embedded in the spirit of this place. Figures 9.8f and 9.8g show the masterplan I developed in 2012. While the design evolved through many transformations, core ideas still remain.

SUMMARY

Geometry helps organize and enhance spiritual and religious experiences. As an architect, I was initially drawn to the fantastic Gothic and Baroque cathedrals such as

9.8
(Continued)

SADDLE VILLAGE
The Saddle Village is located on the ridge and crossroads and represents the Phase 1a and Phase 1b of the program. It includes the Founder's lots, estate lots, one-half and one-quarter lots, more compact Nest-like dwellings, townhomes, a Condo-hotel and Inn. This phase is planned for approximately 250 dwellings and space available in the hotel and inn. The double circle represents a five-minute walking distance to the center and outer edge of the Village Center. The "north wing" is oriented to less permanent residents and visitors, while the "south wing" is oriented to permanent reisdents and the funders.
VILLAGE CENTER
The Saddle Village center is organized by the circle and the square along the cardinal directions. To the north are the Condo-Hotel and Micro-Conferencing Center, to the east are the Summit Series functions (including large dining area, great flexible hall, offices and other support functions), to the south is a facility housing Activities that support the Summit Community, including sound studio, music and bar, game rooms, lounges, and to the west is the ski lodge with attendent functions, such as ski rentals, ski school, etc. The Center circle has a public outdoor plaza which can be covered in the summer with a flexible tent structure. On the west end of the plaza is a circling bridge for group sunset watching. All buildings are connected on the second floor for winter access.
SKIING
This ski lift is designed to provide beginner's skiing and a ski-in and ski-out opportunity for those wanting to ski the slopes or to ski to the Village Center.
1-acre founder's lots
bridge
entrance road
1 acre estate lot
1-acre estate lots
visiting community
parking overflow
parking
large group amphitheater
special place
nest
ski lift
future expansion
hot tubs
hotel
conf
ski lodge
center
plaza
summit
activities
planetarium
morning sun yoga platform
W
E
N
S
group yurt
grocery
recreation
soccer
library in woods
cogeneration
can be 1-acre founder's lots
founder's cafe
photovoltaic farm
PV expansion
greenhouse
community gardens
permanent community
1-acre estate lot
3-5 acre ranchette
shared barn
3-5 acre ranchette
bridle trail
FOUNDER'S CAFE
The founder's cafe and bar is planned to provide a place for more private gathering as well as an entrance to Narnia Park.
june 21, 2012
PHASE 1a and 1b
acre
SUMMIT SADDLE VILLAGE
Eden, Utah
Dr. Phillip Tabb Consultant
College Station, Texas

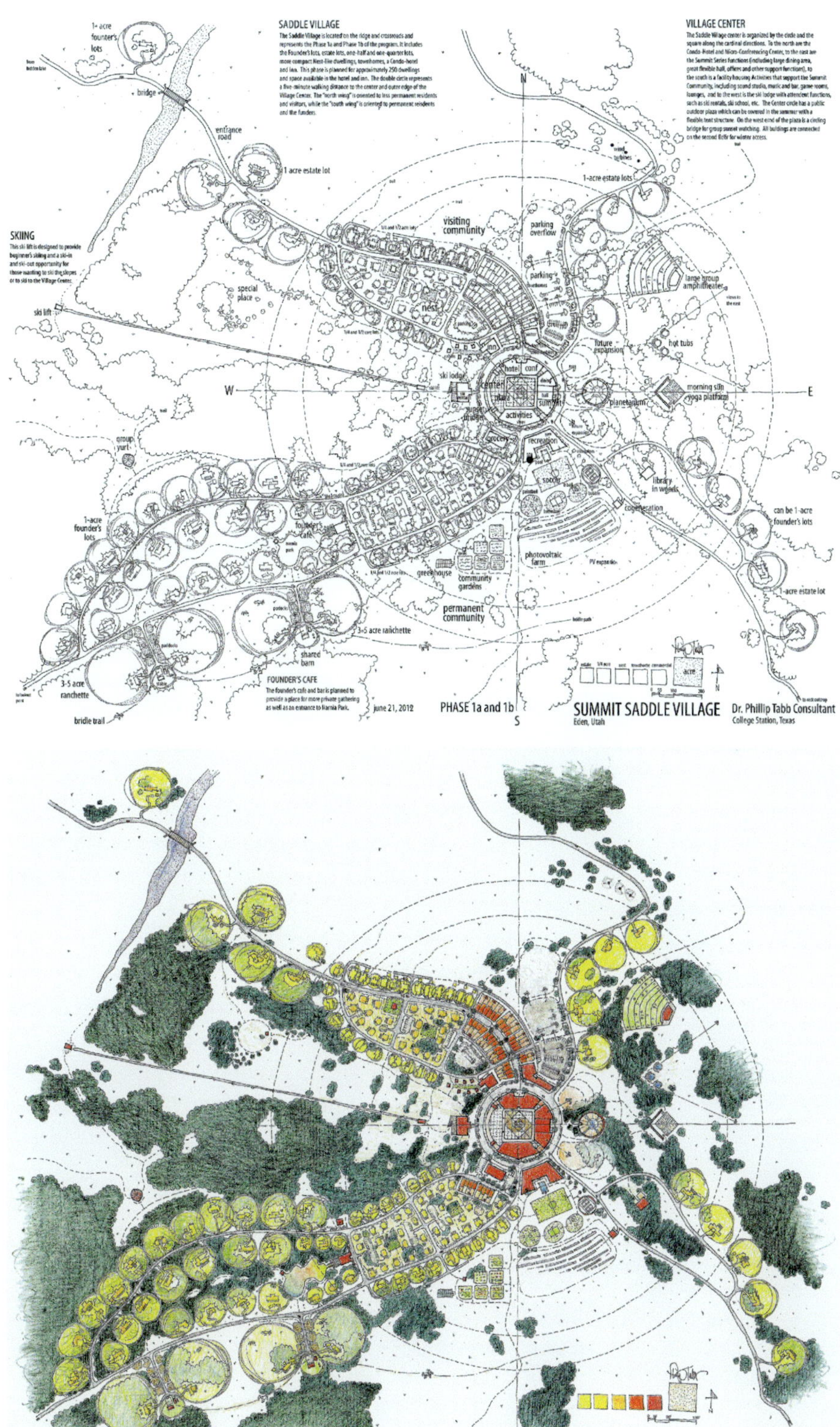

St. Peter's in Rome, Florence Cathedral, Chartres Cathedral, the classical Ottoman Blue Mosque in Istanbul, and the modernist Catalan Sagrada Família in Barcelona. These places are awe-inspiring, with incredible spatial generosity, buttressing walls, qualities of light, stained-glass windows, and beautiful color. However, I must confess, my more remembered spiritual experiences occurred in smaller spaces, most often a quiet, modest parish church. I loved the rural churches in English villages and Italian hill towns. They were soulful, grounded, present, extremely quiet, and relatable on a deep personal level. Plus, afterwards, there was the likelihood of a pub or Italian pizzeria lunch. This brings up the question, "What is the role of geometry in spiritual wellness?" The answer for me is part intention, part execution, and the maintenance of the golden thread.

In sacred geometry, symmetry refers to the balanced and harmonious arrangement of forms, patterns, and proportions.[18] Symmetry also interrelates specific objects with their surroundings, and with us as well. According to Michael Mehaffy, this extended symmetry relates mathematically to the larger scale of urban spaces, neighborhoods, and city regions (and, ultimately, to the whole Earth and even the cosmos beyond). This new understanding of the symmetrical relatedness of buildings and cities rejoins the disciplines of architecture, urban design, and planning within a larger contextual framework.[19]

Spiritual wellness should be accessible and should occur daily. Hence, the geometric triggers or elicitors and their energetic qualities should be readily available and a common part of the environments we occupy. While the physical world is inextricably expressed through geometry, it, too, often obscures it. When our world is truly beautiful, geometry is always there. The role of sacred geometry is to amplify our connections to spiritual wellness. For me, the most valued wellness effects are the calming of my mind, the feeling of being present, the igniting of my imagination, the offering of a physical space to engage my process of drawing, and welcoming the patience to let it unfold and the resultant release of stress. On a spiritual level, drawing, like other spiritual art forms, explores ideas and images of the sacred and divine and helps to bridge the gap between the known and unknown, the secular and the sacred, and the mundane and the ineffable. In relation to the built environment, sacred geometry can contribute to harmonious atmospheres, provide meaningful organizations, promote wellness experiences, create a sympathetic resonance between our bodies and a sacred space, and facilitate spiritual connections.[20]

NOTES

1 Naismith, Robert, *Buildings of the Scottish Countryside* (London, UK: Victor Gollancz, 1985), pp. 141–142.
2 Martineau, John, Ed., *Quadrivium: The Four Classical Liberal Arts of Number, Geometry, Music, & Cosmology* (New York, NY: Walden Books, 2005).
3 Critchlow, Keith, The Platonic Tradition on the Nature of Proportion, in *Lindisfarne Letter 10: Geometry and Architecture* (Stockbridge, MA: The Lindisfarne Press, 1980), p. 14.
4 Lawlor, Robert, *Sacred Geometry: Philosophy and Practice* (London, UK: Thames & Hudson, 1980), p. 22.
5 Pennick, Nigel, *Sacred Geometry* (New York, NY: Harper & Row, 1980).

6 Critchlow, Keith, The Platonic Tradition on the Nature of Proportion, *Lindisfarne Letter 10: Geometry and Architecture* (Stockbridge, MA: The Lindisfarne Press, 1980).
7 Lawlor, Robert, *Sacred Geometry: Philosophy and Practice* (London, UK: Thames & Hudson, 1980), p. 44.
8 Plato with Peter Kalkavage, Trans., *Timaeus* (Newburyport, MA: Focus/R. Pullins, 2001).
9 Lawlor, Robert, *Sacred Geometry: Philosophy and Practice* (London, UK: Thames & Hudson, 1980).
10 Waterfield, Robin, *The Theology of Arithmetic* (Grand Rapids, MI: Phanes Press, 1988), pp. 22–23.
11 Eames Charles, & Ray Eames, Powers of Ten (1977) (accessed December 10, 2024), https://www.youtube.com/watch?v=Ww4gYNrOkkg.
12 Jiddu Krishnamurti (1895–1986) was an Indian philosopher, speaker, and writer considered one of the 20th century's greatest spiritual figures. Krishnamurti established several schools around the world based on his educational philosophy, emphasizing a holistic approach to learning and the cultivation of a free and intelligent mind. He continued to speak and write until his death in 1986. Opening in 1987, after Krishnamurti's passing, the Krishnamurti Study Centre is a retreat center for adults to study his work and explore its relevance to their lives.
13 Timeless Quality. Freedom to Inquire (accessed September 22, 2024), https://krishnamurticentre.org.uk.
14 Nabokov, Peter, and Robert Easton, *Native American Architecture* (New York, NY: Oxford University Press, 1989), p. 71.
15 In the sacred design process, the concept of a "golden thread" represents the essential, unifying principle that weaves through every stage, ensuring coherence and continuity of purpose. This thread embodies the core intention, the spiritual essence, or the fundamental values that underpin the creation. It acts as a constant reference point, guiding decisions about form, materials, symbolism, and spatial relationships. Without this golden thread, the design risks becoming fragmented, losing its spiritual resonance, and failing to effectively communicate its intended sacred meaning. If this guiding principle is diligently followed, the resulting space or object achieves a profound sense of unity, integrity, and a powerful connection to the sacred, fostering a deeper experience for those who interact with it.
16 StarHouse website (accessed August 15, 2021), https://www.thestarhouse.org/events-and-cources.
17 Rubber B, The Meaning of the Omega Symbol (accessed October 7, 2024), https://rubberb.com/blog/meaning-of-the-omega-symbol/#:~:text=Although%20the%20symbol%20of%20the,to%20as%20"Doomsday%20cults.
18 In sacred geometry, symmetry is a fundamental principle referring to the balanced and harmonious arrangement of shapes, patterns, and proportions. It manifests in various forms reflecting the underlying order and unity within the universe. These symmetrical designs, often mirroring patterns found in nature and incorporating proportions generated by Pythagorean and Platonic geometries, are believed to hold symbolic meaning and evoke a sense of aesthetic resonance and connection to deeper cosmic principles.
19 Mehaffy, Michael, The Surprisingly Important Role of Symmetry in Healthy Human Environments (accessed April 10, 2025), https://www.imcl.online/post/the-surprisingly-important-role-of-symmetry-in-healthy-human-environments.
20 Sympathetic resonance, in the context of sacred geometry, refers to the idea that geometric forms and proportions found in sacred geometry are not merely static visual patterns but are also vibrational and resonant in nature. It suggests that these geometric structures possess inherent frequencies or vibrational signatures that can interact and resonate with other systems, both physical and energetic.

10 NARRATIVE VIGNETTE 3

The Value of Mythic Landscapes

INTRODUCTION

Mythic landscapes are imaginary narratives weaving a sense of the spiritual with the landscapes they inhabit, shifting human awareness. As a drawing process, the mythic realms awaken insights, profound deductions, an enlivened presence, and a spiritual wellness. Traditional forms of sacred visual art, such as Thangka painting, Tsa Tsa, icon writing, mandala sand painting, Zen drawing, Vastusutra Upanisad, Persian miniature painting, and Islamic patterning, seem to grow from a focused discipline that includes an integration of mind, body, and spirit. The value of drawing while traveling is twofold. First, I find the drawing process tends to slow time down and contribute to greater presence. And, second, the completed drawing later reminds me of my experience of the place and time.

Broadly, mythological explorations can be renewing and creative when found in drawings as they become what author J.R.R. Tolkien called "mythopoeia," a visual narrative of archetypal themes emerging where the myth-making is closely connected to the experience of a place. Myths are said to take place before a space becomes a place, and this process becomes a sacred narrative that is attached and gives significance to a place. Myths can explain the origins or how the place came to be; they can teach lessons and values; and they can give identity to the place. According to Joseph Campbell, they can evoke a sense of the mystery of existence. They connect us to the larger cosmic context within which all places are situated.[1]

THE VALUE OF TRAVEL

Travel broadens perspectives, fosters empathy, and enriches the soul through firsthand experience of the world's diverse natural and urban landscapes. Encountering breathtaking landscapes, ancient ruins, or diverse cultures can evoke a sense of awe and wonder, reminding us of something larger than ourselves and fostering a connection to the urban places found around the world. Exploring mythic landscapes allows us to physically engage with the power and resonance of ancient narratives. Travel transforms ordinary geography into extraordinary mythic landscapes, imbued with the echoes of past beliefs and spiritual significance.

My journey into mythic landscapes began with my travel, especially in Europe, and my resultant re-engaging with drawing. Throughout the years, my travels were associated with work, teaching, and family connections. My teaching brought

DOI: 10.4324/9781003546085-10

me to Canada, England, and Italy, and my academic research and conference presentations took me to Turkey, Greece, South Korea, Egypt, Italy, and throughout the United States. My family connections were in England and Switzerland. My initial reentry into drawing involved quick sketches in my journal. They were of intriguing and beautiful places such as the Acropolis in Athens, the Forum in Rome, the Duomo in Florence, and Galata Tower in Istanbul. Although the value of travel has been well documented, such as improving cognitive function and introducing one to new customs, cultures, and both urban and natural environments, for me, travel contributes to transformative and spiritual experiences, leading often to the experience that there are things greater than ourselves.

When traveling, I would bring my cameras and drawing materials. Typically, I drew with Micron waterproof pens on a smooth-paper watercolor block. The watercolor block was easy to carry and offered a rigid surface for composing and drawing. I typically carried two sizes. Some of the drawings were re-created from photographs I took while traveling. For example, the drawing of the village of Civitella in Italy was created from a photograph I took while flying over the site in a small airplane (Figure 10.2d). Later, I re-created the image on the watercolor block in my apartment.

THE VALUE OF DRAWING

Drawing, and in particular freehand drawing, cultivates observation skills, fosters creative expression, and strengthens the direct connection between the eye, hand, and the intended image. Further, it provides a process of becoming more present within a place. This vignette explores several pen and ink drawings created in extraordinary places as well as in studio. While in undergraduate architecture school, I took five years of drawing and painting classes; it was not until the early 2000s that I began drawing for pleasure again. I engaged in two basic drawing processes, *in situ* and *studio-enhanced* drawings. Those drawings completed in situ, or while *in place*, offered firsthand and direct experiences of those places. Walking around these interesting places and talking with residents gave valuable insights into their meanings. The *studio-enhanced* drawings allowed for opportunities to research the subjects and spend more time with composing and completing the work. Some of these drawings were drawn in place, usually taking between half an hour to an hour to create. Later, I began to create more serious drawings, many of which were drawn from photographs that I took on site, and I enhanced or added detail to them in my home studio.

In situ sketching is an on-site drawing method where fast sketching techniques are combined with the heuristic of a general perceptual awareness of a place. On one level, it provides immediate immersion and "macroscopic" vision, particularly when traveling through interesting places. On another level, it calls for a gestural feeling for a place and an observational presence with an essential, rapid representational response – converting impulse into image. Most importantly, in situ sketching requires the development of a quick "field" drawing style (*squinting, scanning, culling, quickly composing,* and then *drawing*) where the entire

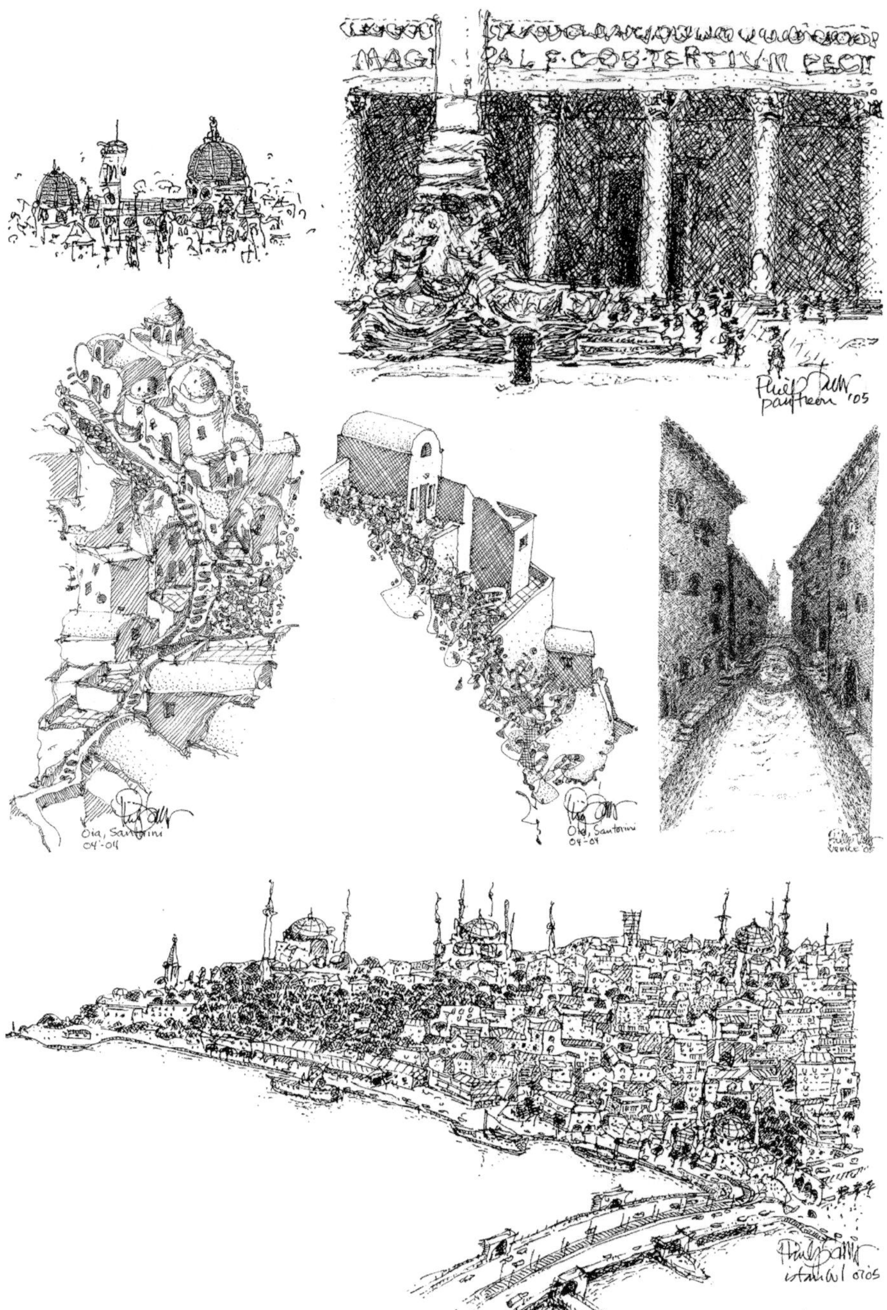

10.1
In Situ Drawings: (a) Florence Duomo, (b) Pantheon Entrance, Rome, (c) Oia, Santorini, Greece 1, (d) Oia, Santorini, Greece 2, (e) Water Steet, Venice, Italy, (f) Istanbul Mosques, (g) Galata Tower, Istanbul, Turkey

composition can be captured in one explosive setting. I drew the *Florence Duomo* with simple and quick line work within five minutes in the Piazzale Michelangelo overlooking Florence (Figure 10.1a). A touch of color was added to the dome to emphasize its function as a place marker. The image of the Pantheon, Figure 10.1b, I did while having lunch in the Piazza Della Rotonda one afternoon.

10.1
(Continued)

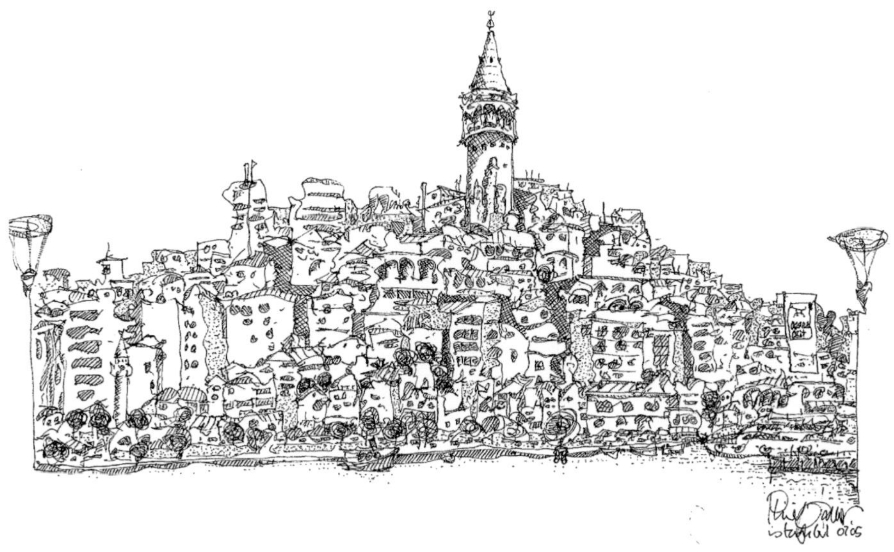

The figures *Oia, Santorini 1* and *Oia, Santorini 2* are an attempt to capture the spirit of place with its complexity, Euclidian forms, fluidity, cascading geometry, and sloping topography (Figures 10.1c and 10.1d). Figure 10.1e is an in situ drawing of a Venice water street sketched while on a vaporetto. In the summer of 2005, I was invited to give a paper at Istanbul Technical University, which happened to coincide with my 60th birthday. I decided to take the day off and spent it walking from my hotel in Taksim Square along the Golden Horn. On my way, I stopped at the Galata Tower and had a coffee high up in the café at the top of the tower. From there, I could see all the mosques and the Galata Bridge, which connected two parts of the city down below. The mosques along the Istanbul skyline seemed to reach to the heavens (Figure 10.1f). The *Galata Tower* sketch was done very quickly on the opposite side of the Golden Horn in an attempt to capture it as a place marker in the context of a complex urban fabric (Figure 10.1g).

Studio-enhanced drawing begins with being present at a site, making initial sketches, and taking subject photographs. Then, the drawing is worked on in the studio environment where it can either be reconstructed or enhanced and developed into a more precise drawing. Dutch artist and author Fredrick Franck suggests that "time stands still," and this drawing technique seems to support this process where multiple drawing episodes allow for meditation, visual research, reflective adjustments, and careful drawing practices. Examples of this process include a studio-enhanced drawing taken along the Via dei Servi connecting the Piazza della Santissima Annunziata with the Duomo. It illustrates simultaneously the human scale of the streetscape and the impressive scale of the Duomo (Figure 10.2a). From one of the courtyards in Pienza, Italy, there is a wonderful view of the Val di Orca and Monte Amiata beyond it. In the drawing, framed by wind-blown Cypress trees, are the Pieve di Corsignano (below) and Monte Amiata (above) (Figure 10.2b). A class visit to Orvieto led to the drawing in Figure 10.2c in which the street framed the view of the west façade of the cathedral which, by

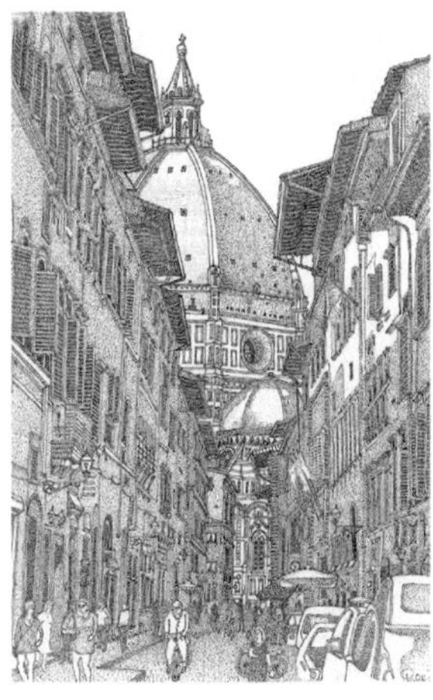

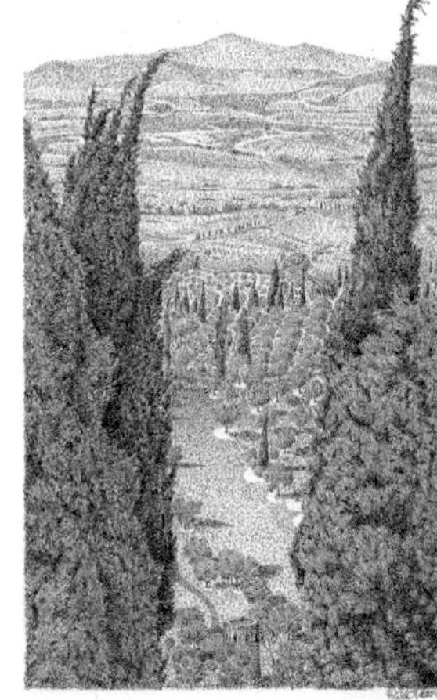

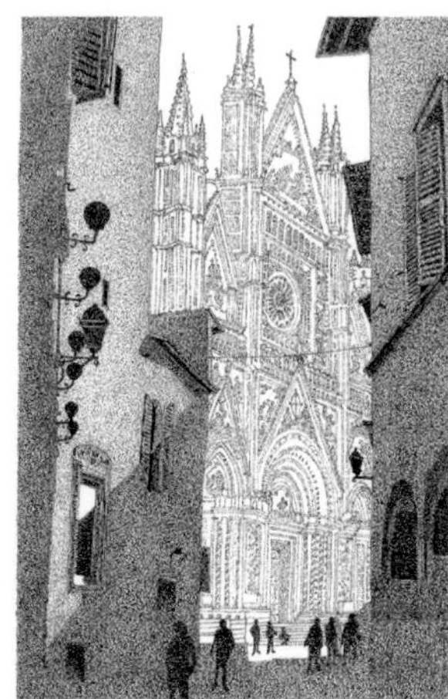

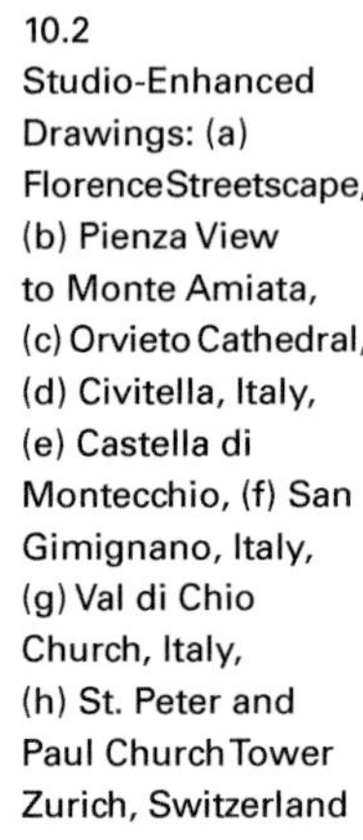

10.2 Studio-Enhanced Drawings: (a) FlorenceStreetscape, (b) Pienza View to Monte Amiata, (c) Orvieto Cathedral, (d) Civitella, Italy, (e) Castella di Montecchio, (f) San Gimignano, Italy, (g) Val di Chio Church, Italy, (h) St. Peter and Paul Church Tower Zurich, Switzerland

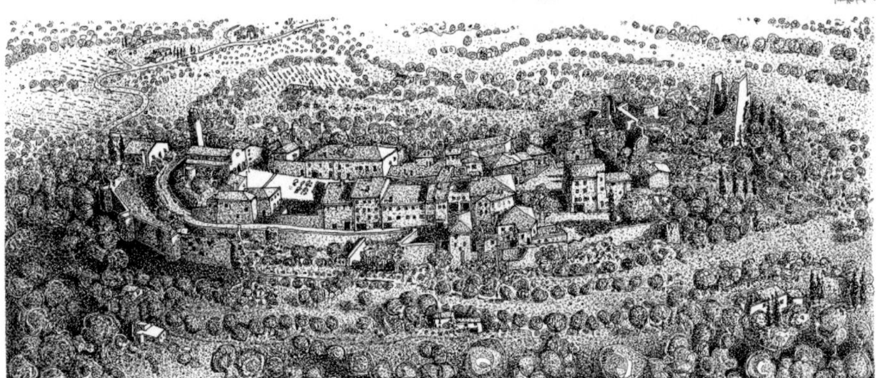

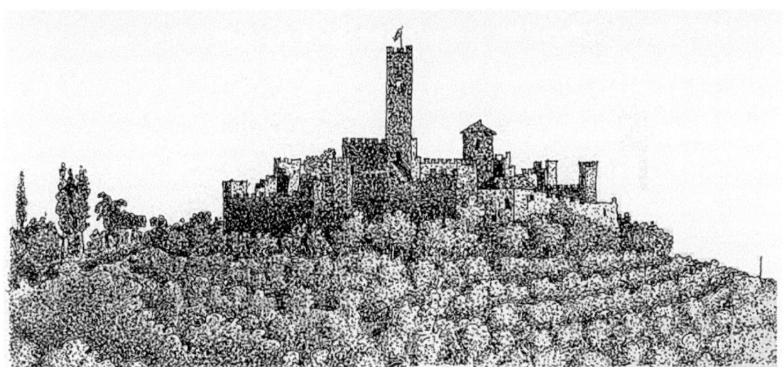

contrast, was drawn as ethereal. *Civitella in Val di Chiana* and *Montagna e Chiesa* show the greater detail and rendering care afforded by more time and controlled studio conditions (Figure 10.2d). The aerial drawing attempts to capture an image of the entire place with a clearly defined boundary and center. Figure 10.2e was drawn from my bedroom balcony at the Santa Chiara Study Centre in Castiglion Fiorentino. The drawing features the Castello di Montecchio on a hill, surrounded by olive trees. At first, my drawings were a bit sketchy and were done quite quickly over five or ten minutes. Figure 10.2f is a quick drawing done after lunch in the Piazza della Cisterna in San Gimignano. Figure 10.2g illustrates the small Val di Chio Church, also drawn

10.2 (Continued)

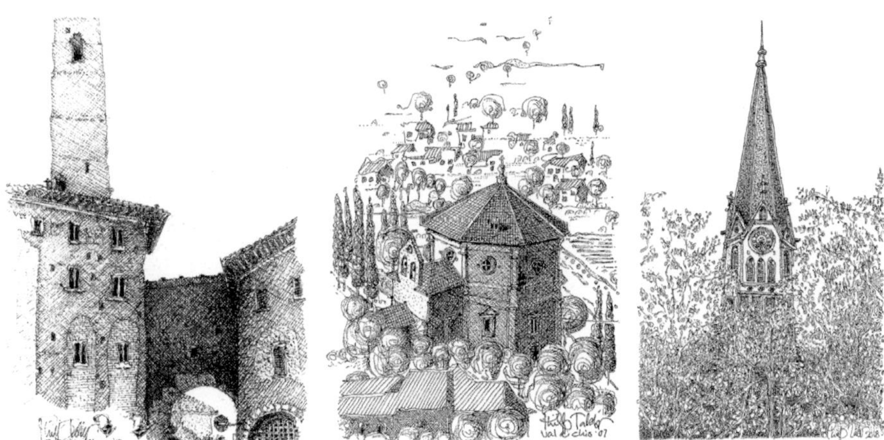

from my balcony overlooking the Val di Chio, with the Tuscan farms, vineyards, farmhouses, and landscapes that float away into abstraction in its background. The church, in the foreground, has more detail, while the landscape and trees behind it are more loosely drawn. And, finally, Figure 10.2h is a drawing of the St Peter and Paul Church tower in Zurich, Switzerland.

Each of the drawings in Figure 10.2, with the exception of 10.2f, drawn on site, were studio-enhanced drawings. Sometimes, initial sketches in pencil were drawn on site, but, for the majority of the drawing, the work was done under more controlled conditions and over longer periods of time. These studio-enhanced drawing took over a month to complete. Once the pencil work captured the image on the watercolor block and the Micron linework was finished, the pencil lines were erased. Stippling was the final part of the process and often took many days to complete. Drawing sizes vary, but most are around 6 inches (15 centimeters) by 10 inches (25 centimeters).

For those who draw, it becomes a meditative process as you are completely lost within the drawing. Pencil lines were drawn from photographs and later replaced by Micron pen lines and then stippled to give a rendered effect. For me, a magical process occurs as line after line and dot after dot go into the drawing, and then it no longer exists as lines and dots on a page but rather is transformed and comes alive. To me, this is a spiritual moment. I have framed and hung many of these drawings in my home, and their presence serves as reminders of the drawing experience and the time spent in these wonderful places.

I have always loved mythic stories and how they ignite the creative imagination. In the early 2000s, as I became interested in myths as a way of informing design and further understanding spiritual concepts, I began creating mythic landscapes. This interest bolstered my desire to expand my drawing to create mythic landscapes.[2]

MYTHIC LANDSCAPES

According to author Robert Samples, a symbolic metaphor exists whenever a visual or abstract symbol is substituted for an object, process, or condition.[3] *Mythic*

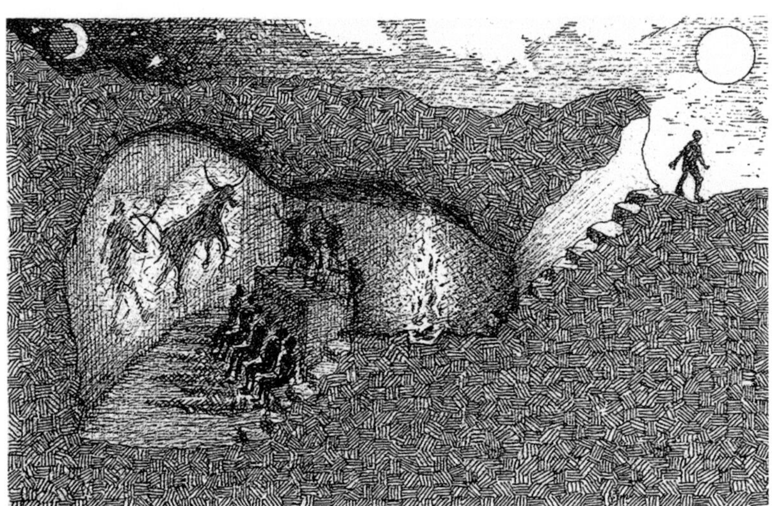

10.3
Mythic Landscapes Vignette: Allegory of the Cave

landscapes are a drawing process, where the mythic realms coexist with the natural or human-made elements of the place. When the myths derive or are created from the fabric and evolutionary process of the place, they are said to be *mythopoeic*.

Twenty-four hundred years ago, Plato wrote one of his best-known works, *The Allegory of the Cave*, in the *Republic*, Book VII.[4] As described by Socrates in a dialogue with Glaucon, Plato's older brother, it describes humans chained with their backs to a stone wall in a cave-like dwelling under the earth. They existed there from early childhood for the duration of their lives. They faced a blank wall upon which illusionary shadows were projected from wood and stone objects passed by puppeteers in front of a fire located behind the chained humans. Consequently, their reality became informed by these shadows, echoes, and the names they assigned to them, all of which were a reflective language and misrepresentation of reality. It was the philosopher (philosopher-king) who broke away from the shackles of imprisonment and emerged from the cave into the outside world to experience the true nature of reality. Eventually, the philosopher no longer saw dim reflections but instead perceived the true light of the fire and, for the first time, saw the sun and the dome of the heavens and experienced the seasons of the year. He saw pure form, the authentic source of truth, and experienced the intelligible world. Figure 10.3 shows the cave, fire, puppeteers, projected images on the back wall, and the philosopher-king climbing the steps into the light of day.

Initially, the light of the fire and direct sunlight hurt the philosopher's eyes. So, the new source of reality was experienced first by looking at shadows, then at reflections in water, and, finally, directly at the sun and night sky. Sense perception in the cave ascended to rational knowledge in the outer world. Problematic for the philosopher was his need and concern for the other prisoners still shackled in the cave. Going back into the cave, he was surprised to find the remaining prisoners reluctant to leave the reality they had become so accustomed to, knowing no other life. He also needed time for his eyes to re-adjust to the darkness of the cave and the distinctions of the image shadows cast on the cave wall. The prisoners did not want to leave their bondage because they could not understand this incomprehensible new reality. Socrates concludes with the notion that the freed philosopher might be silenced and possibly killed by them. And Glaucon concurred.

I found this allegory useful when reflecting upon modern culture today and creating a sketch of the cave. I sensed that the very same forces that chained humans deep within Plato's cave are the same distractions, behaviors, and lifestyle practices that separate us from high-level wellness today. The philosopher-king seems to symbolize connecting to something more authentic, real, vital, and greater than ourselves. More contemporary examples of such connections exist. This mythic story reminded me of a book by Neil Postman which was given to me by a friend. It was called *Amusing Ourselves to Death: Public Discourse in the Age of Show Business.*[5] This is a poignant critique on our fascination with television, digital technology, and today's social media. The spiritual wellness significance of this mythic landscape is in the idea that humanity can be mesmerized, even tranquilized, into certain belief systems, lifestyles, and behaviors that are not healthy or spiritually invigorating. To change, one must transform through all of the wellness pillars to ultimately experience high-level well-being. The process of reading about this allegory and drawing it gave me time to reflect upon it and see how it related to my own life.

I found other myths rich subjects for drawing. The story of Pegasus, according to Dr. Gail Thomas, offers a way of imagining spirit in the making of cities and, in so doing, creates an energy that draws people to it.[6] This magnetic energy seems true for any scale, from a region to a room. The offspring of Poseidon (earth shaker and presider over the deep sea) and Medusa (serpent-haired Gorgon), Pegasus is known for his healing powers. His Greek name, *Pegae*, means geyser; so, when his hoof touches the earth, a healing spring emerges with a strong spirit of place (Figure 10.4).[7] This spirit of place, or *genius loci*, becomes a catalyst for spiritual wellness. I loved this drawing, which seems to be engulfed by the unknown, surrounded by uncertainty, and yet Pegasus, coming from the heavens, touches the earth, and a sacred place is born. The thought of Pegasus descending to a particular place – a new building site, housing development,

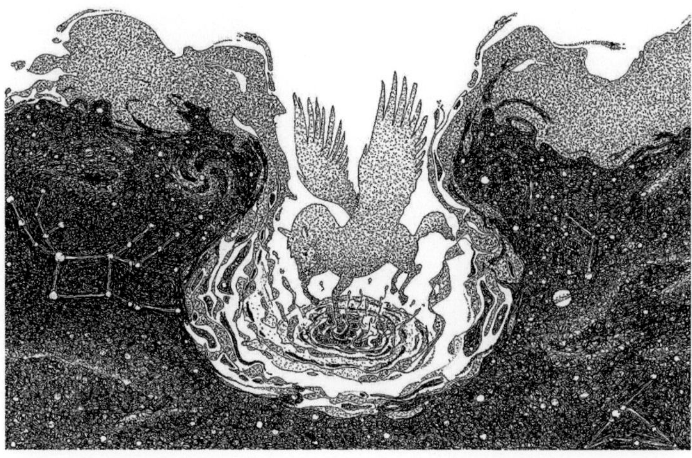

10.4 Mythic Landscapes Vignette: Pegasus Myth

or city – suggests that a vital and healthy spirit of place might be present or at least invited to reside there. The Pegasus image is an optimistic drawing and a reminder of the myth to me.

In another example, the winged lion, Figure 10.5a, was the symbol of Venetian independence, regality, strength, and power. It is the symbol of peace and of Saint Mark the Evangelist and is used as the symbol of St. Mark's Parish. Larger than life and full of celestial images, the winged lion gives protection to the city and its intricate waterways while walking its perimeter. The winged lion is an allegory of Saint Mark, embodying certain characteristics such as the mane as the strength of the republic, the wings as spiritual power, the halo as its holiness, and the tail as its majesty and power. Walking around Venice countless times, I felt the winged lion's presence supporting a kind of spiritual wellness. The lion is also significant in the city of Florence, again for its strength and power. In my drawing with the Ponte Vecchio in the background, the lion is walking along the river Arno and is somewhat transparent (Figure 10.5b). There is a comforting feeling about the idea that the heavenly presence of these two lions in these drawings might originate from a source much larger than us.

Myths reflecting seasons and directions provided other enriching sources for my drawings. The four sacred beasts of ancient China are the *green dragon* (east), *red phoenix* (south), *white tiger* (west), and *black tortoise* (north) and are said to have aided in the creation of the world and give energy to the four directions in feng shui. The white tiger, in Seishuku astrology, occupies seven Western constellations, Orion, Taurus, Aries, and Andromeda (Figure 10.5c). Another animal representing direction and season is the green dragon (Figure 10.5d). The animal symbols and their natures help remind us of the qualities of those directions and seasons. These symbols can be important in the designs of building façades and their abilities to mediate external conditions. They are also reminders of the changing hours of the day, with the passage of the sun, from morning to evening. This effect can be created with healing light qualities occurring throughout the spaces of a building. These myths and drawings act as reminders and invitations to design appropriately. For me, these drawings not only help in emplacing me but they also reflect the seasons and directions within which I live.

I was fortunate to live in Italy over the years and visited Siena many times. One of the most astonishing experiences is walking down the steps into the Piazza del Campo. Surrounding the campo are 17 contrade (neighborhoods or urban wards) that function as a microcosm of the central piazza. Each contrada has a local piazza typically framed by a chapel, museum, and animal symbol reference. They form a particular historic and cultural component of the function and nature of the central campo. The square that forms the central campo was arranged in the 12th century and initially was used as an open marketplace; the shell-like center was divided into nine segments representing the initial nine neighborhoods. There are now 17 neighborhoods, including the original nine.

The view of the campo in Siena in the drawing, Figure 10.5e, is a juxtaposition of the space and animals representing six of the original nine contrade that are surrounding the campo. Moving clockwise from the tower are the elephant

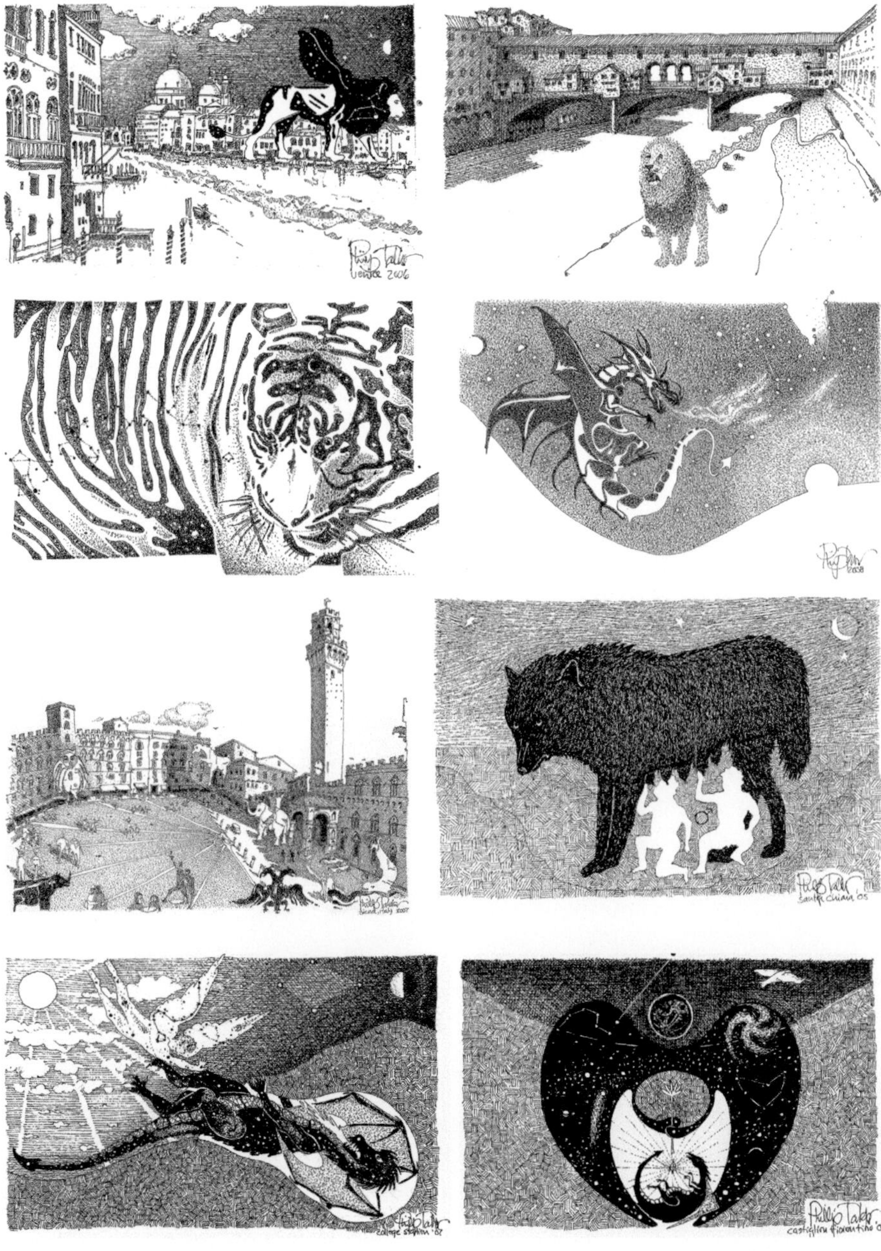

10.5
Mythic Landscapes: (a) Winged Lion of Venice, (b) the Lion of Florence, (c) White Tiger, (d) Green Dragon, (e) Siena Campo, (f) She-Wolf, (g) Archangel Michael, (h) Archangel Gabriel

(Torre), wave (Onda), eagle (Aquila), rhinoceros (Selva), little owl (Civetta), and unicorn (Leocorno). The last time I was there, a local vendor who sold me a flag asked which of the contrade was my favorite. I responded, I was drawn to the Leocorno contrada. I loved the intimate plaza and the fountain that supplied water from the unicorn's horn. In talking to many of the residents of Siena, I found that they have immense pride in their neighborhood. Each neighborhood, in a way, is a microcosm of the whole of Siena, as each has its own church, plaza, museum, animal sculpture, and sense of place. I was told a pink flag flying on the façade of one of the neighborhood's churches signals to residents that another baby had just been born into their neighborhood.

The founding of Rome derives from the 8th-century BC myth in which King Amulius, feeling a threat to his rule, ordered the twins Romulus and Remus to be killed. To save them, the babies were placed in a basket that floated down the River Tiber and were discovered by a she-wolf. The she-wolf, or *lupa* in Latin, was an Italian wolf who suckled and sheltered the twin babies, raising them to adulthood. Eventually, the twins were adopted by a shepherd and grew up guarding flocks of sheep. When grown, they joined their grandfather in killing Amulius and set out to establish their own city. One story tells of Remus jumping over the Palatine Hill wall surrounding the new city on the day of the city's founding; Romulus was furious with Remus and killed him. Romulus was very angry because Remus mocked him and, thus, demonstrated a lack of sensitivity to the sacredness of the containing wall, which broke Remus's divine right to create a sacred city. This story of the founding of Rome served as a powerful narrative tool that linked the city's inhabitants to a divine destiny while providing a model of the virtues and values. While the drawing in Figure 10.5f simply depicts the she-wolf suckling the twins, it is a reminder of Rome's creation myth.

Cycles of change provide intriguing subjects for drawing. The four seasons give us a broader understanding of these changes as climate moves from the extremes of cold in winter to heat in summer (northern hemisphere). The equinoxes yield relatively milder weather that vacillates between warm and cool temperatures. The Druids saw dragons as a way of connecting us to the forces of nature and the turning of the seasons.[8] Dragon lines or earth energy pathways originate from Chinese geomancy and feng shui and are seen to flow within the landscape. Dragon lines are considered crucial for harmonizing the environment with human activity.[9] The archangels Michael, Gabriel, Raphael, and Uriel represent a presiding presence over these periods. In some places, the dragon is a mythical symbol of the Earth or of Earth's energy.[10] Another set of drawings depict the Archangels of Presence: Michael (autumn), Gabriel (winter), Raphael (spring), and Uriel (summer). Two archangels are shown in Figures 10.5g and 10.5h. The symbolic depiction of the Earth's dragon energy is a process of ascending and descending as the solar light increases from the winter solstice and decrease after the summer solstice. Throughout the world, spiritual and religious ceremonies are associated with these seasonal changes.[11] Historically, both architecture and urban designs possess the ability to respond to these cycles of change.

- **Winter solstice**: increase in light, new beginnings, and the nurturing of Earth energies and union with elemental spirits.
- **Vernal equinox**: emergence of Earth energies, an increase in warmth, rising nutrients, and a balance between extremes.
- **Summer solstice**: beginning of the decrease in light, exaltation of Earth energies, festive and outdoor activities, abundance, and active natural processes.
- **Autumnal equinox**: a time of harvest, a time of migration, movement of energies back into the Earth, and a balance between extremes.

Religious depictions show Archangel Michael slaying the dragon as a symbol of the victory of good over evil, the defeat of Satan, and the triumph of righteousness. However, in this drawing, the dragon is seen as earth energy rather than evil, which depicts a different story (Figure 10.5g). The dragon, in certain traditions, is a symbol of earth energy. According to this myth, with the help of these archangels, its energy is transformed as the Earth turns through the seasons. In the northern hemisphere, the energy in autumn is redirected back into the Earth, as exemplified by the falling leaves of deciduous plants and trees. In winter, the energy is protected in the ground by Archangel Gabriel. In Figure 10.5h, Gabriel is seen protecting the dragon energy suspended deep within the Earth. In spring, this energy is drawn upward with the aid of Archangel Raphael, as in the new growth and life of plants.

And finally, in summer, earth energy is united with solar energy and radiance with the help of Archangel Uriel. This depicts a cycle of descending and ascending energy. In religious depictions, Archangel Michael usually kills the dragon, as a symbol of good over evil. Archangel Michael is not killing the dragon but, rather, is redirecting the dragon's energy back into the Earth. Again, these depictions were reminders of the specific energies represented by these times of the year. The drawing of Archangel Michael shows him redirecting the dragon back into the Earth with his hand and not his sword, during winter, rather than killing it. This symbolizes the movement of life energy back into the Earth. These drawings and their associations with the Angels of Presence gave me a deeper understanding of the sacred nature of the changing seasons. Now, in autumn, for example, I am aware of life energy moving back into the Earth with the colder weather and the falling of leaves.

Figure 10.6 is a drawing that illustrates a sequence and arrangement of mythic stories about Apollo, the sun god, and Corvus, his sacred raven. The drawing begins with the myth of the Titans' attack on Mount Olympus and Apollo's shape-shifting into a silver-winged raven. The next story illustrated is the adultery of Coronis the Thessalian princess and the mortal Ischys. Apollo asked Corvus to fetch some water as he watched over Coronis as Apollo and his chariot traversed the sky. Corvus had stopped on his way for the water and saw figs that had fallen to the ground. So taken by the abundance of the figs, Corvus stayed for days, thereby neglecting to retrieve water for Apollo and missing the adultery of Coronis and Ischys. Upon his return to Apollo, Corvus lied, saying he was detained by a large snake (refer to Figure 11.2c, the Hydra with Corvus). In a fit of rage, Apollo's scorching gaze burned Corvus's feathers black; hence the reason why all ravens are black. Apollo then threw him into the heavens, thereby creating the constellation Corvus, consecrating the lie. The Greek Corvus was borrowed from the mythical Babylonian raven, which was usually depicted perched on the tail of a serpent.[12] This medley concludes with the Corvus constellation myth and his embodiment within the chapel at Ronchamp, designed by the architect Le Corbusier. Interestingly, he changed his name from Charles-Édouard Jeanneret to Le Corbusier, which means "raven-like." Perhaps the inclusion of the raven in the lower-tier window of the Assumption wall at the Ronchamp chapel is an interesting coincidence, or, possibly, it is Le Corbusier's signature to the inspiring building.

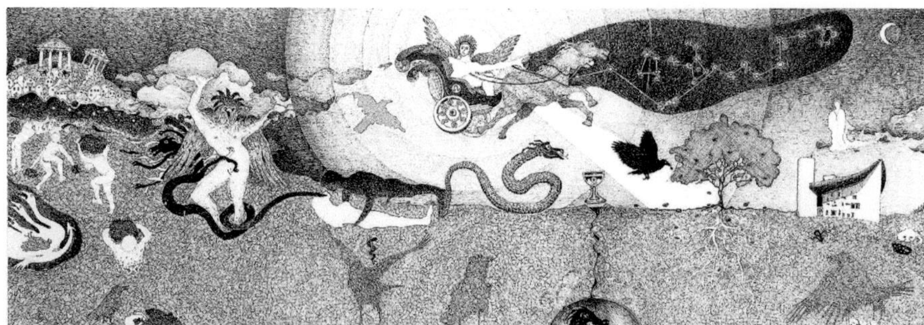

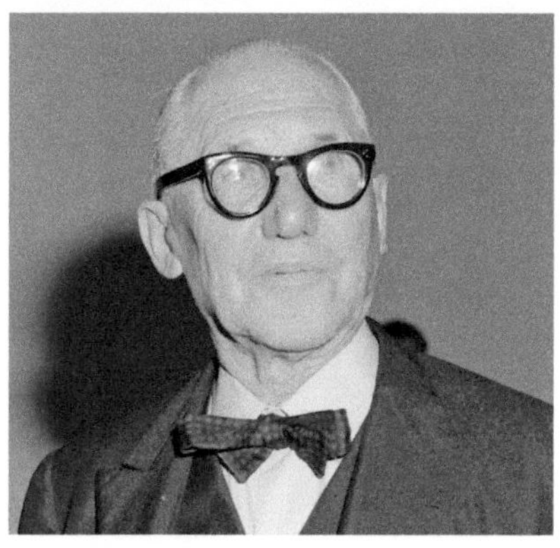

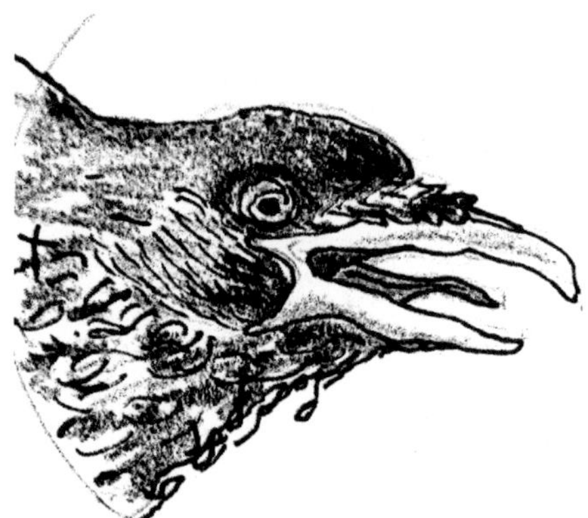

10.6
Mythic Landscapes:
(a) Corvus Myths,
(b) Le Corbusier,
Photograph,
(c) Raven Sketch

Another takeaway for me in creating this visual medley was how myths and their stories can relate to, and even inform, architectural design. The spiritual wellness comes from the spirit and moral content of the stories and, in the context of this work, how the narratives can inform design decisions. Concerning the Corvus myths, the spiritual wellness benefits may occur when facing adversity (the attack of the Titans), transforming with the healing qualities and beauty of nature (shapeshifting into a raven), keeping steadfast with one's purpose (fetching water and guarding Coronis), remembering past mistakes or lessons (Corvus constellation), and seeing hope and light in the face of darkness. Architecturally, this myth might manifest as it does within the chapel at Ronchamp.

The four Roman bronze horses, known as the Triumphal Quadriga, serve as the subject of another one of my drawings. These replicas are placed on the porch of the Basilica of St. Mark. In the drawing, the unique perspective of the foreground horse's legs frame St. Mark's astrological clock tower in the background (Figure 10.7b). The four gilded bronze horses stand on the porch in front of St. Mark's Basilica in Venice, Italy, facing the Piazza San Marco. Many scholars believe they were sculpted in the 2nd or 3rd century AD. However, some say that the evident technical expertise and naturalistic rendering of the animals suggest they were made in classical Greece in the 5th or 4th century BC. The sequence in Figure 10.7a shows the progression of the pointillism drawing from pencil work to stippling of the shapes. This is a sequence of the drawing in progress from pencil line drawing to line inking and, finally, rendering. In the finished drawing, the lower image in Figure 10.7b, the rendering is complete, and, between the front and back legs of the

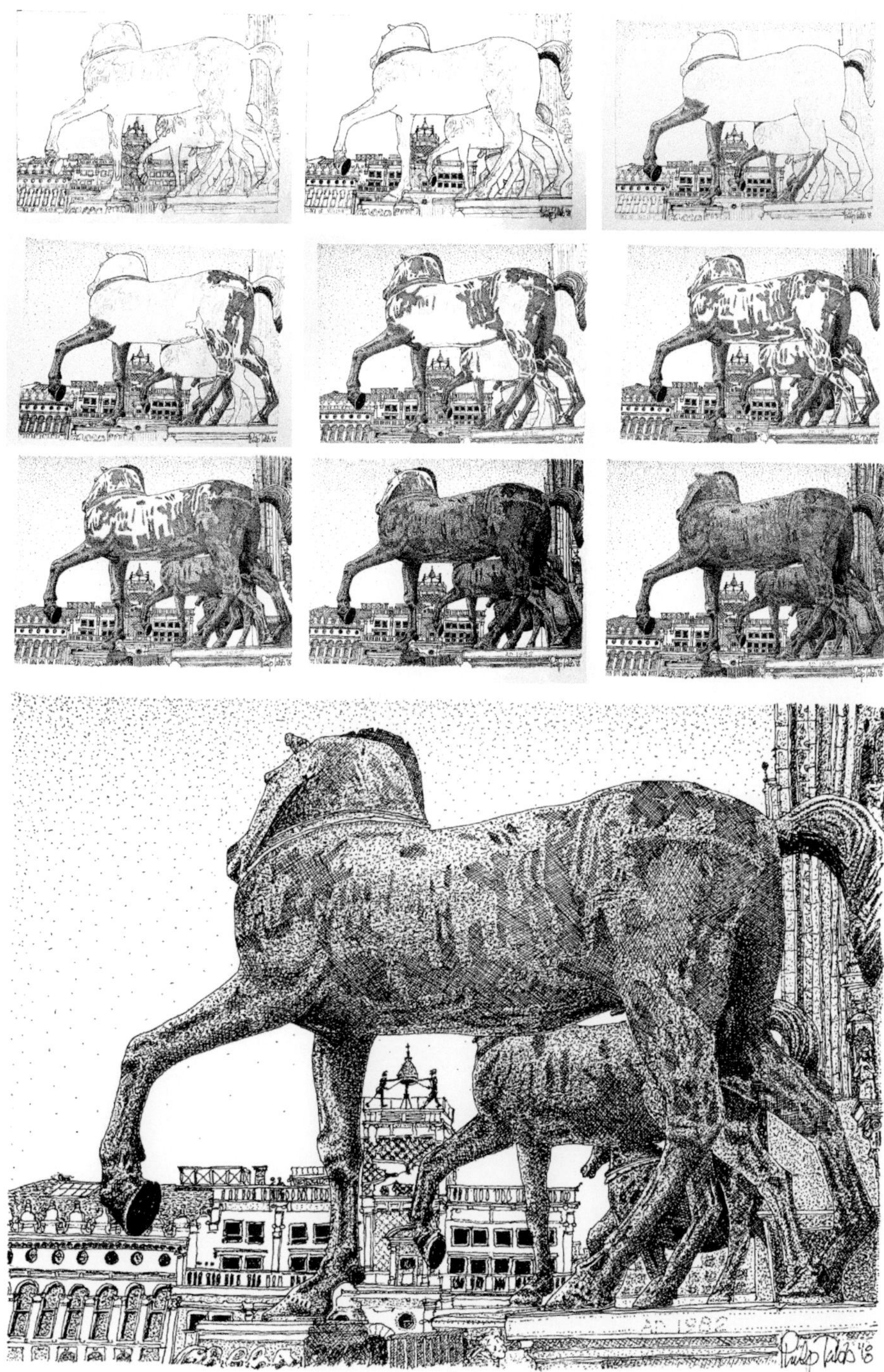

10.7
Mythic Landscapes Vignette: (a) Drawing Sequence for Triumphal Quadriga, Venice, Italy, (b) Final Drawing of Triumphal Quadriga, Venice, Italy

first horse is St. Mark's 15th-century clock tower, with the two great bronze figures striking the bell, and the winged lion on the north side of the piazza. The Micron pen dots are intended to create the illusion of form. The drawing process took nearly a month, accompanied by extended periods of presence, intense focus, mindfulness,

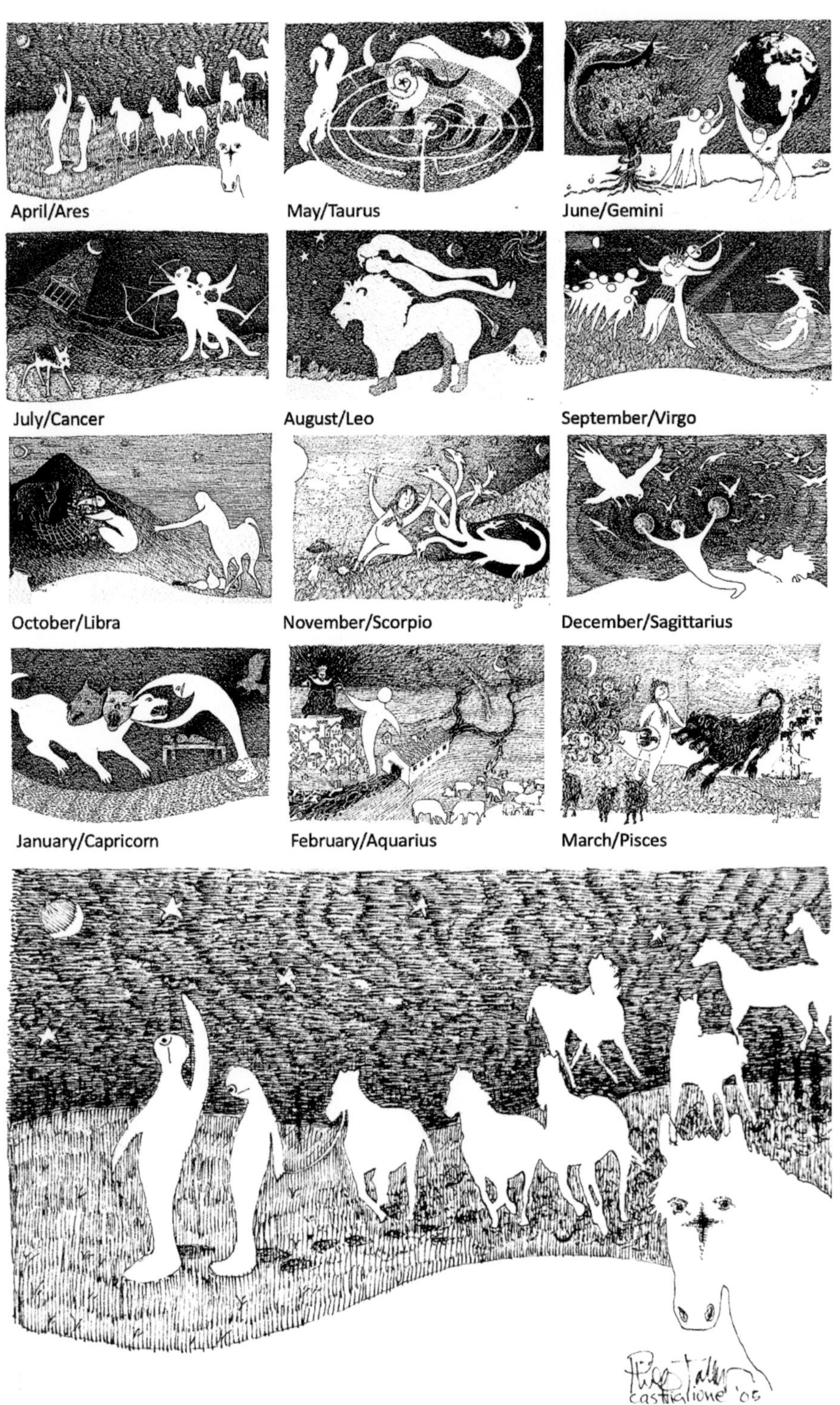

10.8 Labors of Hercules: (a) Twelve Labors Drawings, (b) April/Aries Labor

and contemplative practice (Figure 10.7a). From a spiritual wellness point of view, the process was serene, engaging, and personally rewarding.

Two books, *The Four Seasons and the Archangels*[13] and *The Labours of Hercules*,[14] informed my understanding of the idea of how we perceive yearly changes in climate and weather. These changes result from the Earth's rotation around the sun, as generally measured by the seasons of spring, summer, autumn, and winter. I was interested in how we physiologically and emotionally change throughout the year and how these changes might affect design, especially in architecture. Most modern buildings are hermetically sealed from weather and seasonal changes. However, many older, as well as newer, designs, especially biophilic designs, tend to interact more with the outside and, therefore, promote the experience of these seasonal changes.

I was also interested in a more detailed delineation of the seasons which was provided by a month-by-month division where each season was divided into three months. The Labors of Hercules provided a model for understanding the subtle changes through each season. For example, autumn occurs under the dominion of Archangel Michael and progresses through October (*Libra*), November (*Scorpio*), and, finally, December (*Sagittarius*). This period is characterized in the northern hemisphere by the life energy transferring from the extant ambient environment back into the Earth.

The changes from month to month are a more refined increment of change. For example, the changes from the summer solstice (June) through the vernal equinox (September) involve slowly getting hotter and then slightly cooler. The change is subtle, but perceptible when temperature changes are more dramatic in autumn and spring. Falling leaves and changing colors in autumn and budding trees and new growth in spring are tell-tale signs of these changes. For me, *The Labours of Hercules* was a mythic tale that helped me understand these subtle changes in the form of monthly stories or "labors" that Hercules was to perform (Figure 10.8a). Following is a brief summary of the first labor, associated with the spring equinox, and the story of emergent spring growth and energy. Refer to the image in Figure 10.8b for the labor "The Capture of the Man-Eating Mares." The image reflects Hercules' arrogance at the front of the procession, followed by his friend Abderis, who has tethered the wild mares just before they break away.

> Hercules and his friend, Abderis, went to a land ruled by Diomedes (son of Mars) who raised the horses and mares of war. After roaming the land, they cornered the mares and tethered them. Hercules overjoyed and confident, told Abderis to drive the horses to the Gate. Unable to control the horses, they turned on him and trampled him to death. Saddened by the event Hercules returned to the task of capturing the mares, but it took longer this time giving him time to reflect on his actions. Eventually Hercules caught the mares and carefully drove them to the Gate himself. This labour is related to powerful spring energy.[15]

This labor, given to him by his teacher, illustrates the first gate or test for Hercules. Overconfident and careless in achieving the task, Hercules experiences the death of his friend, Abderis. His lesson was to understand the power of thought, presence, and mindfulness in balance with the tremendous energy and powerful natural forces of spring. A fascinating benefit of reading these stories and creating the drawings was to relate them to what Alice Bailey called the keywords or keynotes. The keynote for this particular labor is "I come forth and from the plane of mind, I rule." This is to suggests that one should think before jumping into action. The keynotes were distillations of the lessons or wisdom associated with each task given to Hercules.[16] Beginning in spring and ending in winter, the path through each of the 12 months was a journey from ignorance and material desire to wisdom and spiritual achievement.[17] Additionally, this journey passed through the 12 signs of the Zodiac. The 12 keynotes for each of the labors, beginning with April and the Aries labor, describe the essence of the lessons learned by Hercules as follows:[18]

- **April labor (Aries)** – I come forth and from the plane of mind, I rule.
- **May labor (Taurus)** – I see, and, when the eye is opened, all is illuminated.
- **June labor (Gemini)** – I recognize my other self and, in the waning of that self, I grow and glow.
- **July labor (Cancer)** – I build a lighted house and therein dwell.
- **August labor (Leo)** – I am that, and that I am.
- **September labor (Virgo)** – I am the mother and the child, I God, I matter am.
- **October labor (Libra)** – I choose the way which leads between the two great lines of force.
- **November labor (Scorpio)** – Warrior am I and from the battle I emerge triumphant.
- **December labor (Sagittarius)** – I see the goal, I reach the goal, and then I see another.
- **January labor (Capricorn)** – Lost in light supernal, yet on that light I turn my back.
- **February labor (Aquarius)** – Water of life am I, poured forth for thirsty men.
- **March labor (Pisces)** – I leave my father's home and, turning back, I save.

The four seasons give me an allegoric understanding of the yearly cycle through the signs of the Zodiac as well as a broader understanding of climatic changes through each month, from the extremes of cold in winter to heat in summer (northern hemisphere). The equinoxes yield relatively milder weather that fluctuates between warm and cool temperatures. Growing up in Washington and Idaho and living in Texas gave me experiences of these extremes. The Druids saw dragons as a way of connecting us to the forces of nature and the seasons' turning.[19] Dragon lines or earth energy pathways originate from Chinese geomancy and feng shui and are seen to flow within the landscape. Dragon lines are considered crucial for harmonizing the environment with human activity.[20] The archangels, Michael, Gabriel, Raphael, and Uriel, represent a presiding presence over these periods of time. This seems more important in climatic contexts that experience more drastic seasonal changes. Most people live in temperate climate zones and are subject to these seasonal changes.

While these are mythic interpretations, they are reminders of the sacred nature of the Earth and the transformation undergone during a solar year. Architectural designs can reflect these changes and provide appropriate ways to respond and interact with them. These myth are also reminders of the spiritual nature of these changing cycles and special moments. My seasonal interactions within my own home serve a pragmatic and sustainable function, but also connect me to something larger than myself. It is important to connect the wisdom of these ancient myths to the presence of our own lives.

SUMMARY

What are important to take from these mythic landscapes are the design implications and the deeper meanings behind the stories. Also important is the way in which they help us understand spiritual wellness through spirit of place, orientation, noetic experiences, ritual and ceremony, momentary transcendence, life purpose, and connections to things greater than ourselves. Mythic landscapes are in part designed to create a vivid and lasting image in the minds of designers and building users and serve as reminders of the spiritual qualities of the spaces we occupy – sacred orientations, changes of the seasons, qualities of light, and the experiences of the spirit of place and wholeness.

The process of traveling to these interesting places, either literally or imaginatively, was both enriching and transformative. While sketching or painting, time stood still, and I became extremely connected to and present within each place. There appeared to be an invitation to escape into a world of the imagination and the landscapes of mythic realms. The spiritual wellness outcomes were difficult to define but certainly contributed to my sense of presence, experience of awe, an overwhelming feeling of calm, and a practice of mindfulness, focus, self-discipline, and appreciation of the landscapes and mythic stories that were the subjects of these exercises.

Drawing is an incredible process that can have spiritual and wellness benefits. Drawing and sketching can lower stress levels, trigger positive emotions, sharpen focus, and enhance creativity and the imagination. In addition to creativity, there are cognitive benefits that help release endorphins and help build neural pathways.[21] Sketching is an exercise for the hand, mind, and eyes, and the activity provides benefits that can be applied to many aspects of one's life.[22] It enhances fine motor skills and can boost self-esteem. I realize that everyone is not confident in drawing, but, regardless of comfort level, I highly recommend travel, learning about new places, particularly mythic ones, and sketching if you are so inclined. Mythic landscapes offer opportunities to see things differently in a bemusing, ordinary life. The value of mythic landscapes is in their reflection of and guidance on important values and character that, in the context of this work, support spiritual wellness. The combination of travel, drawing, and observing the mythic quality of a place deepens a sense of being present and unlocks a richer understanding of its layers and the resonance within oneself. And, finally, sketching new landscapes, capturing cultural experiences, or simply doodling during downtime can enhance the overall travel experience and can broaden perspectives of one's understanding of the world around us.

NOTES

1 Campbell, Joseph, *The Masks of God*, Vol. 1. (Hammondsworth, UK: Penguin Books, Primitive Mythology, 1991).
2 Tabb, Phillip James, Mythopoeia: Drawing, Myth and Remembering, *2A Magazine*, Spring 2011 issue, Dubai.
3 Samples, Robert, *The Metaphoric Mind: A Celebration of Creative Consciousness*, (Boston, MA: Addison Wesley, 1978).
4 Hamilton, Edith, & Huntington Cairns, Trans., *Plato: The Collected Dialogues*, Book VII, *The Republic* (Princeton: Princeton University Press, 1961), pp. 575–844.
5 Postman, Neil, *Amusing Ourselves to Death: Public Discourse in the Age of Show Business* (New York, NY: Penguin Books, 1985).
6 Thomas, Gail, Ed., Pegasus: When the Hoof Hits the Ground, in *The Muses* (Dallas, TX: Dallas Institute Publications, 1994).
7 Thomas, Gail, Ed., Pegasus: When the Hoof Hits the Ground, in *The Muses* (Dallas, TX: Dallas Institute Publications, 1994), p. 5.
8 Nisha Designs, Earth Dragon (accessed August 6, 2024), https://nishadesigns.com/portfolio/earth-dragon/.
9 Dragon lines or ley lines are the veins in the Earth that are intricate energy pathways that crisscross the globe, often running through and connecting ancient and sacred sites.
10 Steiner, Rudolf, *The Four Seasons and the Archangels* (London, UK: Rudolf Steiner Press, 1996).
11 Purucker, G. de, *The Four Sacred Seasons* (Pasadena, CA: Theosophical University Press, 1979).
12 Corvus Constellation (accessed November 20, 2024), https://www.constellation-guide.com/constellation-list/corvus-constellation/.
13 Steiner, Rudolf, *The Four Seasons and the Archangels* (London, UK: Rudolf Steiner Press, 1996).
14 Bailey, Alice A., *The Labours of Hercules* (New York, NY: Lucis, 1974).
15 Bailey, Alice A., *The Labours of Hercules* (New York, NY: Lucis, 1974), pp. 27–38.
16 The keynotes are statements that the Teacher said to Hercules upon his completing a labor and represent the essence of the wisdom embodied within the particular labor. The labors correspond to the changing of the seasons and the evolution of the year from March, the beginning of spring, through February, the end of winter. For designers, these lessons are reminders of how buildings and places may respond to the variable external natural progressions and conditions.
17 Bailey, Alice A., *The Labours of Hercules* (New York, NY: Lucis, 1974).
18 Bailey, Alice A., *The Labours of Hercules* (New York, NY: Lucis, 1974), pp. 210–214.
19 Nisha Designs, Earth Dragon (accessed August 6, 2024), https://nishadesigns.com/portfolio/earth-dragon/.
20 Dragon lines or ley lines are the veins in the Earth that are intricate energy pathways that crisscross the globe, often running through and connecting ancient and sacred sites.
21 Invaluable, The Science-Backed Ways That Sketch Drawing Improves Mood (accessed September 6, 2024), https://www.invaluable.com/blog/sketch-drawing/.
22 Invaluable, The Science-Backed Ways That Sketch Drawing Improves Mood (accessed September 6, 2024), https://www.invaluable.com/blog/sketch-drawing/.

11 NARRATIVE VIGNETTE 4

The Importance of Pilgrimages

INTRODUCTION

Pilgrimages are generally intentional journeys undertaken for spiritual purposes and directed to places of spiritual, historical, or health and wellness significance. According to the Global Wellness Institute, a pilgrimage is a metaphor for the path to enlightenment, engendering slow, meditative travel and facilitating deeper engagement with our surroundings to foster a sense of awe.[1] It also produces unexpected encounters with strangers that lead to a deeper perspective on the place of our "self" in a very big world. There are pilgrimages offering wellness programs that incorporate journeys between sacred sites.[2]

Pilgrimages across the world include the Hajj pilgrimage to Mecca, Saudi Arabia, pilgrimages to the Western Wall in Jerusalem, the Camino de Santiago, Spain, Kumano Kodo, Japan, Chartres Cathedral, France, and the Char Dham pilgrimage circuit. They even include treks to places such as Chimayo in New Mexico, the Aztec pyramids at Teotihuacan, Mexico, and the Inca Trail to Machu Picchu, Peru. According to Eric Wilson, pilgrimages are a revised wellness trend especially occurring worldwide following a post-pandemic gloom. Pilgrimages offer health benefits from walking and purposeful connections to nature and, more broadly, serve as a metaphor for a path to enlightenment. For example, nearly a half of a million people completed the Camino di Santiago, Spain, in 2023.[3] In contrast to seeking thrilling adventures or traveling to a mass tourism destination, the slow travel movement emphasizes greater personally meaningful experiences, such as seeking wellness or spiritual renewal.

THE IMPORTANCE OF PILGRIMAGES

Pilgrimages hold deep significance across cultures and throughout history, serving as powerful journeys of faith, devotion, and self-discovery.[4] While both traveling to other places and going on pilgrimages can broaden one's horizons, pilgrimages often offer a deeper, more transformative benefit rooted in spiritual or cultural significance, fostering a sense of inner reflection and connection that goes beyond the simple enjoyment of new experiences. The act of physically traveling to sacred or significant sites often involves sacrifice and intentionality, fostering a heightened sense of spiritual focus and connection to the divine or to deeply held beliefs. These journeys can provide solace, inspire reflection, and strengthen communal

DOI: 10.4324/9781003546085-11

bonds among fellow pilgrims who share similar aspirations. By stepping outside of ordinary life and immersing oneself in a sacred landscape or tradition, individuals often return from pilgrimages with a renewed sense of purpose, clarity, and a profound understanding of their place within a larger spiritual narrative. Even without religious connotations, non-religious pilgrimages to sites of natural beauty or historical, cultural, or personal significance can offer profound opportunities for reflection, connection, and a deeper understanding of oneself and the world.

My first pilgrimage was an architectural adventure to Notre-Dame du Haut in Ronchamp. The second was a spiritual pilgrimage to Normandy in 2000, when I traveled around a series of cathedral towns over a period of a week. My third pilgrimage was to the small fortified hill-hamlet of Castell di Gargonza in 2007, with my son David. On subsequent visits in 2009, 2011, and 2013, I took my design students from the Santa Chiara Study Centre there for the day. The visits included a guided tour, a lecture on the history of the place by the owner, time for drawing and water coloring, and lunch at their fabulous restaurant. My fourth was a visit to the Republic of Ireland in 2023 on a quest to experience sacred places so common there, which I refer to as a thin place adventure. In differing ways, each pilgrimage provided me opportunities to revisit the meaning and purpose in my life, to expand my perspective on the world, and to ultimately spark meaningful transformations. The pilgrimages' first task was facing apprehension, opening to the unknown, and finding meaning and applying it to my life.

THE NOTRE-DAME DU HAUT CHAPEL AT RONCHAMP PILGRIMAGE

During the 1960s, it was most architectural students' dream to visit Europe and, in particular, the chapel at Ronchamp. As an architect interested in extraordinary sacred architecture and landscapes, several places strongly called me. When I finally got to visit Europe, I could not wait to visit London, Paris, Barcelona, Stonehenge, St. Paul's Cathedral, the Sacré-Cœur, and Antonio Gaudí's Sagrada Família. And, finally, I was excited to visit Notre-Dame du Haut in Ronchamp, which I visited twice, in 1977 and 2007. The first time I visited Ronchamp, it took quite a while to drive to the town of Ronchamp in east-central France, about 200 miles from Paris and on the same latitude as Zurich. When I arrived in Ronchamp, I saw the chapel high on the Bourlémont hill overlooking the town, a beautiful site. It was not clear how to drive up to the chapel, but I was finally able to get there. Its form was heroic, and it had a confident presence, intellectual intrigue, spatial generosity, dramatic use of light, sparkling truncated glass windows, and creative use of concrete.

Ronchamp was designed by Le Corbusier in 1950, and construction was completed in 1955. Scholars consider the chapel one of his most important buildings, and it has been added to the UNESCO World Heritage List of internationally significant architectural sites. The overall sculptural form of the building is dynamic and creates "ineffable space," as architectural historian Charles Jencks calls it.[5] The anchor on the floor and crab-form roof visually connect the three primary defining walls into a single unity. The dark roof contrasted to the slightly distorted white walls and sensuous towers all respond to one another. Taken together, its expressionist form suggested a metaphoric whole – sometimes a monk's hood, a ship's prow, or, perhaps, even a celestial vessel (Figure 11.1b). According to Robert Coombs, the two towers to the west brought light down into two small prayer rooms, one dedicated to God the Father (southwest) and the other to the Virgin Mary (northwest). During rain, the large sloping roof directs the roof water to a single scupper located between these two towers, thereby creating a column of water falling into an oval pool below.[6] This column of water serves as a thin veil between the realm of the holy and the secular. This is an example of architecturalizing mythic or religious ideas.

The second time I visited Ronchamp, in July 2002, I was particularly intrigued by the religious and celestial references and I wanted to delve deeper into its symbolic layers. Architect Le Corbusier (known as Charles-Édouard Jeanneret prior to 1917), one of the most important architects of the 20th century, began designing the current chapel in about 1950. The name Le Corbusier derives from the meaning of "crow-like" and is associated with "observing from a bird's-eye view." Architectural historian Robert Coombs published a book in 2000 titled *Mystical Themes in Le Corbusier's Architecture in the Chapel Notre Dame Du Haut at Ronchamp: The Ronchamp Riddle.*[7] The book was based on research that he did at the Foundation Le Corbusier and the Bibliothèque Nationale in Paris. This work became an informative lens for my second visit.

Coombs speculated on several mystical concepts behind the design. First was an analysis of the south entrance door panel in which he reported that the lower black and white portion of the door was about the New Testament of the Bible, with the serpent located in the lower left. The red left hand in the central panels of the door represented Gabriel, and the slightly lower, blue right hand represented the Virgin Mary. The door is divided into eight panels. The left-side three panels are of the heavenly realm, while the right-side three panels are related to Mary and the secular realm. And, finally, the top panels show the sky and spiritual transformation, with the blue and red clouds co-joined (Figure 11.1a).

The second observation was that there were the three symbolic Marian programs (Annunciation, Assumption, and Coronation) formalized within the building form. You can produce the essence of the floor plan by drawing these three walls (Figure 11.1e). The Annunciation wall is to the west, joining what Coombs called the "God-the-Father tower or the Heavenly tower" and the "Mary tower." Between these two towers, on the roof, is a large scupper that funnels all the rainwater off the roof into an oval basin below – a metaphor for the Annunciation and the column between Gabriel and Mary (Figure 11.1d). The Assumption wall is the truncated wall to the south, with recessed windows (Figure 11.1c). To Coombs, the pattern of windows and the sparkling light which flowed through it reflected constellations in the sky. This was a metaphor for the Virgin Mary being "assumed" into the heavens. The two constellations he identified were Virgo above and Hydra below it. The Coronation wall is to the east and wraps around to the north, forming the Red or Christ tower. The east portion of the wall separates local religious services conducted on the inside from pilgrimage services that occur outside.

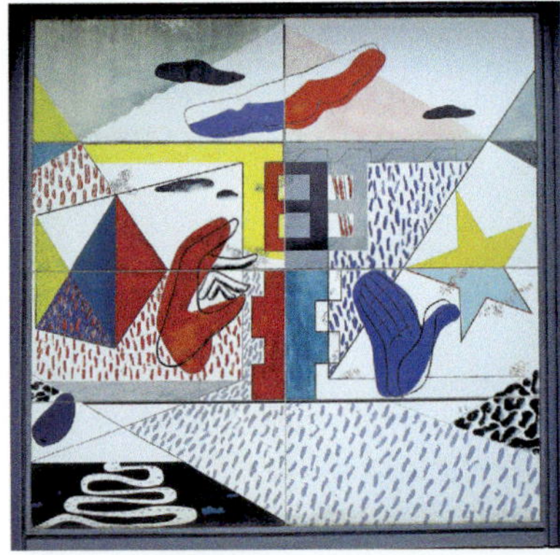

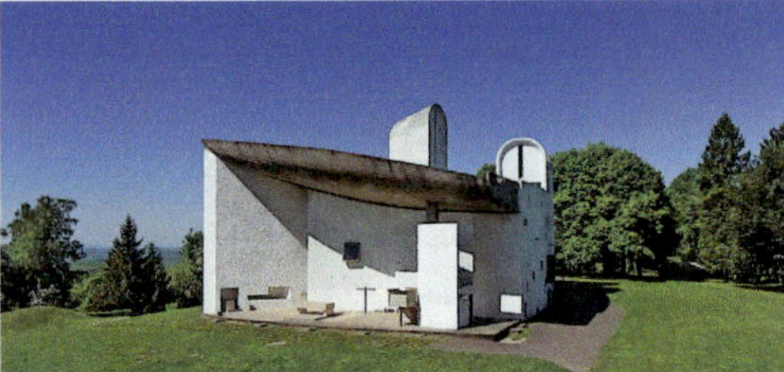

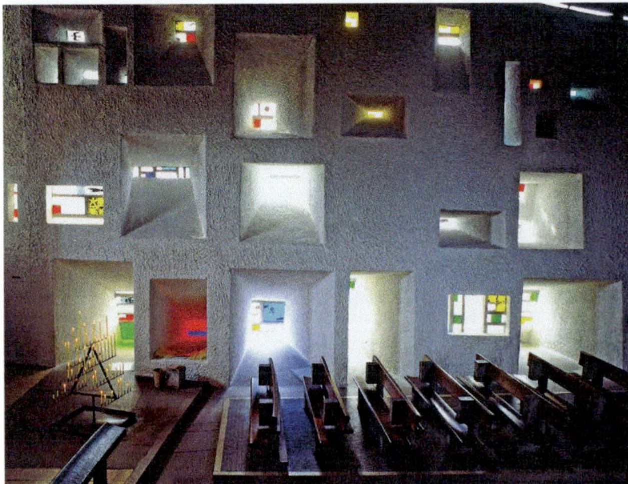

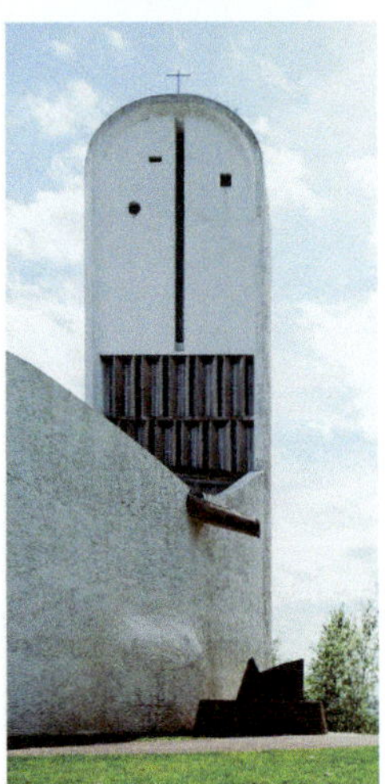

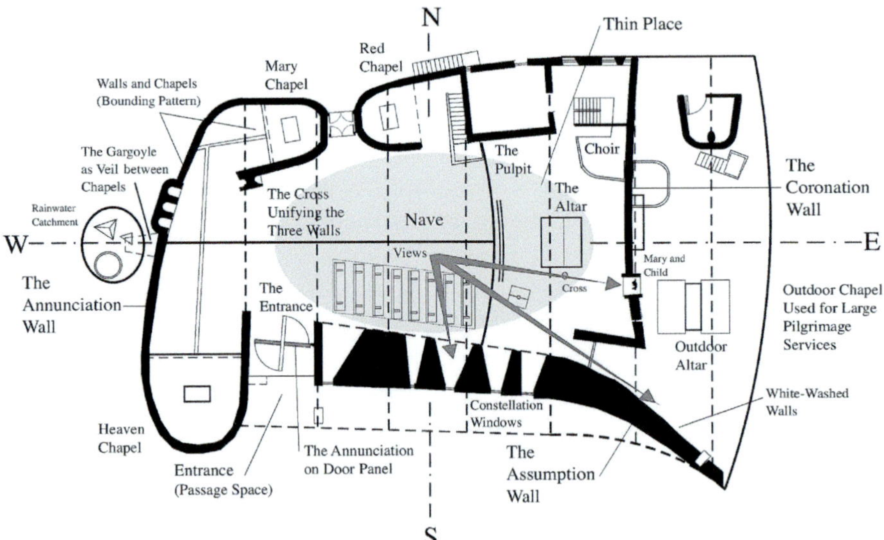

11.1
2002 Ronchamp Pilgrimage: (a) Ronchamp Chapel Entrance Door, (b) Ronchamp Chapel East View, (c) Ronchamp Chapel Interior, (d) the Scupper, (e) Ronchamp Chapel Plan

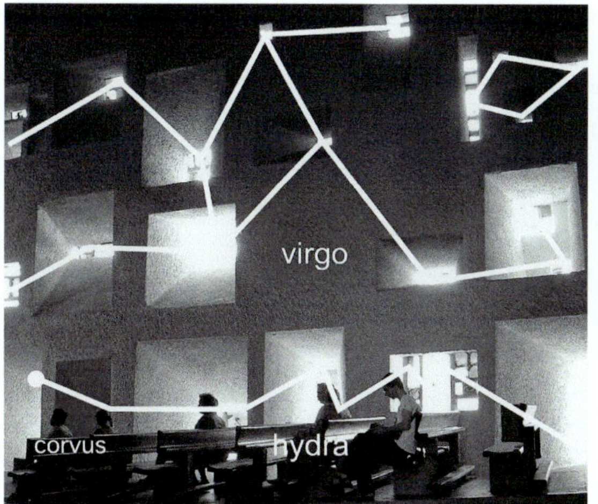

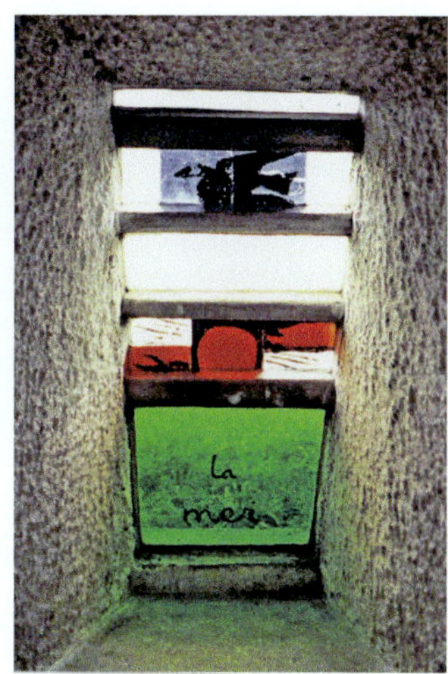

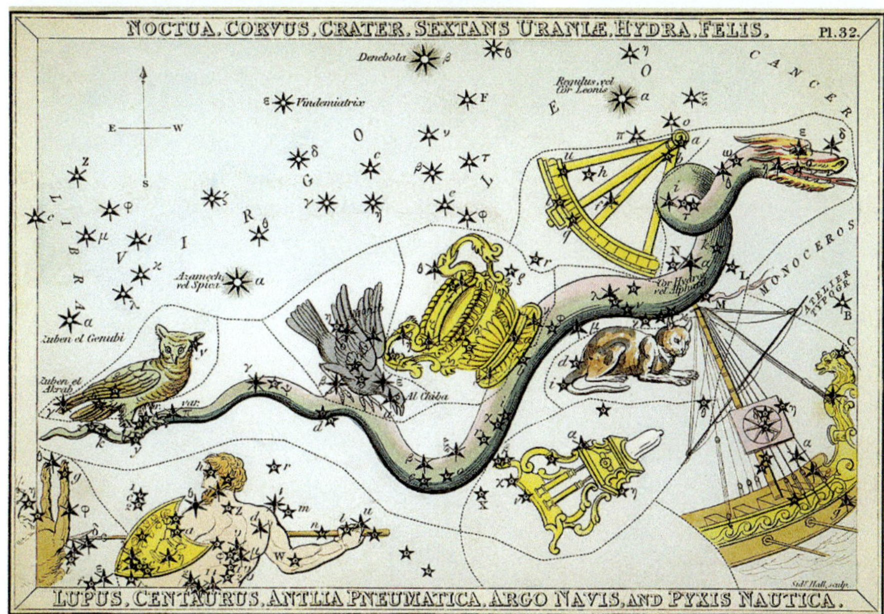

11.2 2002 Ronchamp Pilgrimage: (a) Virgo and Hydra Constellations Superimposed on the South Façade of Ronchamp Chapel, (b) the Corvus Window, (c) Painting of Hydra with Corvus on the Tail

Coombs's third speculation concerned the design of the south wall with its recessed and truncated glass windows. Rather than being an abstract composition of window patterns with no apparent meaning, Coombs referred to them as the constellations of Virgo and Hydra having examined drawings he obtained from Le Corbusier's archives.[8] He also showed several other elevations, with the constellations Libra (Le Corbusier's birth sign) and Corvus. I played around with the elevation of this south wall's interior and confirmed a plausible correspondence between the pattern of windows and the constellations of Virgo (on top) and Hydra (beneath). However, I showed the figures placed in opposite directions (Figure 11.2a).[9] This was purely speculation on my part, but I found the possibility of Le Corbusier's interest in astronomy interesting.

Even though we were not allowed to photograph inside the chapel, my son, David, videotaped the exterior as I surreptitiously photographed the interior where I was able to get images of the south wall and each of the punctuated glass windows. I created a photograph and drawing library of each of the south windows. In addition, the drawings of each window identified their colors and iconic subjects – sun, moon, stars, clouds, seas, flowers, and ravens. Located in the lower tier of the Assumption wall is a three-paneled colored window with green (water), a red sun, and a black raven. Assuming symbolic intentions by Le Corbusier, it is my observation and speculation that this lower glass window, located on the tail of the Hydra constellation, is Le Corbusier's signature for the building and homage to the raven and his namesake (Figure 11.2b).

My spiritual wellness experiences in this place were profound. I was uplifted emotionally and noetically. The pilgrimage, approach, entrance, and spatial experience inside filled me with the numinous. It transported me in a heavenly way, and I felt the tremendous spirit of place that elicited a more profound spiritual perspective. I transformed from a powerful sense of awe approaching and entering the chapel and then to a calm feeling of serenity after sitting quietly inside. I loved unfolding the mystery as Robert Coombs had done decades before. After I sat quietly in the chapel space, mesmerized by the flickering candelabra near the altar, I refocused my gaze on the Assumption wall and its joyful light pouring into the space. I recognized the Virgo and Hydra constellations and imagined them as real far beyond this chapel, beyond this small French town, and beyond our planet, far into the unknown in outer space. It was then that I really felt a powerful connection to something much more significant than myself.

CATHEDRAL TOWNS OF NORMANDY PILGRIMAGE

My second pilgrimage was to a series of cathedral towns in Normandy, France, in the summer of 2000. My week-long pilgrimage exported me to another world both literally and spiritually. I spoke only a little French and experienced the cathedral towns alone. I usually drove to a new town arriving early in the morning, excited to experience the place and wondering what might be revealed. Each day, after thoroughly observing and photographing, I typically found a local café in which to sit, reflect, and enjoy a wonderful French lunch or dinner with a glass of wine. I often chose a corner table, had a coffee, and wrote in my journal.

Traveling through northern France, I followed up on observations made by a French monk more than 75 years ago. He posited that a remarkable similarity existed between the location of a series of cathedral towns in Normandy and the configuration of the major stars in the constellation Virgo. This raises assorted questions about the interaction of religion and celestial cosmology in medieval France. In a 1966 book by Louis Carpentier, I discovered the identity of 12 cathedral towns, each of which has a major cathedral dedicated to the Virgin Mary (Notre Dame).[10] According to Carpentier, the major cathedral towns corresponded to the 12 major stars in the constellation: for example, Vindemiatrix for Amiens, Spica for Chartres, Porrima for Paris, and Zavijah for Rheims.[11] These constituted the focus of my attention on this brief trip. I visited the towns in a specific order – Amiens,

Rouen, Bayeux, Evreux, Sees, Alençon, Chartres, Paris, L'Épine, Rheims, and Laon. This order progressed in a counterclockwise direction, beginning in the north, or at the top of the constellation, and relates to the temporal movement of the plan of the Zodiac. I spent anywhere from half a day to a day and a half in these cathedral towns looking for signs in the building form and iconography within each cathedral. I thoroughly observed, photographed, journaled, and sketched, so that, subsequently, I might have sufficient data to confirm, refute, or at least test the monk's speculation that these cathedral towns formed the constellation Virgo.

Although these Gothic cathedrals were constructed around the same time (11th and 12th centuries) and dedicated to the Virgin Mary, I discovered there were slightly different designs and details in relation to their sacred signs, symbols, ornamentations, and icons. For example, Amiens Cathedral has a southeast orientation of the apse and cruciform plan, symmetrical towers, a strong sense of entry, and abstract ornamentation (Figure 11.3c). Rouen Cathedral has a southeast orientation of its apse, toward the winter sunrise, and three different towers, and the one on the left has a large gold sun (Figure 11.3e). Bayeux Cathedral has a southeast orientation of its apse, symmetrical towers, and abstract ornamentation (Figure 11.3d). Evreux Cathedral, has a northeast orientation of its cruciform plan and unsymmetrical towers, with the right one unfinished (Figure 11.3f). Paris's Notre Dame Cathedral has a southeast orientation of its cruciform plan, symmetrical, unfinished towers, and Virgin Mary and angel iconography (Figure 11.3h). And Rheims Cathedral has a northeast orientation of its apse and cruciform plan and many angels on all façades (Figure 11.3g).[12] Other cathedral towns I visited, not illustrated here, included Beauvais (dedicated to St. Peter), La Ferté-Macé, Alençon, Sées, L'Épine, and Laon.

Chartres proved the most intriguing cathedral of all. Louis Carpentier stated that, on the map, Chartres corresponded to the brightest star in the Virgo constellation, Spica.[13] In depictions of the Virgo figure, this star is located at the center of a shaft of wheat being held in her hand. While approaching Chartres, I noticed wheat fields surrounding it, and I can see why it was considered to be in the "breadbasket" of France (Figure 11.4c). This seemed to emphasize the importance of this place, so I spent a couple of days there. Some of what I observed from the visit included the fascinating differences between the lunar (south) and solar (north) towers, built centuries apart. The labyrinth was beautiful, worn, and full of soulfulness. According to John James, the labyrinth was not a maze but, rather, a single way to the six-petal rose in the center and an important symbol of man's way to God on Earth.[14] At the crossing of the cruciform plan of the cathedral, I noticed the color difference between the southern and northern portals. The north portal had an iconic program dedicated to the Virgin Mary, with a dominant blueish color. The south portal's iconic program was dedicated to Christ, with a dominant reddish color. I did not visit the Sous Terre crypt housing the holy relic (*Sancta Camisa*), Mary's veil, speculated to have been worn at Christ's birth, for which Chartres is most known as a pilgrimage site (Figure 11.5c). This holy relic was given as a gift from the Byzantine Empress Irene to Charlemagne and later given to Chartres by King Charles the Bald in 876. I did manage a photograph from the main cathedral into the adjacent St. Piat's Chapel.

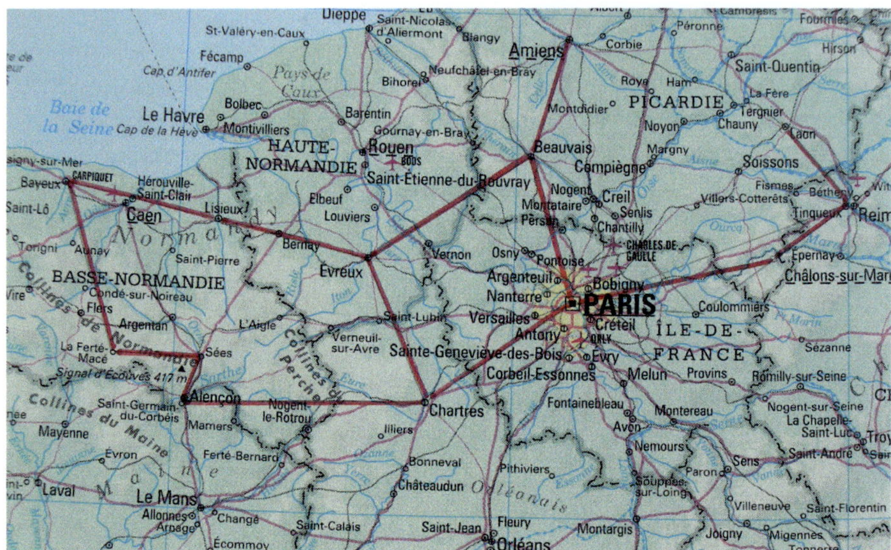

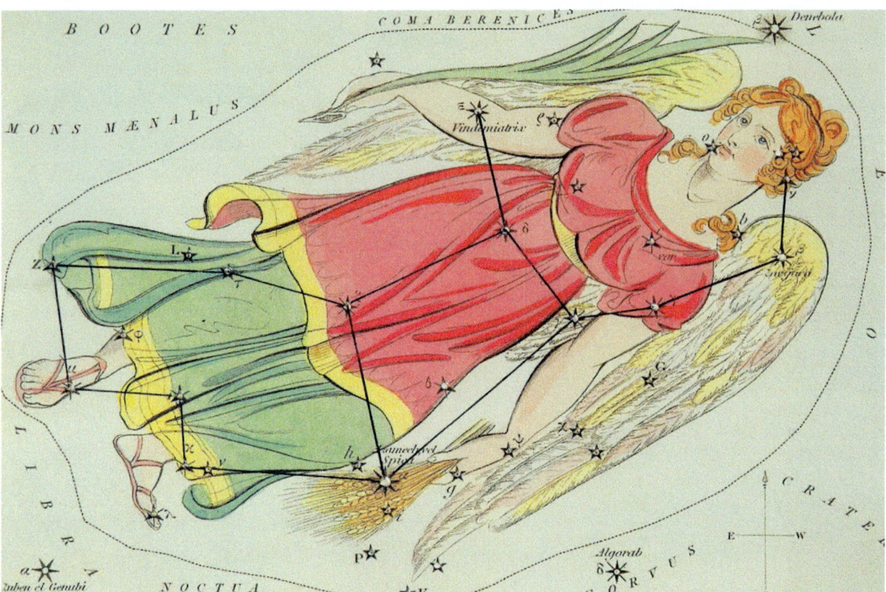

11.3
2000 Normandy Cathedral Town Pilgrimage: (a) Normandy, France, Map, (b) Painting of Virgo Constellation, (c) Amiens Cathedral, (d) Bayeux Cathedral, (e) Rouen Cathedral, (f) Evreux Cathedral, (g) Rheims, Cathedral, (h) Notre Dame, Paris, Cathedral

The cathedral was oriented with the apse pointing to the northeast and the sunrise in summer. The drawings of Chartres indicate that the plan shape seemed to be organized by the vesica piscis or √3 geometry, as seen in Figure 11.4a, and a correspondence between the plan and west elevation, Figure 11.4b. The western stained-glass rose window aligns with the labyrinth. The lunar tower height corresponds with the center of the roundpoint in the apse. The solar tower marks the circumference of the roundpoint. The lunar south tower and spire, completed in 1221 at the end of the initial rebuilding, had an iconic symbolism and are simple and elegant in design. They represent the feminine principle. The solar spire, built

11.3
(Continued)

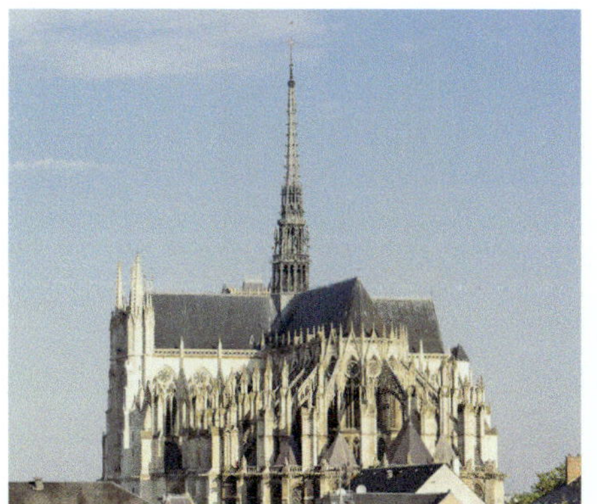

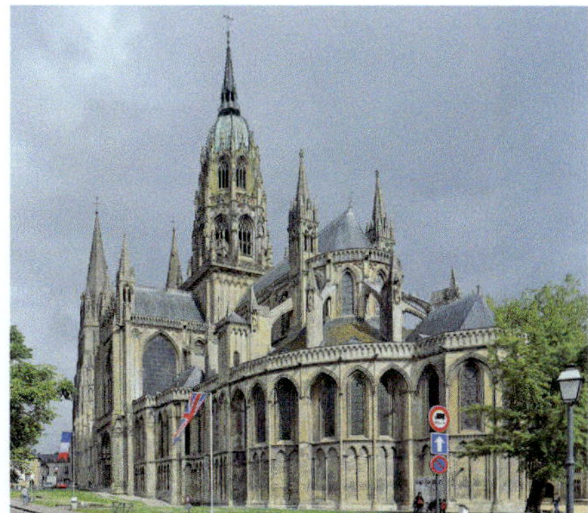

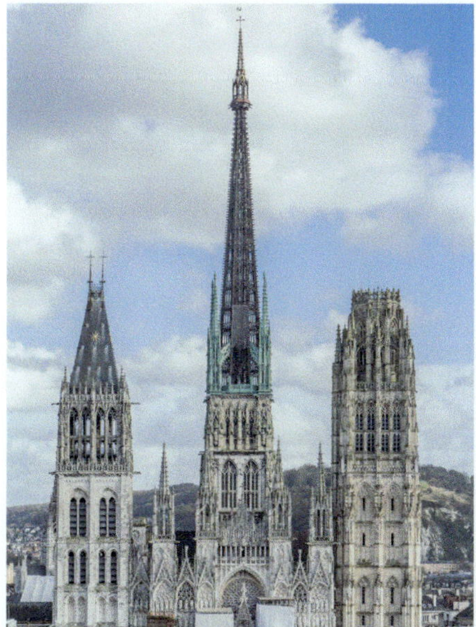

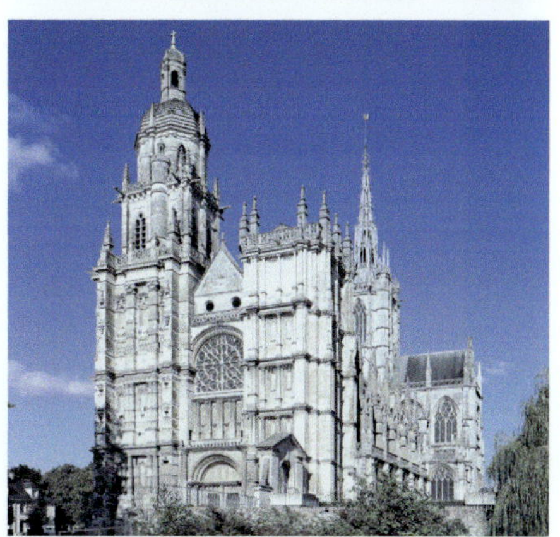

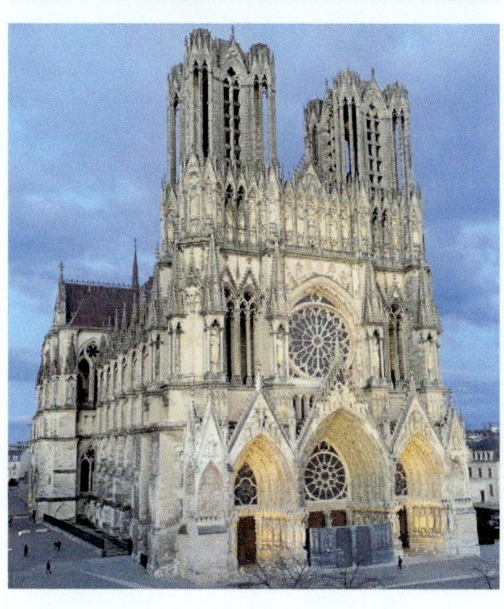

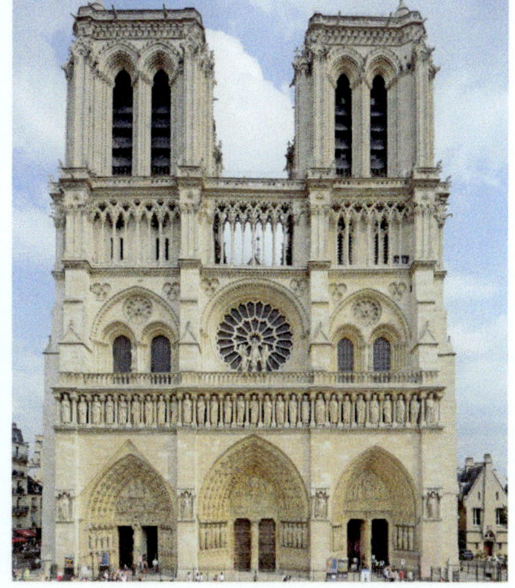

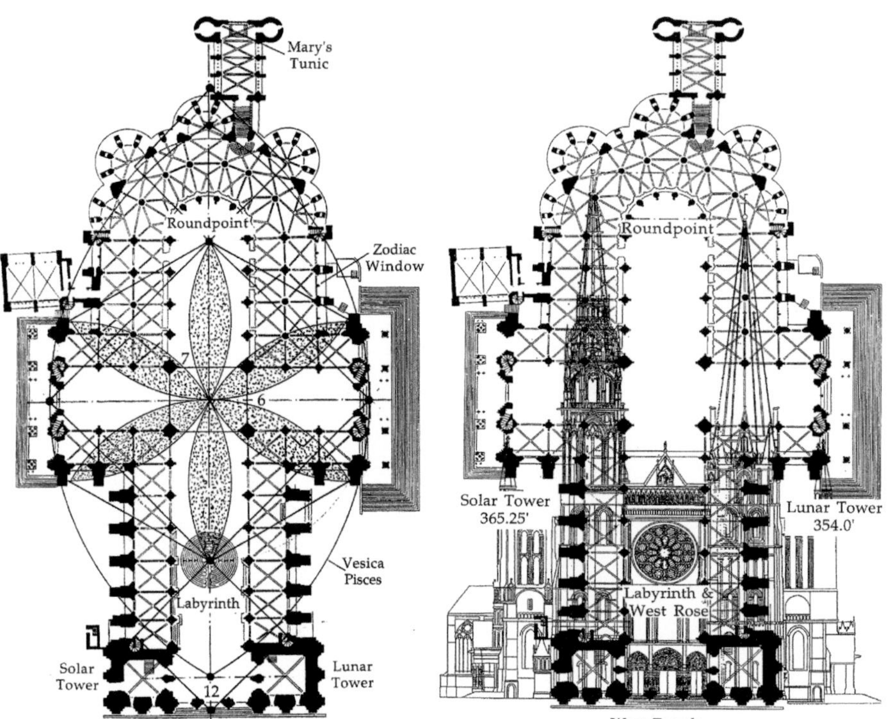

11.4 Chartres Cathedral: (a) Chartres Cathedral Plan with Vesica Piscis, (b) Plan with West Façade Superimposed

three centuries later (1513), rises higher, has far more expressive ornate detailing, and represents the masculine principle. According to René Querido, in his book *The Golden Age of Chartres: The Teachings of a Mystery School and the Eternal Feminine*, the location was originally a sacred Druid site and later an early Christian site. After the fire of 1194, the reconstruction embodied the Seven Liberal Arts, astronomy, and Christian programs in the form of the building, anticipating a shift of knowledge centers from religious to secular university sites such as Bologna and Padua in Italy and Paris in France.[15] Its physical form became a concretization of the knowledge and wisdom of these times. It was important for me to have these lenses to understand the place.

While I was painting the west façade in the courtyard, I met a young French woman, Blandina, who was also sketching. We spoke for a while and shared our work. She grew up in Chartres and had worked in the Chartres archive. Now living in Paris, she had just sat for her exams in Classics. She invited me to join her to ascend the King's Tower, and we had four distinct 20-minute conversations as we walked around the tower balcony. On the south side, she spoke of her upbringing in Chartres and pointed out her home and things and places from her childhood. She said, "I am a Virgo," words that stayed with me the rest of my trip. She also said how she loved the wind. On the east side, I spoke of my understanding of Archangel Michael, who stood prominently over the intersection of the crossing roof form, and his influence on the building. On the north side, she spoke of her work at the archive, and, finally, on the west side, she recalled the suicide of a

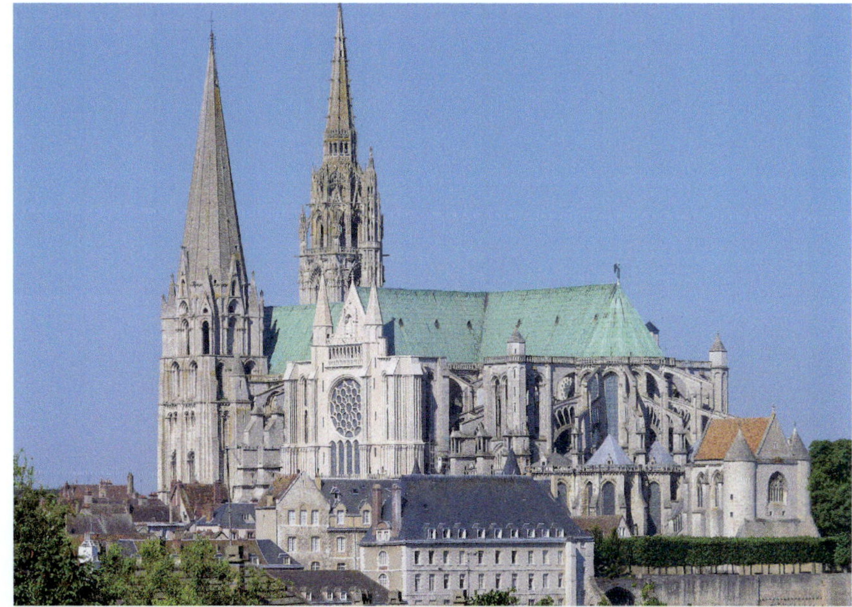

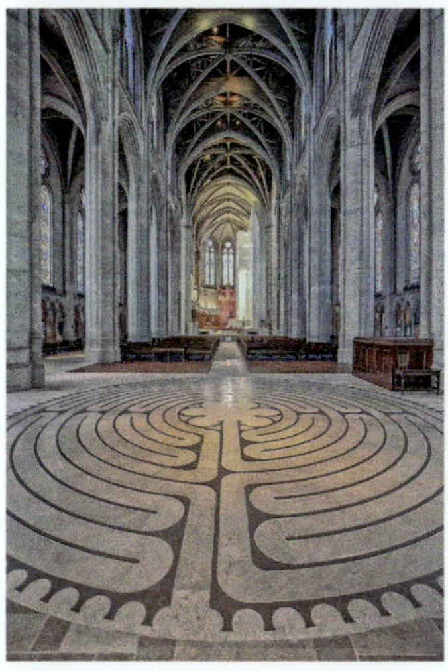

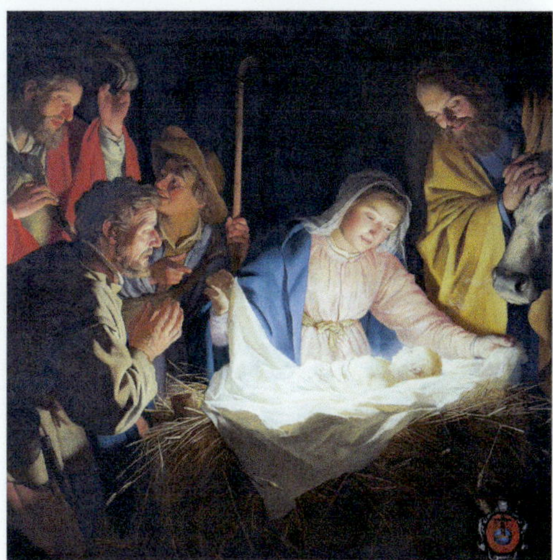

11.5
(a) Chartres Cathedral, (b) Chartres Interior, (c) Adoration of the Shepherds

resident who jumped off the tower. She mentioned how she says a prayer every time she walks by there. On that sad note, we descended, and she went to the train station to go back to Paris. I spent the rest of the afternoon photographing and preparing for my drive to the next cathedral town.

Driving to Paris after Chartres and Alençon proved to be quite stressful as traffic was hectic closer to the city center. I eventually found the quaint Saint Paul's Hotel on the Left Bank. It had one room left, and I had a quiet evening. The next morning, I awoke early and headed to Notre Dame Cathedral. There was a full moon on this Sunday morning. I entered the Place du Parvis Notre-Dame, and it was empty. I photographed a little and began walking around the cathedral when I noticed a small group of people going through the north-side entrance. So I followed. We were ushered into the small ambulatory chapel near the tip of the nave where a Sunday morning service was being held. The service was in French, and it was poignant seeing the morning light and listening to the hymns in French. An hour later, we were escorted out the front doors into the plaza, and that hour had made such a difference with the increasing activity.

The plaza was filled with visitors and tourists. Many were in groups with their group leaders holding their guide flags. I moved to the center and waited for a sign. I noticed the pigeons swooping in and out, and the homeless sitting on perimeter benches were entirely in tune with the place. They saw every movement. The tourists, however, seemed to be oblivious to the goings-on of the place as they were obsessed with taking selfies with their iPads and cell phones. After waiting awhile, I closed my eyes and felt this breeze wash past my face. I recalled Blandina's words about the wind, so this was a sign to move on. Off to Rheims and Laon I went.

Throughout the journey, there were spiritual, iconographic, and architectural differences between the cathedrals, although each was constructed at a slightly different time and each was dedicated to the Virgin Mary. Some cathedrals were entirely free of symbolism and iconic references, such as Evreux. In contrast, others were full of angels, such as Rheims, references to the Virgin Mary, such as Paris, or celestial references, such as Rouen and Chartres. I experienced the spiritual wellness dimension as a cocktail of differing experiences, partly defined by the overall journey and partly created by my individual visits. In regard to the original purpose of the pilgrimage to confirm the intention of the cathedral towns and their echo of the constellation Virgo, I remained unsure, but did believe there was a strong correspondence.

While I found little direct evidence linking the cathedrals to the Virgo constellation, except the dedication to the Virgin Mary, I did discover the beauty of the Beauce plains and the cathedral towns it contained. The wellness benefits consisted of positive physical and emotional experiences. The spiritual experiences that undoubtedly stood out were the feeling of how these magnificent buildings, their histories, and their celestial references were so much greater than mine. The incredible sense of place and a feeling of oneness accompanied these feelings. Traveling alone like that was very reflective, allowing for experiences and time for reflection. For me, the huge take-aways of this week-long sojourn were the realization of an inner tuition and reunited self-love.

CASTELLO DI GARGONZA PILGRIMAGE

My third pilgrimage was to Castello di Gargonza, located in Tuscany, Italy, about 16 miles (25 kilometers) from Cortona as the crow flies. A great deal further by car is the little *borgo* of Gargonza, just up the secluded Apennine hill from Monte San Savino. I first became aware of this borgo, or hamlet, in a delightful book by Donlyn Lyndon and Charles Moore called *Chambers for a Memory Palace.*[16] In fact, on the cover of this book is a small watercolor of a bird's-eye view of the borgo, and I have always wanted to visit this place. When I went on my first faculty-led semester in

Castiglion Fiorentino, I discovered that Gargonza was a short drive on the other side of the Val di Chana. With my teaching in Italy every other year from 2005 through 2017, I visited it several times each trip and became quite familiar with its history and quality, beginning with my first visit there in 2007.

More like a castle whose walls contain a perfectly preserved 13th-century hamlet, Castello di Gargonza is a 1,235-acre (500-hectare) estate with a dominating prospect above the Val di Chiana from the center of its wooded site.[17] It was known as an agricultural community dedicated to cultivating the forest as well as wool production. Later, it became a sharecropper farm with 33 farmers' homes. It was also an outpost settlement a day's horseback ride from Siena. The hamlet had a parish church, school, an olive oil mill, stables, and bread ovens. It is reported that, owing to a power shift, Dante Alighieri and other Florentine exiles fled to the hamlet around 1302 in the wake of the trouble between the Guelphs and the Ghibellines.[18] The village proper is surrounded by tapered stone walls and cypress trees.

The hamlet of Gargonza is completely car-free. Vehicles can drive around the exterior of the outside walls to the main entrance for deliveries and drop-off; however, there are only stone and gravel footpaths inside. The central plaza is located near the northeast boundary wall and is defined by the Romanesque church of St. Tiburzio and Susanna, the castle tower, hotel reception, and several of the attached cottages. The plaza's center is a small village green with stone pavers and surrounds a stone well. Spread throughout the village are gardens and green areas. A vegetable garden exists along the southeastern edge, within the fortified walls. Stands of cypress trees line the southwestern side of the village. While the hamlet's center is quite dense, the village is generally punctuated by many green areas and open spaces.

Managers of the hamlet often accompanied my students and me during our class visits. They took us to the conference facilities and many of the apartments. At the end of each class visit, we went to the La Torre di Gargonza Restaurant, the crown jewel of Castello di Gargonza, open for guests of the local bed and breakfast. The stone and wood interior has a high vaulted ceiling, and the dining areas are surrounded by large windows with commanding views of the surrounding forests and hills. A large, protected terrace accommodates up to 170 guests and boasts breathtaking views framed by the cypress trees. The menu consisted of authentic traditional Tuscan cuisine and local wines. The long Italian lunch was a highlight of our visit.

Our trips to Gargonza usually happened near the end of the semester, and we would take a large bus across the valley and up the hills where we could park in a remote lot a short walk from the village. The approach and experience had every element of a sacred pilgrimage. We walked around the perimeter canted-stone foundation wall counterclockwise until we reached the other side. A small stone opening in the wall led to an entrance passage space leading to a small plaza with a well in its center. Surrounding the plaza was the church, the guest facilities, and the tower. On one of our visits, we had the opportunity to meet with the count who owned the hamlet, and he gave us background information on the history of Gargonza and his intentions for its revitalization.

After spending time in Gargonza, I could see how its location was strategic. Later, it became a sharecropper farm with 33 farmers' homes. It was also an outpost settlement a day's horseback ride from Siena. High on the Arezzo hills, there were clear views east to the Val di Chiana where invaders from the south might have come. Its protected boundary and high perch served both as a strong prospect and a refuge. It was like a hidden treasure. I often went alone and spent the morning sketching and photographing. While there, I could tune into its presence, solitude, and silence. It was such a contemplative place, and I enjoyed many intimate moments there.

In 2015, I had the opportunity to go up in a Cessna airplane with Paolo Barucchieri, the program director at Santa Chiara where I taught. It was an unbelievable experience, flying several hundred feet above the beautiful Italian landscapes. The hill towns and small villages had such interesting geometry and patterns. I photographed as much as I could while on the plane. One of the photos I took was of Gargonza (Figure 11.6a), which shows the heart-shaped plan, tower, gridded interior cottages, and the stone retaining wall around its perimeter. Figure 11.6b shows one of my student classes in the Lemon Garden, and Figure 11.6c shows the octagonal well beneath the tower.

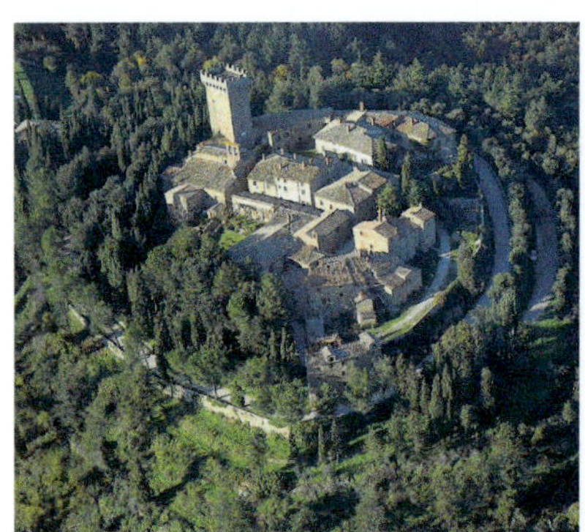

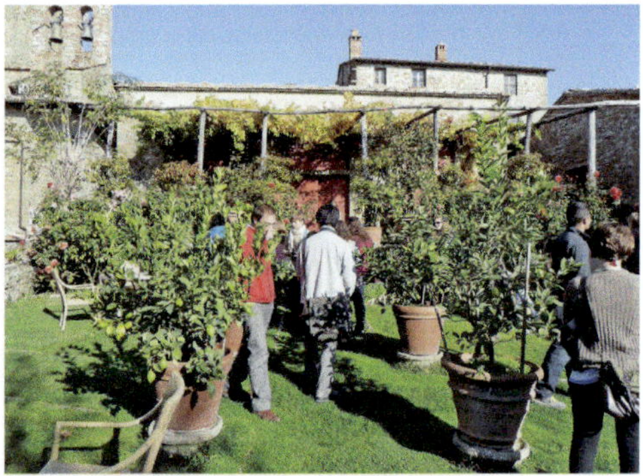

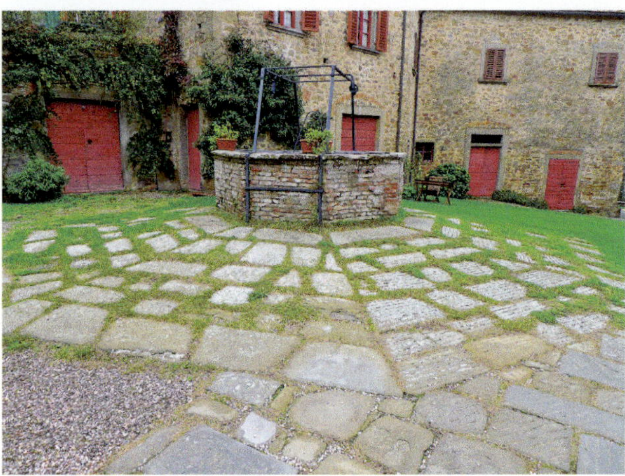

11.6
2011 Italy Pilgrimage: (a) Castello di Gargonza Aerial View, (b) Lemon Tree Garden, (c) Hamlet Well, (d) Castello di Gargonza Hamlet Plan, (e) Cottage 1, (f) Cottage 2

11.6 (Continued)

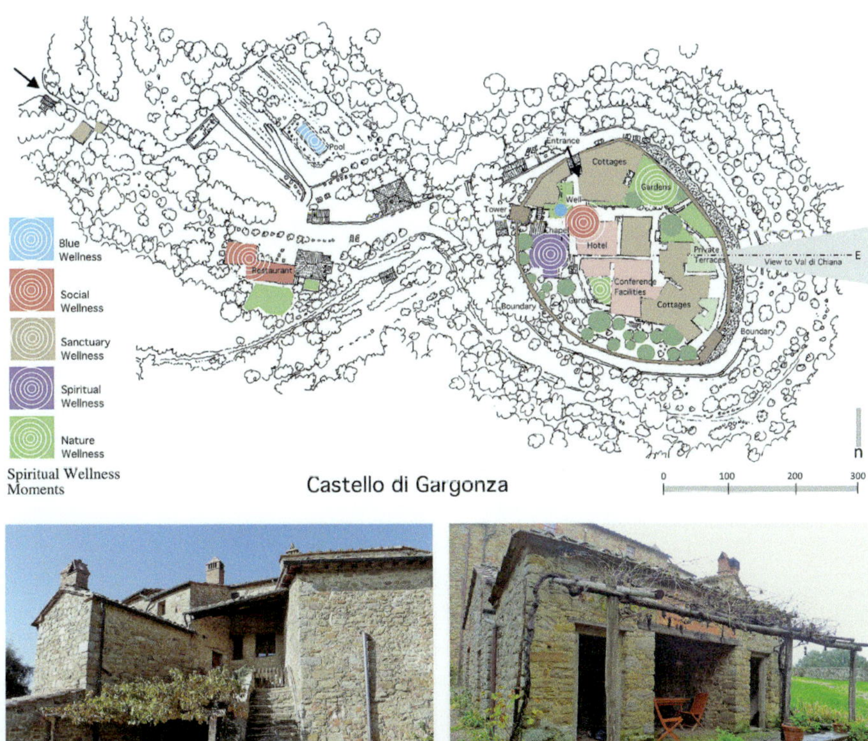

There are many health, wellness, and spiritual qualities in experiencing and reflecting on Castello di Gargonza as a personal pilgrimage site. Although the plan has an enclosing boundary, dominant tower, and strong prospect, I found the place extremely introspective (Figure 11.6d). It has a quiet demeanor that supports reflection. While physically it gave me a sense of calmness, I did feel a gentle spirit and something greater than myself. I felt awe and wonder, but not in the vast sense described by Dasher Keltner.[19] For me, the awe experiences at Castello di Gargonza came as a strong sense that activated all my senses, giving me a sense of place. There was a vast sense of silence. The experience was elevational, yet grounded. Afterward, I felt the need to accommodate or make sense of the experience, which usually occurred with the 45-minute drive back to the study centre. I loved sharing this place with family and friends as it appeared like a jewel tucked away in the Tuscan hills.

IRELAND'S WEST PENINSULA PILGRIMAGE

My fourth pilgrimage was in the fall of 2022 to Skellig Michael Island, Ireland. This pilgrimage was to understand thin places and sacred landscapes better. I visited

Ireland to experience firsthand the thin places that reportedly existed there – in some cases, for millennia. In addition, I wanted to take photographs, carry out research, and conduct interviews with residents as background for my book *Thin Place Design*.[20] For several months before my trip, I solicited recommendations from neighbors, friends, and colleagues worldwide about places to visit in Ireland. I received suggestions for dozens of places to experience and formulated my week-long itinerary. I traveled around a large circle in the Republic of Ireland to Dublin, Newgrange, Cork, Dingle, the Skellig Islands, Limerick, the Hill of Uisneach, St. Patrick's Holy Well, and many pubs and other thin places along the way. In and around Dingle, I went on a tour of thin places including several beehive hillforts, the Dunbeg Fort, Gallarus Oratory, Cill Mhaoilchéadair, the Blasket Centre, Dunquin Pier, the Holy Stone, and Brandon Head. I experienced each site, individually photographed them, identified the physical patterns and characteristics each possessed, and brought a daybook for documenting my emotional responses.

It was the Gallarus Oratory, an Early Christian church on the Dingle Peninsula, that began to speak to me in thin place terms with its geometric order, sacred form, and beautiful stonework preserved as it may have been 1,500 years ago. It was considered a spiritual oratory or place of prayer for foreigners and pilgrims wanting sanctuary and for others before departing to the Americas. It is considered dark and confining inside a narrow, thick threshold. A small opening facing east seemed to be a window back to the past. After prayers, visitors would proceed outside, moving westward from relative darkness to openness, fresh air, and light.

From my own experiences of this Gallarus Oratory, many questions arose. As a historical landmark, it functions as such with admissions, information video, and a tour bus car park. Consequently, hundreds of people visit the site simultaneously throughout the day, making it difficult to experience as a sacred space. Once the place was vacated and quiet, I could edit out the noise and my previous encounters with the space, pause, and reenter it. After tuning into the space, I could experience the difference between inside the space, its cut sandstone threshold, and back again to the outside enclosure space. I felt a stillness and serenity inside the space and a real compression at the threshold. When I emerged from the building, the sea breeze refreshingly hit my face, and the sky's light was uplifting. I felt propelled into a sense of optimism and joy. My back was to the past as I faced the future. This was undoubtedly a numinous experience for me (Figure 11.7).

Just to the north of the oratory is a burial site of a flattened stone bed, and at the eastern edge of it is a small standing red stone as a marker for the space. A circle with an equal-armed cross is at the curved top embedded in the stone. This iconographic symbol has fascinated me for years since I came across a similar one at the top of St. Francis Cathedral in Assisi, Italy. It has several meanings, including the union of heaven and earth, male and female, and, as an astronomical symbol, it represents the planet Earth. The circle represents the round celestial sky, and the cross represents the four corners of the known world. Finding it at Gallarus Oratory was a revelation, as I experienced this edge of the world and heaven beyond as a spiritual wellness thin place (Figure 11.7a).

Skellig Islands are two small but steep rocky islands lying off the west coast of Ireland. They are also a UNESCO World Heritage Site. The larger of the two islands, with its characteristic two peaks, is known as Skellig Michael, Great Skellig, or Skellig Rock Great. According to Horn, Marshall, and Rourke, these peaks were once conquered by people "who searched fearlessly for ways to reach God."[21] Located at the western edge of the land mass at the tip of Iveragh Peninsula, about 12 kilometers from Bolus Head, Ireland, is this early monastery that served as a place of refuge and repentance, a place to withdraw from civilization that was void of distractions, where the monks could live solitary lives of prayer.

My visit to the island in 2022 culminated in my experiences of thin places in Ireland. For visitors, the island is beautiful and wonder-filled. Its relative remoteness evokes mystery and fascination around the filming of the final scene of *Star Wars: A Force Awakens*, which was filmed in part there. Part of the intention of this monastic way of life was refuge, sanctuary, and the ability to experience silence and to experience a closer connection to God. This silence, for both predecessors and present-day visitors, may be the language of spirit, God, or the unknown. The rough life had compensations. Asceticism gave an intensified response to the smell of flowers, the texture of stone, the feel of rain or sun or wind, and the flight of birds. When the monks emerged from their dark cells, their spirits must have lifted to heights rarefied beyond our experience.[22] The hike up the mountain to the ridge called "Christ's Saddle" and further up to the monastery site was challenging (Figure 11.7a). The stone path was narrow, steep in places, and often without handrails (Figure 11.7b). I felt at home once I arrived at the monastery site, which had beehive huts, a garden, and a small plaza. I laid down in one of the beehive huts, closed my eyes, and imagined what it might have felt like to have lived there among all that beauty (Figure 11.7d). For a moment, experiences of the numinous, awe, serenity, unity, and the unknown consumed me. Spiritual wellness involved my sense and recollection of the larger universe of which I was a part, the peacefulness of this place, my connections to family, friends, and community, and a feeling of wholeness.

The Early Christian monastery and beehive-like stone huts remain intimate in scale. I was curious to find that this island was occupied as a spiritual and religious site in the 6th-century monastery. This was eight centuries before Christopher Columbus discovered that the Earth was not flat, even though earlier Greek philosophers mentioned the concept of a spherical Earth. This suggests that these early Skellig residents sought the end of the Earth and a place closest to the unknown.[23] Survival was extremely difficult for the 12 monks. Still, the spiritual wellness they likely experienced must have been profound. Refer to Figure 11.7e for the Skellig Michael site plan indicating the location of the hermitage, monastery, and spiritual wellness attributes. The hermitage located on the southeastern edge has prospect to incoming visitors and protection from the northerly winds. The hermitage located on the south peak and facing west must have been truly transformative and seen as the nearest place on Earth to the unknown or heaven.

Preserving cultural and historical sites and natural reserves is important as a memory of the past and lessons for the future. Although many, if not most during

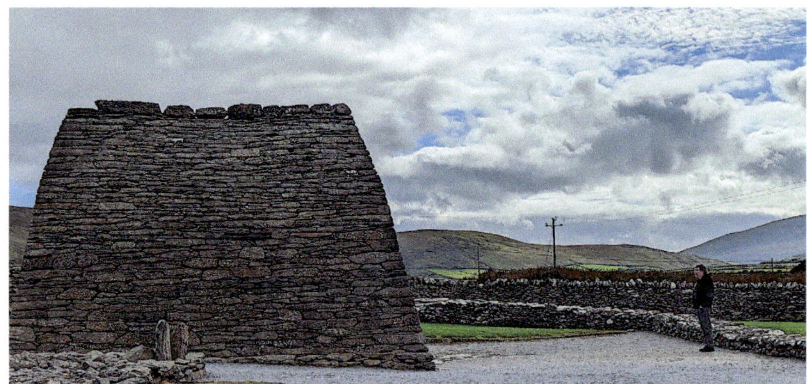

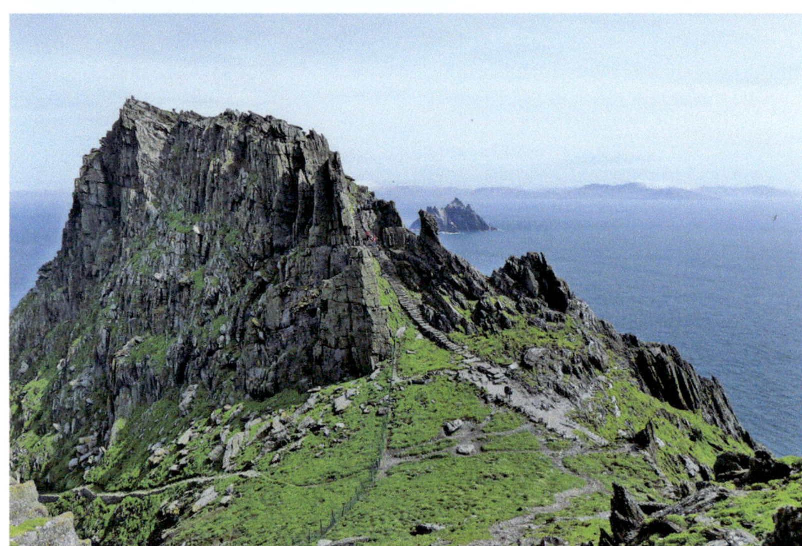

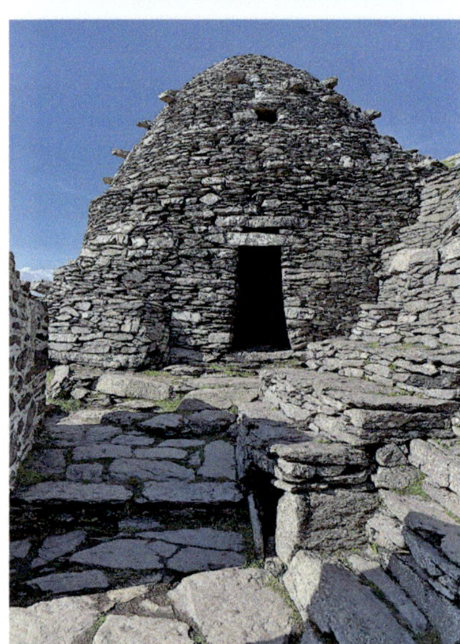

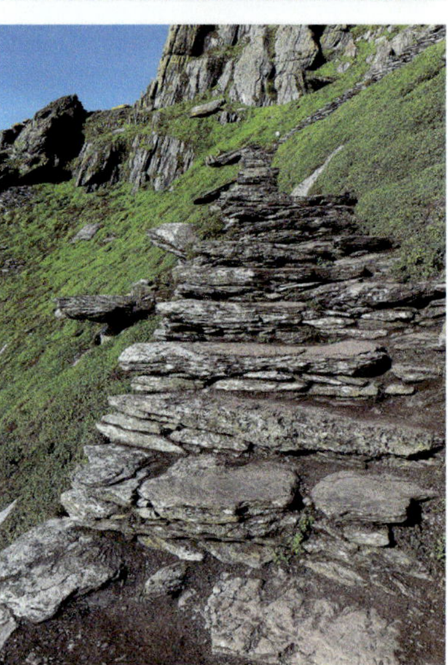

11.7
2022 Ireland Pilgrimage: (a) Gallarus Oratory, Dingle Peninsula, Ireland, (b) Skellig Michael, Christ's Saddle, (c) Skellig Michael, Pathway to Monastery, (d) Skellig Michael, Monastic Beehive Dwellings, (e) Skellig Michael Site Plan

11.7
(Continued)

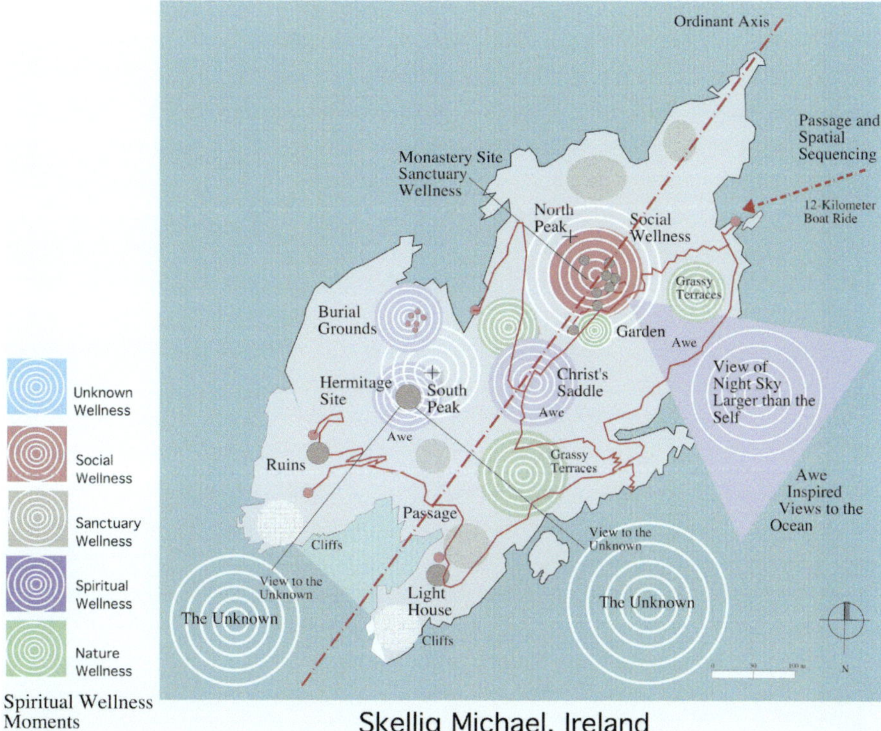

Skellig Michael, Ireland

their prime use, did initially function as thin places, such as community wells, burial grounds, fortified settlements, stone calendrical monuments, chapels, and even ancient cities, today they appear to be frozen in time. The physical remains are still there, but the vital activities that seemed so intertwined with them seem to have vanished. They no longer function as thin places as originally intended. During my travels, it became clear that Irish thin places were changing in function and place with time. I did not encounter the end of the rainbow, leprechauns, Pan, angels, nature spirits, or other spiritual apparitions. However, I did receive moments of spiritual wellness from the hearts of the Irish people I met and a connection to the land they call Eire.

SUMMARY

Pilgrimages have been practiced for centuries and provide a host of physical, mental, emotional, and spiritual benefits. The value of these pilgrimages contributed to my spiritual wellness. They were physical, emotional, social, and environmental and, above all, were transformative, feeding my intellectual and spiritual growth. They were generally outside my everyday life routines, and I was rejuvenated from visiting and analyzing Ronchamp Chapel and discovering its hidden treasures. Trekking around the cathedral towns of Normandy as a visitor in a foreign country, I surrendered to the unexpected and became open. My pilgrimage to Ireland was rich as I searched for the mysteries of sacred places and the spirit that occupies them. I was inspired and humbled. Taken together, these pilgrimages added to my understanding of sacred places and the role that planning and architecture can play within them, especially toward spiritual wellness.

There are numerous spiritual and wellness outcomes of pilgrimages, and many involve experiences within the built environment. For me, these included the extraordinary architecture and mysteries of the chapel at Ronchamp, the many Normandy towns and cathedrals dedicated to the Virgin Mary, the enchanting borgo of Castello di Gargonza, and the monastery at Skellig Michael in Ireland. Each of these created awe experiences and, with them, a strong sense of presence, meaningful orientations, noetic experiences, feelings of unity, and a sense of participation, ritual, and ceremony with the spirit of each place. These experiences served a sense of purpose and, at times, moments of sanctuary and transcendence. Indeed, they formed connections and feelings about things greater than myself. The wellness outcomes were stress-relieving, calming, filled with positive emotions, and accompanied by enriched experiences of nature and extraordinary architecture. While travel to new places is invigorating and healthy, pilgrimages offer a journey with another layer of experience. Going on a pilgrimage is not simply visiting a place to admire its treasures of nature, art, or history; it means going beyond and stepping out of ourselves to encounter and experience spiritual connections, renewal, and wellness. Pilgrimages are important in the journey to experience something different, beyond our daily routines, that further awakens spiritual wellness.

NOTES

1. Global Wellness Institute, Wellness Travel Trend: Pilgrimages and "Epic Walks" See Further Momentum (accessed August 28, 2024), https://www.globalwellnesssummit.com/trendium/wellness-travel-trend-pilgrimages-and-epic-walks-see-further-momentum/.
2. McGroarty, Beth, Global Wellness Summit Releases 10 Wellness Trends for 2024 (accessed July 5, 2024), https://www.globalwellnesssummit.com/press/press-releases/gws-trends-2024/.
3. Wilson, Eric, Global Wellness Trend: The Power of the Pilgrimage (accessed October 20, 2024), https://www.youtube.com/watch?v=2bjDG7J6Phg.
4. Wikipedia, Pilgrimage (accessed April 4, 2025), https://en.wikipedia.org/wiki/Pilgrimage.
5. Charles Jencks, *Le Corbusier and the Tragic View of Architecture* (London, UK: Allen Lane, 1973), pp. 151–153.
6. Coombs, Robert, *Mystical Themes in Le Corbusier's Architecture in the Chapel Notre Dame Du Haut at Ronchamp: The Ronchamp Riddle* (Lewiston, NY: Edwin Mellin Press, 2000), p. 29.
7. Coombs, Robert, *Mystical Themes in Le Corbusier's Architecture in the Chapel Notre Dame Du Haut at Ronchamp: The Ronchamp Riddle* (Lewiston, NY: Edwin Mellin Press, 2000).
8. The drawings for the constellation Virgo superimposed on Ronchamp's south wall are from Robert Coombs's book, obtained from drawings by Le Corbusier, the Artists Right Society (ARS) NY/ADAGP,PARIS/F. In this image, the Virgo constellation's shape and position on the south wall were adapted by Phillip Tabb.
9. When analyzing the constellation wall at Ronchamp, I used several astronomy books that contained images of the dominant stars in Virgo and Hydra. They also showed the Grail and Corvus constellations. I drew these constellations on tracing paper and superimposed them onto the interior of the south wall. With Virgo above and Hydra below, I was able to

associate the position of Corvus with the lower-left stained-glass panel with the raven on it. My speculation is that this window is the signature of Le Corbusier on this building.

10 Carpentier, Louis, *The Mysteries of Chartres Cathedral*, trans. Ronald Fraser (Wellingborough, UK: Avon Books, 1966), pp. 27–29.

11 Carpentier, Louis, *The Mysteries of Chartres Cathedral*, trans. Ronald Fraser (Wellingborough, UK: Avon Books, 1966), p. 29.

12 The details about these Gothic Normandy cathedrals were taken from my personal journal written in July 2000.

13 Carpentier, Louis, *The Mysteries of Chartres Cathedral*, trans. Ronald Fraser (Wellingborough, UK: Avon Books, 1966).

14 James, John, *The Master Masons of Chartres* (Sydney, AU: West Grinstead, 1990), pp. 86–87.

15 Querido, René, *The Golden Age of Chartres: The Teachings of a Mystery School and the Eternal Feminine* (Hudson, NY: Anthroposophic Press, 1987).

16 Lyndon, Donlyn, & Charles Moore, *Chambers for a Memory Palace* (Cambridge, MA: Massachusetts Institute of Technology Press, 1994).

17 Tabb, Phillip James, *Biophilic Urbanism: Designing Resilient Communities for the Future* (New York, NY: Routledge, 2021), pp. 77–84.

18 Tabb, Phillip James, *Biophilic Urbanism: Designing Resilient Communities for the Future* (New York, NY: Routledge, 2021), pp. 77–84.

19 Keltner, D.J., & J. Haidt, Approaching Awe, a Moral, Spiritual, and Aesthetic Emotion. *Cognition and Emotion*, 17(2), 2003, 297–314. https://doi.org/10.1080/02699930302297 (accessed October 4, 2021).

20 Tabb, Phillip James, *Thin Place Design: Architecture of the Numinous* (New York, NY: Routledge, 2019).

21 Horn, Walter, J.W. Marshall, & G.D. Rourke, The Forgotten Hermitage of Skellig Michael (accessed July 28, 2022), https://publishing.cdlib.org/ucpressebooks/view?docId=ft1d5nb0gb;chunk.id=0;doc.view=print.

22 Horn, Walter, J.W. Marshall, & G.D. Rourke, The Forgotten Hermitage of Skellig Michael (accessed July 28, 2022), https://publishing.cdlib.org/ucpressebooks/view?docId=ft1d5nb0gb;chunk.id=0;doc.view=print.

23 Replogle Globes, The Shape of the Earth: Who Discovered the Fact that the Earth Is Spherical? (accessed October 27, 2023), https://replogleglobes.com/blog/the-shape-of-the-earth-who-discovered-the-fact-that-the-earth-is-spherical/.

12 SPIRITUAL WELLNESS SUMMARY

INTRODUCTION

Woven throughout the discussion of spiritual wellness are certain concepts that, when combined, form a rich vision and pathway toward both individual and planetary health and well-being. They include connectedness, wholeness, purposefulness, transcendence, renewal, luminosity, and things larger and more significant than ourselves. At the individual scale, they can contribute to high-level wellness. And, at a larger scale, they form a powerful vision and principles that could positively shape our future. It is interesting that the extremes of these two scales are intrinsically connected. Most will agree that individual wellness is a desirable outcome. The spiritual dimension, however, elevates wellness and broadens inclusiveness. Spiritual wellness is being linked to something greater than yourself and having a set of values, principles, morals, and beliefs that provide a sense of purpose and meaning in life. Then, spiritual wellness becomes a guide to actions.

Wellness and spiritual strategies can be applied at all scales. Yet, post-pandemic, wellness has been targeted to what is being called home-centric wellness hubs and the wellness real estate market. This includes digital-first work cultures, homebody lifestyles, out-of-clinic care, and technological advances.[1] The home is not simply a place of shelter and refuge. Still, there is a shift in consumer attitudes about the function of living spaces augmented as multifaceted domestic health hubs supporting health, wellness, and spiritual renewal.

THE NEED FOR EVERYDAY SPIRITUAL WELLNESS

In contrast to extraordinary architecture and intentional pilgrimages, spiritual wellness is experienced more casually through everyday life. Everyday sacred places are often domestic, individualistic, personal, authorless, soulful, and normative and are often developed from lived everyday experiences. This chapter recounts my everyday experiences within my community, home, and walled-in garden. My home is a modest size of 1,650 square feet, with three bedrooms, office-studio, living and dining areas, kitchen, and three bathrooms. The most interesting features are the vaulted roof, with 35 photovoltaic panels, the Tesla Powerwall, and the large south-facing passive solar glazing and distributed thermal mass.

My home was the realization of a dream I have had for a long time. I wanted a place of my own that was modest in scale, sustainable, connected to nature,

DOI: 10.4324/9781003546085-12

and responsive to my daily routines. In addition, I wanted a unique design, something that fit into the Crossroads neighborhood – a design that was an appropriate representation of the community's town plan. I wanted it to be special, but not self-indulgent. In 2009, I purchased a beautiful, wooded estate lot in the Crossroads neighborhood with all white houses. I completed the design and built a scale model in Italy in 2013 (Figure 12.1a). Construction began in 2015 and was completed in 2016. I do not have a conventional lawn. My home is sited at the edge of the Crossroads neighborhood and is on an estate lot, surrounded by southern pine, sweet gum, white oak, and red maple trees. In my detached garage is an electric car, golf cart, and Vespa scooter, all charged by my photovoltaic system.

The quality of light in my home is changeable, especially from early morning throughout the day and from season to season, when the sun's position in the sky rises and lowers. In winter, the low-altitude sunlight passes into the house, penetrating deep into the northern rooms. In summer, the roof overhang and operable shades block the high-altitude sun. Sunlight reflecting off the surface of the garden pond shimmers in rhythmic waves. At certain times of the year, warm, mystical light casts shadows through the nine windows onto my interior walls. Additionally, there is an intentional light intensity gradient that decreases in natural light from the light-filled living space to the south, to the office and library with moderate light in the center, and to the more cave-like master bedroom to the north.

Woods surround my house on three sides, and to the east is a neighbor's house, close enough for them to see into my home. I do have a stand of trees between us, but I am more exposed in winter when the leaves are gone. To create privacy and not have to use shutters that block out the light, I commissioned my neighbor, Diane Cuttler, to make two stained-glass pieces to be placed in the two windows on that side of my house (Figures 12.1g and 12.1h). I chose the

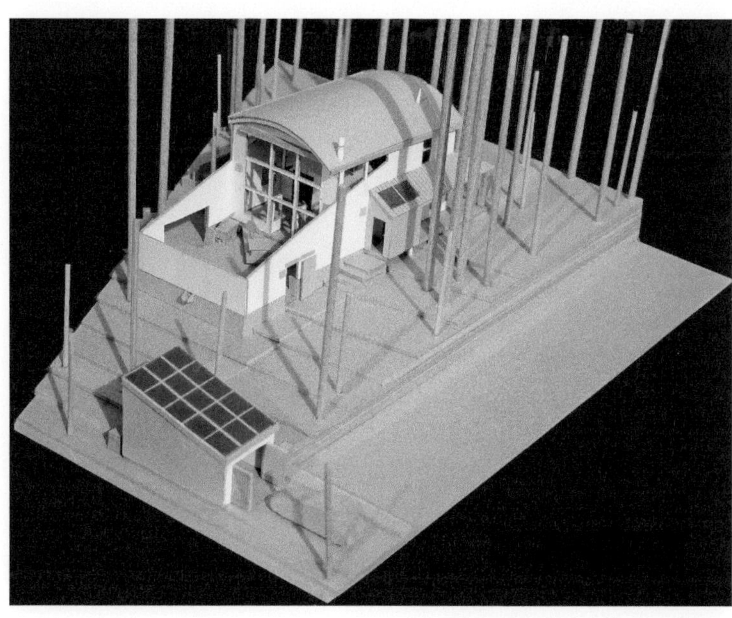

12.1
Tabb Residence: (a) Architectural Model, (b) North–South Section, (c) Garden View, (d) Interior View, (e) Rear View and Matini Hut, (f) Walled-in Garden, (g) Stained-Glass Mandala, (h) Stained-Glass Spiral

Photovoltaic Array
Flue
Air Handler
Glu-lams
Vaulted Roof
Screen
Fan
Solar Wall
Bathroom
Living Space
Garden Wall
Cross-Ventilation
Sliding Gate
The Maple Trees
Master Bedroom
Walled-in Garden
Deck
Trellis
Boardwalk
Insulated Slab
Thermal Mass
Pool
Natural Grade
Geothermal System

North-South Building Section
N 0 2 4 8

12.1
(Continued)

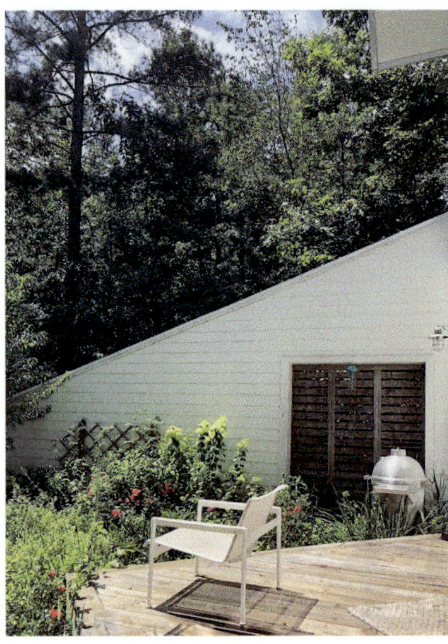

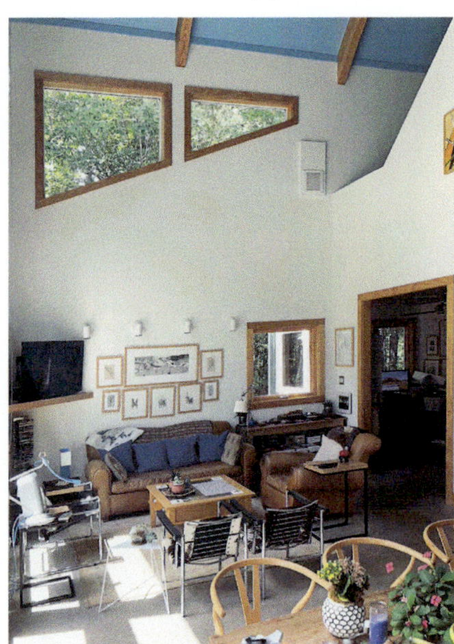

geometry of expanding and radiating squares and four √2 spirals, and she did the rest. Together, they provide visual privacy while allowing natural light to delight my internal spaces, especially in the mornings.

The night view from the garden features the nine-fold window arrangement, the triangular balcony walls, and the blue-painted vaulted ceiling (Figure 12.2a). In the photograph, my home office is on the ground level to the left, and the kitchen is to the right. Above, on the upper floor, are two guest bedrooms that overlook the main living space. When I took the photograph, it was Christmas, so a large Frasier pine was in the center, next to the French doors. Note that all the walls are painted white because of the numerous framed drawings and paintings. Each room ceiling has a different color – the main space is blue, the office is maroon, the kitchen is yellow, the master bedroom is indigo, and the master bath is moss green. I love preparing food in my kitchen, with herbs and a few vegetables from my garden and others from Serenbe Farms.

12.1
(Continued)

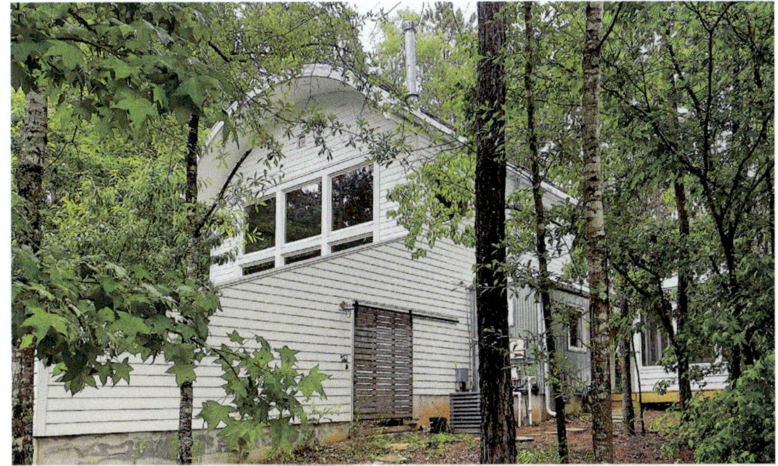

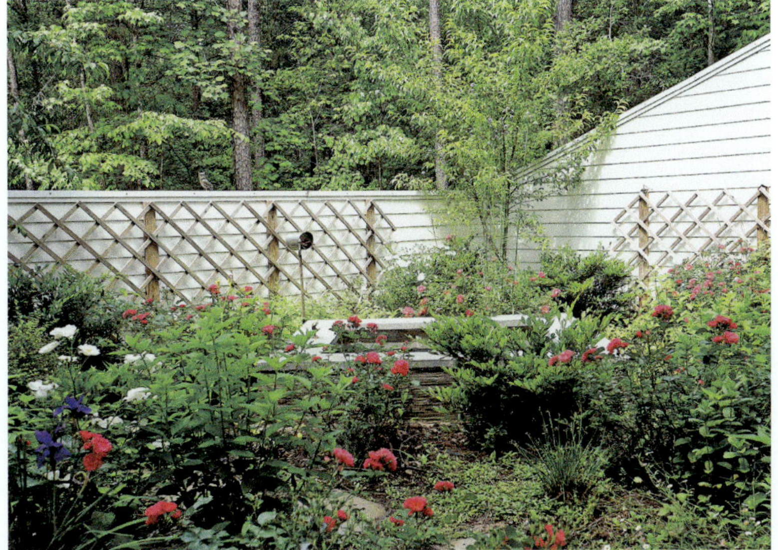

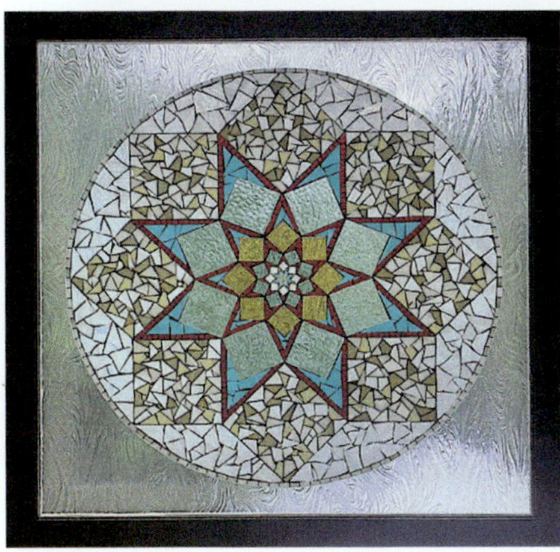

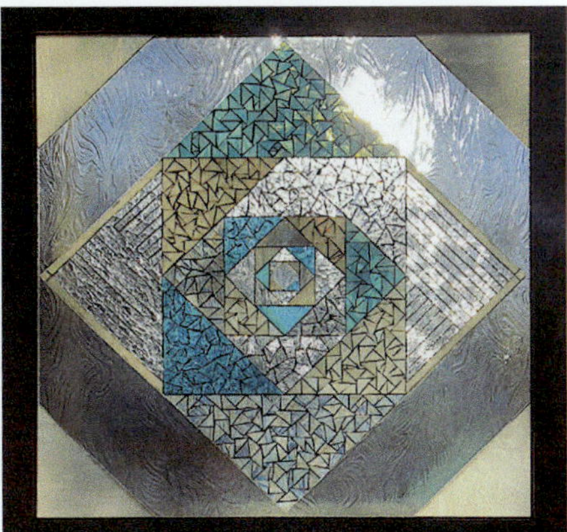

The nine-fold shape of the windows is quite common; for example, it is used in tic-tac-toe and in sudoku, but, for me, it is the ancient symbol of the "square of Saturn." In this square, the numbers one through nine can be placed in such a way that each column, row, or diagonal of numbers add up to 15. This Sun through Saturn conjunction symbolizes profound shifts, personal growth, discipline, and transformations and apparently is prominent in my astrological birth chart.[2] From within my living space, I peer out through this conjunction at my beautiful garden, which gives me promise and delight. Looking from the garden into the house (Figure 12.2a) shows the nine-fold glazing pattern, the triangular wall behind it separating the private functions from the more public ones, and the two upper guest bedrooms. These guest bedrooms have views of the sky-colored vaulted ceiling, the two-story living space, the south façade, the garden, and the woods beyond. The photograph in Figure 12.2b shows the interior wall with the shadow of the Saturn square and a small, 12-inch-square glass block skylight above it with the most amazing amber light. In winter, the light is projected on the triangular wall on the north side of the living space, reminding me of the low angle of the winter sun. In summer, the sun is high, especially at midday, and is blocked from entering my primary living space.

My kitchen is small and functional. It has an Italian espresso maker, Viking range, barn sink, juicers, wok, and other cooking utensils within easy reach. The sink faces the southeast and has morning light. In my kitchen, I prepare on average 10–12 meals a week. The dining table is within the two-and-a-half-story living space and looks out over the garden. Two Turkish floor carpets become place markers for this space's dining and living areas. I spend countless hours in the garden, either attending to it or simply observing and enjoying it. With the geothermal heating and cooling system, there is no AC condenser, and, therefore, it is silent. The garden is quiet except for the natural soundscapes of bird calls.

The garden measures 24 feet (7.3 meters) by 24 feet. The square garden is oriented along the ordinal or intercardinal axis, which parallels the direction of the slope of the land. The garden is bounded by walls that slope down from 14 feet (4.3 meters) to 4.5 feet (1.4 meters) at the end wall. This protects the garden from

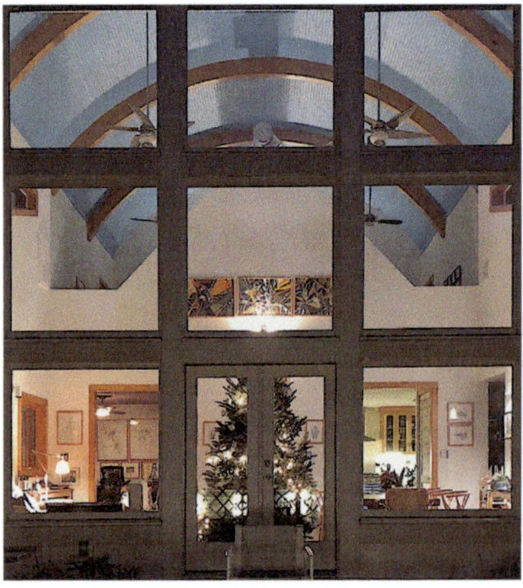

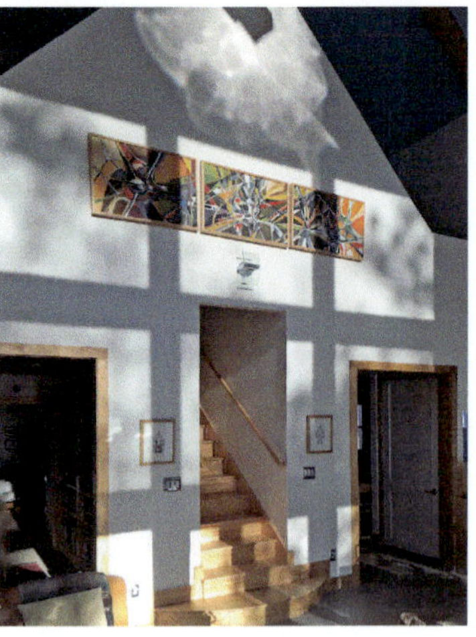

12.2
Tabb Residence: (a) Night View of South Façade from Walled-in Garden, (b) Interior View of Shadow of the Nine-Fold Squares

unwanted wildlife and weather elements and gives a well-defined refuge and sense of place. In the center of the garden is a 7-foot (2.1-meter) square pool which acts as a focal point for the garden. The pool is constructed with concrete and field stone walls and has two small waterfall jets giving it gentle natural sounds. Two sliding gates on both sides of the garden provide soothing sounds from the wind chimes and cooling by the gentle breezes during warm summer weather. In the garden are herbs (rosemary, parsley, thyme, basil, and mint), flowering plants (roses, hydrangea, purple majesty sage, whirling butterfly gaum, blue vervain wildflowers, and iris verna), and various ground cover plants.[3] Two diagonally woven trellises provide visual interest and a backdrop for raspberries, tomato plants, and climbing vines. Bumblebees, butterflies, dragonflies, fireflies, hummingbirds, cardinals, wrens, frogs, eastern box turtles, red-tailed hawks, owls, squirrels, a chipmunk, and the occasional eastern kingsnake visit the garden. In the southeast and southwest corners of the garden are two peach trees that reflect the natural wonder of greening in spring, bearing fruit in summer and losing their leaves in autumn. Next to the garden is a 3-foot compost cube.

I have found that personal spaces are extremely important, given that we typically spend as much as 90 percent of our time indoors. This is particularly desirable for those in retirement and who work at home. Since my retirement from teaching and moving to my new home, I am equally busy, but on my own terms. It is as though my home is an elaborate design studio for the art of living. So, personal space for me is not so much directed to health issues or problems, or crossword puzzles, but rather to planning, thinking, meditation, processing emotional matters, socializing, and functioning creatively. I find moments for spiritual wellness throughout the day within any of these spaces and activities. I love the silence, nature's soundscapes, and connections to my neighbors. Further, I have created sitting areas in the garden, a "man-cave" as part of my home office, seating on a screened-in porch looking out into the adjacent woods to the west, and a front porch facing the neighborhood. Several years ago, I even created a semi-attached screened-in social space that I call the "martini hut," for family, friends, and neighbor gatherings. Needless to say, it has quite a reputation within the community (Figures 12.3a and 12.3b).

The importance of everyday spiritual wellness cannot be understated. For me, especially within the context of my home and community. I am both appreciative and blessed. I awake in the mornings with beauty and silence around me. Daily, I have a renewed self-awareness and experience of the larger world around me. Everyday spiritual wellness can occur by sitting in my sun-filled window seat, working in my garden, or sitting quietly in a comfortable chair. Also, I love it when friends and family are here and enjoy with me the tranquil environment. For me, these experiences are often encountered and routinely followed in my daily activities. Since I work at home, I need to pause and take breaks, and, mainly, it is easy for me to experience the biophilic, wellness, and spiritual aspects of this place.

I view my house not as a traditional home but as a studio with a various spatial preferences. This suggests that my daily life is a flow of creative activities from morning through the evening. My home office has a wall of books, two computers, four screens, a printer, a scanner, and views of the adjacent woods to the west. It is

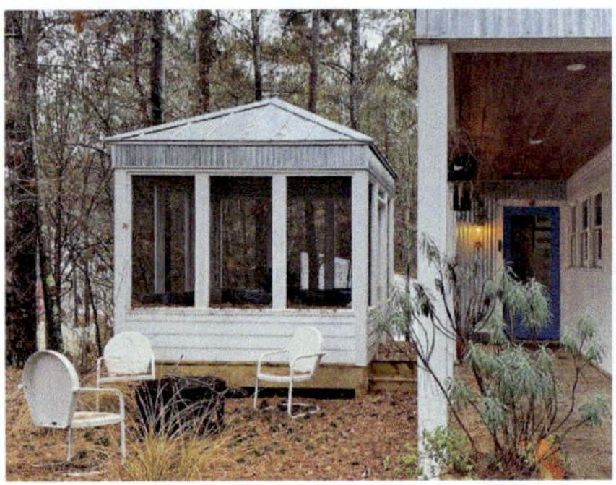

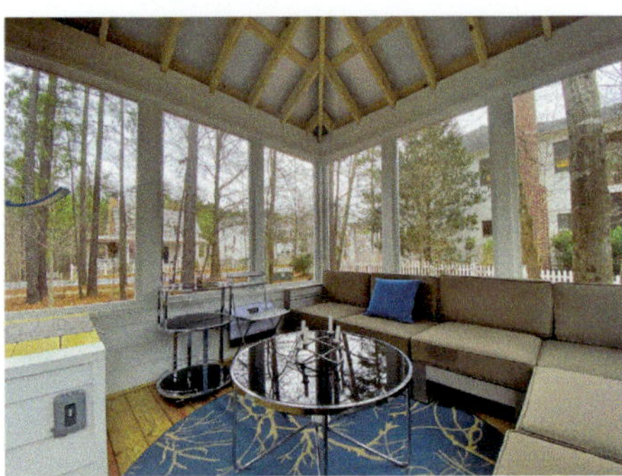

12.3
Tabb
Residence: (a) the Martini Hut Exterior, (b) the Martini Hut Interior

common for birds, squirrels, deer, and even a red-tailed hawk sitting on a branch to check me out. I enjoy food preparation, working in the garden, writing, drawing and painting, and socializing throughout the day. As described previously, most of the spaces in my house are specialized around these activities. Punctuated between many of these activities are my break times, my times to stop, reflect, and enjoy the moment. These pauses occur on my screened-in side porch looking directly into the adjacent woods, in my walled-in garden viewing the afternoon sun and attuning to nature, or in the martini hut with friends in early evening. It is as though I can experience a forest walk by simply moving from one room to another. In these places, there is silence and the beauty of nature around me, only to be punctuated by the soundscapes of birds and insects. And, when I see a butterfly, woodpecker, or deer move into my orbit, I am transfixed (Figure 12.4).

The floor plan shown in Figure 12.5 documents some of the spiritual wellness moments occurring at the ground level. First is the prominence of the walled-in garden and its sense of place. Its relationship to the living functions of the home is highly visible. The pond offers a view and soft sounds of running water, and there are two seating areas for quiet contemplation of the pond and garden. At each of the pond's edges are located bronze animals representing the four directions in feng shui. At the far corners of the garden are two peach trees that yield fruit each year and two dogwoods for spring color (Figure 12.1f). The large windows facing the garden allow for clear views of the garden and its seasonal changes. The living and dining areas are open to one another and have a high ceiling formed by the vaulted roof, expressing spatial generosity (Figure 12.2b). The kitchen receives morning light, and the home office is oriented to the western afternoon light and views to the adjacent woods. The views to the outside offer relief from hours of computer work. Also, the space serves as a "man-cave," with a comfortable leather chair facing a large, wall-mounted entertainment screen. The martini hut is separate from the main house, is screened on all four sides, and faces a fire pit and the street for potential social interaction. The master bedroom is to the north and is more refuge-like, yet has a screened-in porch facing the woods for quiet contemplation. The bed is oriented along the cardinal directions with the head to the north. These design considerations combine to contribute to a spiritual wellness lifestyle.

Living here, I feel somewhat like Emerson, who lived at Waldon Pond surrounded by woods, except my home is connected to a community. Crossroads

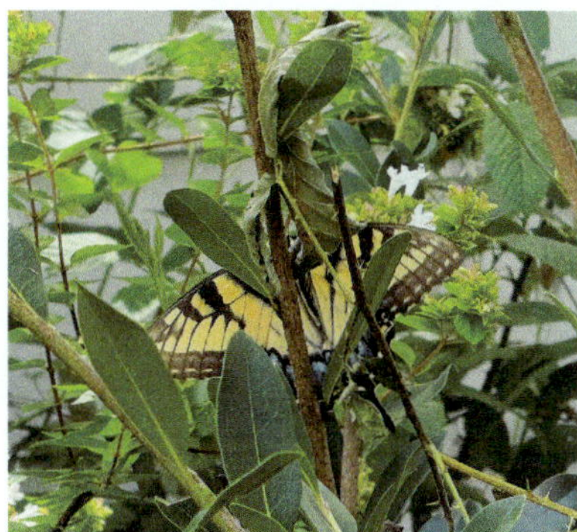
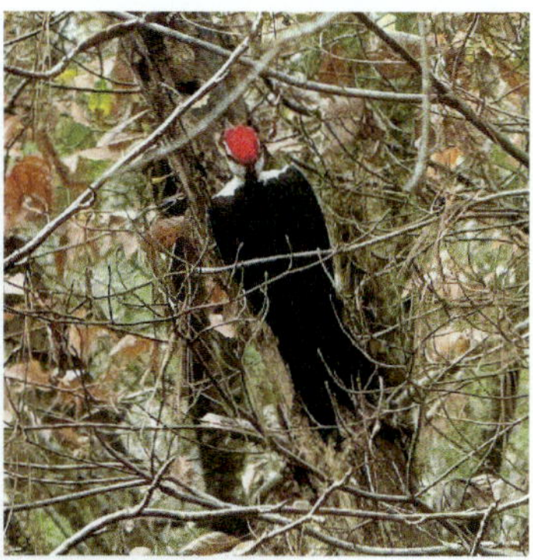
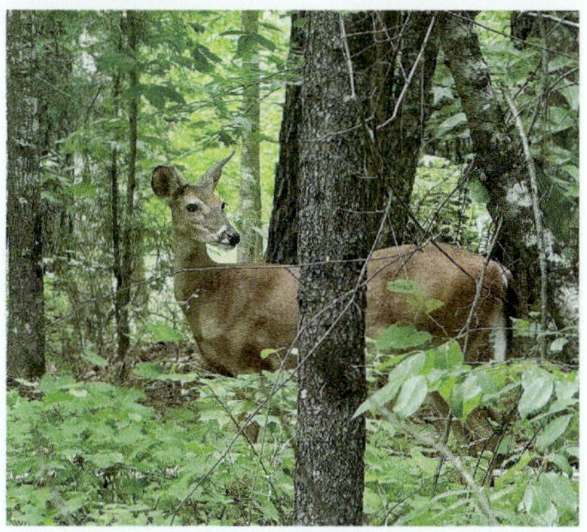

12.4 Resident Encounters: (a) Butterfly Enjoying the Garden, (b) Red-Headed Woodpecker, (c) White-Tailed Deer in the Woods next to my House

neighborhood is located in the geographic center of Serenbe community and comprises 24 homes surrounded by forests. My home is situated on an estate lot at the southwest corner of the neighborhood. Three sides of my property are wooded, with the fourth connected to the street and neighborhood. Figure 12.6a is a view from the front of my property looking east to the neighborhood. It has been long known that social factors can positively affect well-being. They also can elicit spiritual wellness. Several factors contribute to positive social wellness, including regular contact, experiencing quality time, engaging in meaningful interactions, joining interest groups, and participating in family, neighborhood, and community events. I know all my neighbors, and living so close to them gives me constant contact (Figure 12.6b). Our neighborhood is part of a larger constellation comprising multiple hamlets with more than a thousand residents, all within walking distance.

While my home is on the edge of Crossroads, one the smallest neighborhoods, and I live a somewhat introverted life, I am in the middle of a larger, active community. I can choose to participate on multiple levels with a myriad of social opportunities. There are five restaurants all within walking distance. The Saturday morning Artists' and Farmers' Market is always an active social event. Even within my neighborhood, I know everyone, and we have block parties several times a year. I typically encounter someone while I pick up my mail at the neighborhood mail pavilion. I am still engaged in planning work with Serenbe Development, which keeps me involved

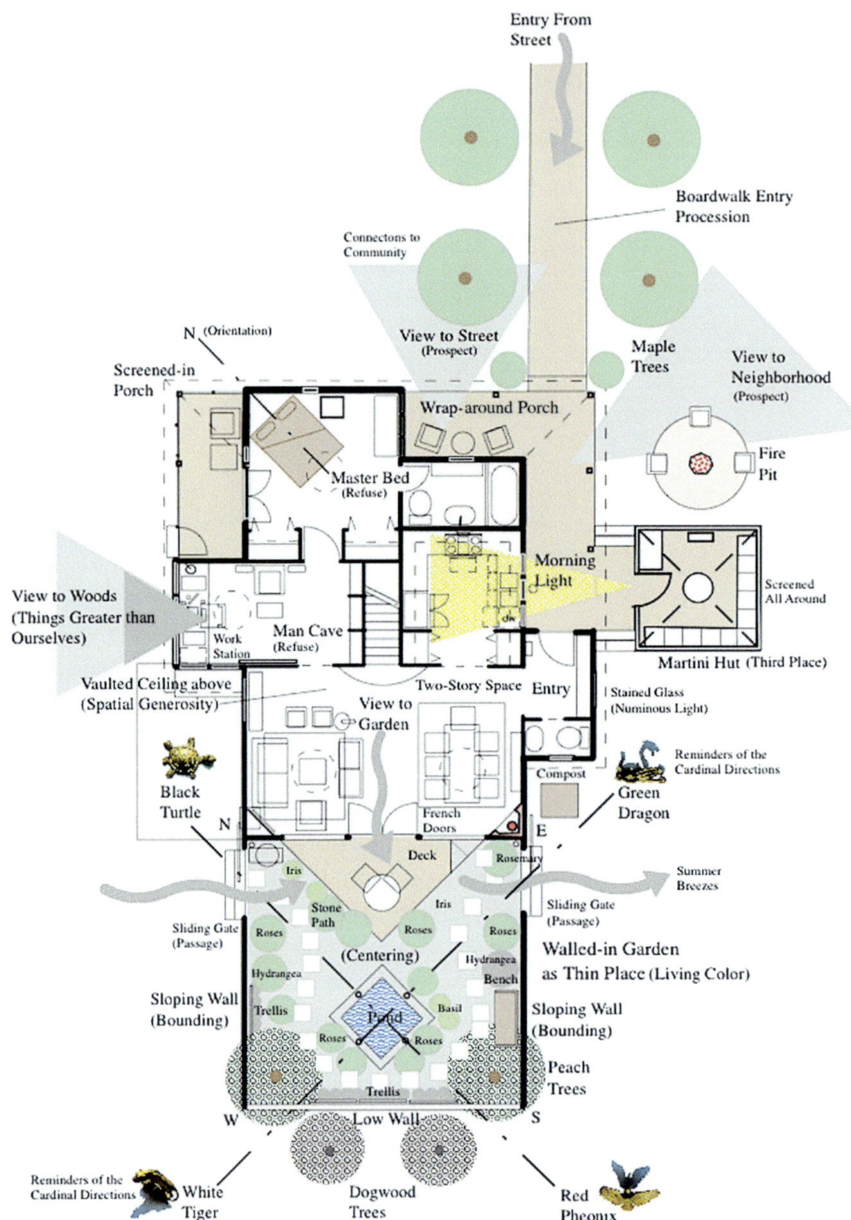

12.5
Tabb Residence Floor Plan Illustrating Spiritual Wellness Features

and connected. I am constantly giving tours of Serenbe to friends, students, and people interested in the community. I have more friends here than any other place I have lived. Every day, I walk through the woods and end up at my mail pavilion to collect my mail. This walk is a mile-long forest bathing experience through a quiet, enchanting landscape. I am blessed to have a serene, naturally beautiful, and socially rich life here. Through my research into wellness, I have realized the spiritual value of social networks and interactions. Finally, I am reminded of one of the Labors of Hercules: "I build a lighted house and therein dwell."[4]

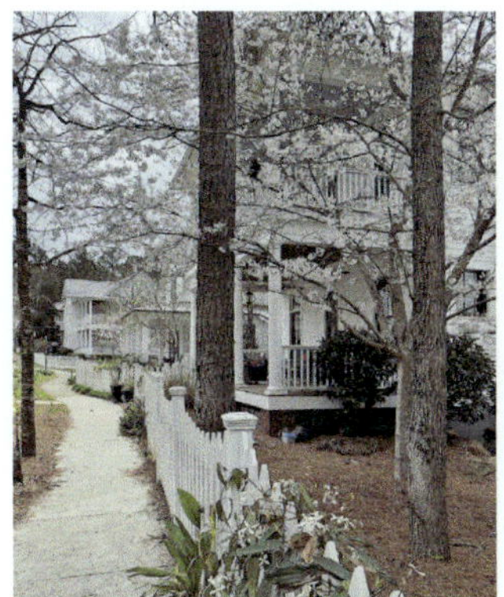

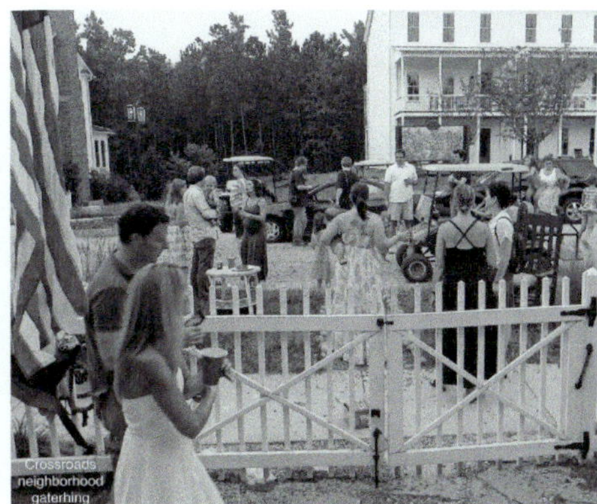

12.6
Serenbe Crossroads Neighborhood: (a) Sidewalk and Houses Next Door, (b) Neighborhood Block Party

Everyday wellness spaces can be awe-inspiring or soulful. Everyday spiritual wellness places vary in type, scale, purpose, and location. In his work *The Re-enchantment of Everyday Life*, Thomas Moore describes enchantment as the inflow of spirituality in everyday activities.[5] Everyday spiritual wellness places, especially within domestic settings, usually occur as intimate humble settings supporting ceremonial participation (meditation, quiet moments, and special family gatherings) and are considered, in Michael Brill's words, to be "embraced places."[6] The spiritual values and daily practice guide a more purposeful life. The following are everyday wellness characteristics:[7]

- Most often they occur within intimate spaces.
- They are places with a personal past.
- They are usually well defined or bounded.
- They are safe from harm and places of refuge.
- They are found or created in unique locations.
- They are part of everyday living.
- They often contain personal symbols.
- They are modest and authentic.
- They have soulful qualities.
- They have qualities of calm, grace, and respect.
- They elicit introspective and contemplative responses.
- These places tend to be private rather than public.
- The wellness spaces are easily accessible.
- They are often individual experiences.
- They also are small group experiences.
- There is a ceremonial connection or ritual.

It seems that everyday spiritual wellness readily occurs in the natural flow of one's life, from morning to night, where opportunities to experience nature, family, friends, and even a quiet moment are present. To Thomas Moore, daily spiritual wellness is about connecting and reconnecting, incorporating concepts of place, story, activity, and ritual.[8] Important is the perpetuating access to the spiritual wellness strategies in terms of frequency (*how often*), duration of exposure (*how long*), and intensity (*how much and the quality*) of the experience. Like the blue zone residents, those spiritual wellness lifestyles are part of the everyday flow of activities that can offer great rewards. They can be simple rituals such as making the bed, watering house plants, weeding the garden, preparing a home meal, meeting friends at a café, having mindful pauses throughout the day, and walking or riding a bicycle to work.

The four vignettes previously covered in Chapters 8–11 describe interests I have pursued over the years in my professional and personal lives. They include solar energy, sacred geometry, mythic landscapes, and pilgrimage trips abroad. And, finally, there is the daily flow of spiritual wellness occurring through the realization of the community I designed and the home I created. Both have been opportunities to realize and practice these principles in my everyday life. The need for spiritual wellness is a revitalizing response to the sometimes hectic everyday modern lifestyles we currently have. Yet, for me, it has been easier because of the beauty and quality of the built environment within which I live. It seems an ever-evolving process of being in place, being present, and being aware of the spiritual wellness opportunities and experiences.

A CULTURE OF RENEWED VALUES AND VISION

Spiritual wellness occurs in tandem with changes in values, behaviors, and lifestyles. Before the positive changes are realized, an intent must precede an action. The *value–action gap* must be reduced or eliminated for the most comprehensive results to be consistent between the wellness intentions and the eventual physical designs. For spiritual wellness to be most effective, each scale must be addressed, from personal space to regions and beyond. The concept of places of light or inspiration provides glimpses of spiritual wellness that focus on models larger than individual buildings. Moreover, shared experiences can contribute to synergy and a more direct expression of the value–action intention. In some ways, they are islands containing a blend of shared sustainable, biophilic, financial, agricultural, spiritual, and community-oriented intentions.

Places such as the Findhorn community in Scotland, Auroville in India, Singapore Neighborhoods, the Cannery in Davis, California, Prairie Crossing in Illinois, and Almere and Aardehuizen in the Netherlands, and Serenbe Community in Georgia all have common characteristics of interconnectedness, regeneration, inclusion, and holistic design principles. Often set in serene locations, these communities offer a sanctuary from the chaos, promoting physical fitness, socialization, and overall balanced, sustainable living. The Global Wellness Institute defines them as groups "living in close proximity who share common goals, interests, and experiences in proactively pursuing wellness across its many dimensions," including spiritual wellness.[9] There are currently very few spiritual wellness communities, but there are communities directed toward all wellness pillars, including the spiritual wellness pillar. However, the emergence of wellness communities provides the opportunity to experience the full range of wellness principles, which can include the spiritual dimension, through shared experiences and values.

MANIFESTATION PATHWAYS

The pathway to natural and built healthy environments requires vision and action. If there is a clear intention, then manifestation is much easier. According to Buckminster Fuller, "In order to change an existing paradigm you do not struggle to try to change the problematic model. You create a new model to make the old one obsolete."[10] This is easier said than done; for example, the modern urbanized world we have created depends on fossil fuels. There is a thread that is an important principle to remember. Change occurs through the expression of values that, in turn, inform intentions. Intentions lead to strategies that eventually lead to implementation.

Architects have an infatuation with signature buildings that wow, entertain, and elicit awe emotions. Often, what is forgotten is the role of and need for "background buildings" that are functional and contribute to creating an urban unity. While the signature buildings seem to draw attention to their heroic forms, innovative technologies, and use of exotic materials, they could instead promote biophilic principles, sustainable practices, and health and wellness outcomes. At the other end of this spectrum are many ordinary suburban buildings that are typically automobile-oriented and have little aesthetic value. They, too, could benefit from more socially and environmentally conscious building; at the planning scale, monolithic suburban sprawl, automobile-dominant infrastructure, and lack of adequate green spaces could also be redirected to support more wellness-oriented urban design.

All areas of the built environment, from personal space to cities, could benefit from spiritual wellness. What is needed is understanding of spiritual wellness considerations within the design fields, the attributes that define them, their health and wellness benefits, and strategies that are manifestation pathways to their realization. Hopefully, what will likely follow are reinvigorated behaviors and lifestyle choices that lead to a state of greater holistic health. Prioritizing wellness as a central concept in the planning and design process can play a significant role in ensuring built environments sustain people living in cities, villages, and rural regions, regenerating and revitalizing these built areas. Spiritual values can further expand wellness outcomes, especially if they are seamlessly integrated at all scales.

SUMMARY OF SPIRITUAL WELLNESS PLANNING AND DESIGN STRATEGIES

Each of the three scales has ten planning and design strategies. In some instances, the strategies cross over the scales, especially those related to natural experiences. Tables 12.1–12.3 illustrate the three categories of spiritual wellness attributes (place, experience, and process) and desired outcomes against the three application scales (personal, architectural, and urban design). Within the cells is a description of the design strategy according to the attribute and scale. The tables enable one to see overall patterns across all the application scales. Spiritual wellness gives us renewed values and vision for implementing pro-individual, pro-spiritual, and pro-environmental designs accessible at all scales of the built environment. The planning and design strategies at the three scales, discussed in previous chapters, follow. Also, the tables show the spiritual wellness attributes and the planning and design strategies at these same scales.

The personal space scale:

1. Designing for an intimate scale.
2. Accessibility to everyday sacred wellness spaces.
3. Creation of sanctuary spaces.
4. Bounded safe places.
5. Sensory connections.
6. Use of color.
7. Subtle use of light.
8. The tactile importance of the space.
9. Encouraging personal expression.
10. Design for silence.

The architectural scale:

1. Spatial sequencing and passage.
2. Use of sacred geometry.
3. Orientation responses.
4. Design for climate.
5. Creating spatial generosity.
6. Design for luminosity.
7. Incorporating water and blue spaces.
8. Responses to celestial phenomena.
9. Design for de-materiality.
10. Biophilic design connections to nature.

The urban design scale:

1. Preservation of ecological zones.
2. Urban spatial structures.
3. Integration of nature within the urban fabric.
4. Creation of community agriculture and gardens.
5. Circular regenerative infrastructure.
6. Zoning for mixes of use and intergenerational living.
7. Planning for solar energy.
8. Creation of gathering, ceremonial, and third places.
9. Creation of human streetscapes and walkable communities.
10. Incorporation of significant spiritual and civic sites and buildings.

It should be noted that place-based attributes more closely reflect the built environment with specific physical planning and design strategies. In contrast, experience-based and process-based attributes are more subjective and qualitative

ATTRIBUTE	PERSONAL SCALE	ARCHITECTURAL SCALE	URBAN DESIGN SCALE
Spirit of Place	Encouragement of personal expression, use of color, places that evoke meaning or tell a story, and opportunities for spiritual connections to nature and the experiences of sacred places	Design for climate; planning for solar energy; response to natural features of the place; sensitivity to historic, cultural, and spiritual characteristic of the place; and dramatic use of light	Integration of nature within urban fabric; design for climate; preservation of ecological zones; reinforcement of natural geography; creation of a community identity
Biophilic Places	Small-scale nature within; incorporation of water and blue spaces; encouragement of interactions with all the senses; prospect and refuge; provision of intimate encounters	Orientation responses; connections to things greater than ourselves; filled with diversity of shapes, forms, patterns, and colors found in the living natural world; quiet spaces; dramatic use of light	Human streetscapes and walkable communities; regenerative infrastructure; creation of community agriculture; water and blue spaces; access to parks and greenspaces; support for renewable technologies
Thin Places	Design for intimate scale; creation of gathering and ceremonial places; bounded safe places; connections to nature; places with earth energies	Design for luminosity; tactile importance of the space; responses to celestial phenomena; creation of sanctuary spaces; spatial generosity	Urban spatial structures; integration of nature within urban fabric; creation of spatial generosity; creation of special historic public spaces and plazas
Third Places	Bounded safe, familiar, & social places; opportunities for intimate interactions; easily accessible; in the home, places for family gatherings; in neighborhood, places frequently visited	Gathering, ceremonial, and meeting places; community building; fostering of integration; often colorful playful environments; inclusion of coffee shops, pubs, theaters, gyms, cafés, bars	Zoning for mixes of use and intergenerational living; creation of easy access; provision of both indoor and outdoor third places; creation of public spaces, plazas, and meeting places
Sanctuary Places	Design for climate; bounded safe places; quiet places; places that can be isolated; provision of nurturing, comforting, therapeutic protection and a safe haven	Design for climate; provision of nurturing, comforting protection for a variety of building types and functions (home, work, school); protection with zoning and buffers	Zoning for mixes of use and intergenerational living; provision of safe places during inclement weather and natural disasters; creation of safe neighborhoods
Healing Places	Places full of life and vitality, containing medicinal plants; sensory connections; acessible connections to nature; safe and bounded	Creation of healing gardens; orientation responses; use of sacred geometry; incorporation of healing water; use of non-toxic materials; connections to nature	Creation of community agriculture, water, and blue spaces; provision of recreation and walking trails for physical activity; reduction of night sky pollution
Religious Places	Use of color; bounded safe places; subtle use of light; spaces that are quiet; soulful and inspirational qualities; use of symbolism; designs with view discrimination	Spatial sequencing and passage; design for luminosity; orientation responses; use of sacred geometry and spatial generosity; designs for view discrimination	Incorporation of significant spiritual and civic sites and buildings within cities; preservation of historic sites; use of geometry significant to special sites; integration of cemeteries
Ritual Places	Places that are personal, intimate, and accessible; encouragement of personal expression; use of personal symbolism	Creation of gathering places and third places; responses to celestial phenomena; use of sacred geometry; encouragement of community involvement	Incorporation of significant spiritual and civic sites and buildings within community; urban spatial structures as processions to sacred sites

Table 12.1
Place-Based Attributes and Design Strategies

ATTRIBUTE	PERSONAL SCALE	ARCHITECTURAL SCALE	URBAN DESIGN SCALE
The Numinous	Design for de-materiality; making sensory connections; design for luminosity; creating spaces that are tranquil and mysterious; designs that have indeterminate qualities	Creating spatial generosity; design for luminosity; design for de-materiality; design for otherworldly, ineffable architectural space; designs that are mysterious with fascinating content	Incorporation of significant spiritual and civic sites and buildings; creation of spatial generosity; connections to things greater than ourselves; preserving natural wild places
Awe Experiences	Connections to nature; connections to things greater than ourselves; connections to unusual environments; interiors with exceptional beauty; spatial exaggeration	Creation of spatial generosity; orientation responses; design for de-materiality; responses to celestial phenomena; buildings that are exceptionally unique and beautiful	Connections to things greater than ourselves; creation of spatial generosity; connections to vast landscapes, cityscapes, and skyscapes; design for unusual architecture
Serenity Experiences	Designing for present centeredness, intimate scale, acceptance, inner haven, and trust; design for silence; subtle use of light; connections to nature	Designing for intimate scale; designing for silence; subtle use of light; tactile importance of the space; designing with harmonic materials	Preservation of ecological zones; creation of human streetscapes and walkable communities; creation of gathering, ceremonial, and third places; planning for parks
Synchronicity	Design for de-materiality; connections to deep-seated awareness of interconnectedness; designs for ambiguous spaces and shapes	Creation of meaningful patterns; connections to things greater than ourselves; creation of ambiguities; architectural elements can be designed for double meaning and meaningfully coincident	Making personal connections to larger contexts; urban elements can be imbued with symbolic meanings; spatial sequencing throughout urban fabric
Noetic Experiences	Connections to things greater than ourselves; design for de-materiality; designs with cognitive content and a certain amount of complexity	Design for de-materiality; design for otherworldly, ineffable architectural space; overall form designed with clarity and identity; interior wayfinding	Incorporating significant spiritual and civic sites and buildings; city-scale wayfinding; clarity of spatial structure and significant sites
Transcendence	Design for silence; use of color; designs that evoke meaning or tell a story; designs that are symbolic portals; designs for prospect and refuge	Creation of spatial generosity; designs for luminosity; designs fostering de-materiality; use of symbolic triggers; increased scale for awe experiences	Incorporating significant spiritual and civic sites and buildings; planning for nature and natural environments; preservation of clarity of night sky
The Unknown	Connections to things greater than ourselves; design for de-materiality; design emphasizing open-endedness	Orientation responses; design for de-materiality; design for the mysterious and uncertain; spaces with ambiguous meanings; designs with negative space	Biophilic design connections to nature; reinforcing of cosmic connections; reduction of night sky pollution; maintaining of some mystery
Unity Experience	Use of color; use of sacred geometry; design for de-materiality; creation of harmonic interiors; designs for human scale; designs for simplicity	Design for luminosity; design for de-materiality; use of sacred geometry; building elements dissolve into a single expression; design for coherence	Urban spatial structures; gathering, ceremonial, and third places; zoning for mixes of use and intergenerational living

Table 12.2
Experience-Based Attributes and Design Strategies

ATTRIBUTE	PERSONAL SCALE	ARCHITECTURAL SCALE	URBAN DESIGN SCALE
Mindfulness	Sensory connections; connections to nature; tactile importance of the space; spaces that are intimate, human-scaled, and experienced daily; design for silence	Design for luminosity; design for places of pause; design for wayfinding, to minimize distractions, and view discrimination; design for silence	Preservation of ecological zones; creation of natural places of refuge; creation of identity; preservation of sacred and memorial sites; reduction of night sky pollution
Existential Issues	Design of spaces that are serene, quiet, and foster reflection; spaces that reflect personal identity; spaces that connect to nature	Design for climate, inclement weather, and natural disasters; design buildings for healing and wellness; designs fostering solitude; designs for luminosity	Design for climate; respect for historical narrative; planning for beautiful memorials and easily accessible cemeteries
Greater Connections	Inward focus; connections to nature; sensory connections; responses to celestial phenomena; outward discriminating views; connections to things greater than ourselves	Biophilic design for connections to nature; planning for solar energy; creation of gathering places and community agriculture and gardens; spatial generosity; encouragement of indoor-outdoor connections	Gathering, ceremonial, and third places; zoning for mixes of use and intergenerational living; incorporation of significant spiritual and civic sites and buildings; reduction of night sky pollution; planning for solar energy
Intentionality	Accessibility of everyday sacred wellness spaces; sensory connections; creation of sanctuary spaces; creation of healing gardens	Ethical and moral practice; designs for low income; use of sacred geometry; designs for inclusiveness; designs that nudge to wellness choices; use of sacred geometry	Zoning for mixes of use and intergenerational living; significant spiritual and civic sites; respect for historical and cultural narratives; inclusion of nature; planning for social equity
Ethical Practice	Design for spaces that are gender-specific; design of safe spaces; respect for personal spaces; provision of affordable spaces; creation of sanctuary spaces	Design for climate and vulnerable sites; universal designs for all building occupants; designs with transparency and authenticity	Zoning for mixes of use and intergenerational living; planning for climate and vulnerable sites; respect for neighborhood character; creation of human streetscapes and walkable communities
Life Purpose	Connections to things greater than ourselves; spaces that reflect self; design for luminosity	Spaces that encourage contemplation and reflection; buildings that support life-long learning and spiritual development	Connections to things greater than ourselves; planning for diversity; creation of human streetscapes and walkable communities
Life Satisfaction	Creation of personal spaces that are comfortable, supportive, and contribute to self-actualization	Accessibility of everyday sacred wellness spaces; creation of spatial generosity; design for luminosity	Appropriate balance between urbanized and natural landscapes; incorporation of water and blue spaces
High-Level Wellness	Opportunities for physical activity, social interaction, access to nature; intellectually stimulating; experiences of mysteries; daily integration of wellness behaviors; maintenance of healthy lifestyles	Design for open-ended, shared, and multifunctional spaces; creation of gathering places; buildings that encourage physical movement; use of color; buildings that are non-toxic	Planning for coherent, safe, accessible, nature-filled urban fabric; planning for safe and clean resources (water, air, energy, food); planning for sacred sites; creation of community agriculture and gardens

Table 12.3
Process-Based Attributes and Design Strategies

and relate to behaviors and lifestyles. The combination of these three dimensions is intended to inform architecture and urban design for spiritual wellness outcomes. For example, the place-based attributes of healing places and third places are more physical than the experience-based attribute of noetic issues or the process-based attribute of existential issues. Refer to Tables 12.1–12.3.

According to theologian Belden Lane, a set of principles are phenomenological categories of "mythogenesis."[11] These characters of experience or axioms of sacred places pre-exist our encounter with spiritual wellness places. They understand how these places ignite the imagination and provide an interesting way of understanding the nature of sacred places. The first axiom is that *a spiritual place is not chosen, it chooses*, a place-centered origin (opposite of solipsism). Sacred places are not determined by human-centered perspectives or in deterministic ways but are selected by the land, genius loci, or a higher presence. While design intentions are important, they do not guarantee connections to this higher presence. The energy and presence of an otherworldly, unknown, or divine source seek us out.

The second axiom is that *places can be ordinary but ritually made extraordinary*, where ritual acts are performed that set them apart from secular space. This suggests a different state of mind and participatory respect for the place, and the fact that sacred places are abundantly located everywhere. That they exist everywhere means that many of the environments that have been destroyed or devalued can be revitalized.

Third, *sacred places can be trod upon without being entered*, and recognition can be existentially discerned. This means that sacred places are related to increased levels of openness and elevated consciousness. The good news is that many sacred places are not yet recognized and can exist for future experiences. The combination of many factors, including our reverent participation, re-initiates the sacredness of a particular place.

The last axiom is that *the impulse within these places is both centripetal (local) and centrifugal (universal)*, and the sacred nature of the space is not confined to a single locale. This axiom allows for serene moments at the intimate scale and cosmic experiences at the larger scale. It also suggests that a divine source can be expressed locally, such as a beautiful flower or flickering candle, and, according to Lane, it can be simultaneously larger and smaller, never confined to a single locale, such as a colorful sunset, rainbow, or starlit night sky.[12] These axioms are a reminder that spiritual wellness is a reciprocal process between that which is sacred and ourselves.

As has been demonstrated in this book, there is a fascinating relationship between spirituality and wellness. Spirituality expands a sense of purpose, gives meaning, helps guide moral and ethical behaviors, helps deal with existential issues, and supports our interconnectedness to the world around us. Wellness focuses on physiological dimensions, eliciting individual health benefits toward more holistic well-being. In the 1990 film *Mindwalk*, the character Thomas Harriman, played by actor John Heard, says, "Healing is an inside job."[13] This suggests that the desire for spiritual wellness is an inward process that progresses outward.

Recently, the wellness movement has made tremendous progress, and there are pockets of really great examples worldwide. One such project, the Forest Temple located in Tobermory, Ontario, was designed by Tye Farrow (Figure 12.7). The beautiful lattice structure is so resonant with the forest, expressing harmony and spiritual wellness.[14] In addition, we need to initiate further changes at each of the actualization scales with systemic reach. For me, spiritual wellness has been a calling, and writing this book has been part of fulfilling my long-term purpose. I have always felt that architecture and design are more than mere building, but they also possess the possibilities of embodiment of higher ideals. This journey has led me to a career in architecture and urban design, design education, creating biophilic and wellness communities, and designing my own spiritual wellness home. These are the legacy I leave to my family – a hope that the world becomes healthier as my four grandsons grow older.

Is it not remarkable that the combination and coincidence of the Sun's size, intensity and distance, atmosphere, and axial tilt, the rotation of the Earth, and the Moon's size, distance, and rotation are such that life flourishes here? If any of these parameters were to change, it would critically affect our very existence (Figure 12.8). Further, Earth's Moon is about 1/400th the diameter of the Sun, but it is also 1/400th as far from us, making the Sun and the Moon perceived as being the same size in the sky. This coincidence uniquely allows for photogenic total solar eclipses.[15] The science is incredible. Still, it also leads one to wonder about the magical and spiritual nature of this planet on which we live. The celestial dance of the majestic Earth, luminous Moon, and radiant Sun, in their profound and predictable rhythms, serves as a timeless inspiration for spiritual wellness, reminding us of the interconnectedness, cyclical nature, and awe-inspiring power. This awe experience is something larger than ourselves and a reminder of what is at stake if we do not heed the destructive signs and act comprehensively.

Spiritual wellness encompasses a broad range of beliefs, values, and practices that provide a sense of meaning, purpose, and connection. It involves exploring

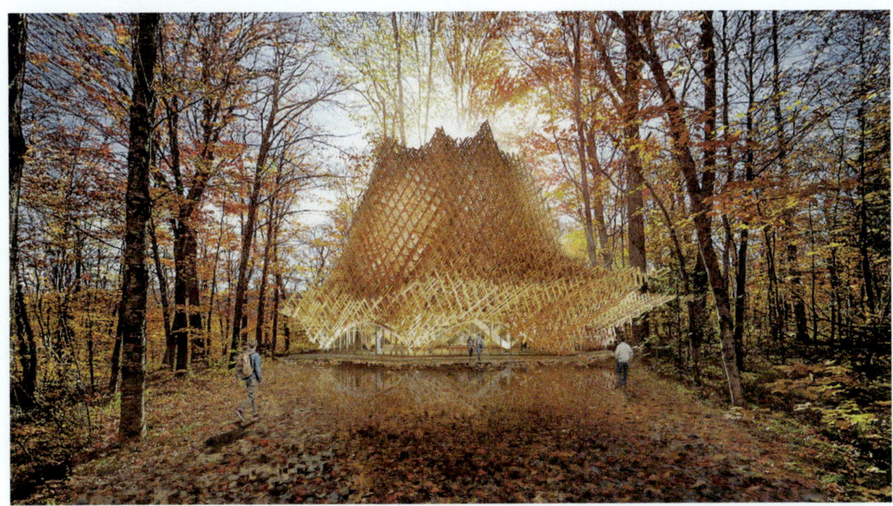

12.7
Forest Temple, by Tye Farrow Partners Architects, Tobermory, Ontario

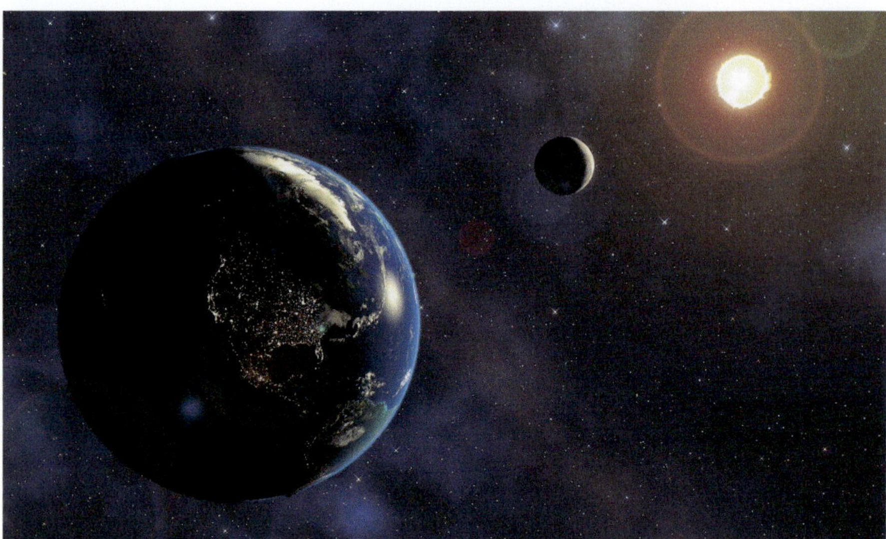

12.8
Sun, Earth, and Moon Spiritual Wellness

questions about existence, morality, and the human condition. This may include engaging in spiritual practices, spending time in nature, meditating, or simply reflecting on one's values and how they guide one's life choices. The built environment has the potential to either support or obstruct individuals' spiritual journeys by shaping their experiences and influencing their moods, emotions, actions, and lifestyle choices. Ultimately, spiritual wellness is a personal journey toward understanding oneself and one's place in the world, fostering inner peace and a sense of fulfillment.

NOTES

1 Houghton, Olivia, & Jessica Smith, The Home as Highest-Tech-Health-Hub (accessed October 20, 2024), https://www.youtube.com/watch?v=vYc470b_5-Y.
2 This Sun–Saturn relationship was discussed in a reading by Caroline Casey in the 1990s and verified in her tape collection: *Inner and Outer Space: The Astrological Language of the Psyche* (1996).
3 Tabb, Phillip James, *Elemental Architecture: Temperaments of Sustainability* (London, UK: Routledge, 2019), p. 159.
4 Bailey, Alice A., *The Labours of Hercules* (New York, NY: Lucis, 1974).
5 Moore, Thomas, *The Re-enchantment of Everyday Life* (New York, NY: Harper & Collins, 1996).
6 Brill, Michael, *Sacred Places and Embraced Places: Using Design-as-Inquiry to Understand the Difference* (Self-published, September 25, 1985).
7 Tabb, Phillip James, *Thin Place Design: Architecture of the Numinous* (New York, NY: Routledge, 2024), p. 152.
8 Moore, Thomas, *The Re-enchantment of Everyday Life* (New York, NY: Harper Perennial, 1997).
9 Global Wellness Institute, Wellness Lifestyle Real Estate & Communities (accessed July 20, 2024), https://globalwellnessinstitute.org/what-is-wellness/what-is-wellness-lifestyle-real-estate-communities/.
10 Fuller, R. Buckminster,

11 Lane, Belden, *Landscapes of the Sacred: Geography and Narrative in American Spirituality* (Baltimore, MD: Johns Hopkins University Press, 1988), p 19.
12 Lane, Belden, *Landscapes of the Sacred: Geography and Narrative in American Spirituality* (Baltimore, MD: Johns Hopkins University Press, 1988), p 19.
13 Capra, Bernt Amadeus, *Mindwalk* (IMDb: Release date 1990).
14 I met Tye Farrow at the April 2025 Biophilic Leadership Summit in Serenbe, Georgia, and witnessed his brilliant presentation that included this Forest Temple. The project is in the design phase, but represents a wonderful example of both biophilic and spiritual wellness design. What Tye Farrow says about this design is "what I like about where we are at, is it has a very simple, buildable envelope, that protects the structure within, with a wood nest feature inside hung off the structure, and a self-supporting nest structure on the outside."
15 Tyson, Neil deGrasse, Quotable Quotes (accessed August 10, 2024), https://www.goodreads.com/quotes/8624109-earth-s-moon-is-about-1-400th-the-diameter-of-the#:~:text="Earth's%20Moon%20is%20about%201%2F%20400th%20the%20diameter,system%2C%20allowing%20for%20uniquely%20photogenic%20total%20solar%20eclipses."

Glossary of Related Terms

Accommodation – *Keltner & Haidt's process of adjusting cognitive structures that cannot assimilate a new experience*

Affective responses – *the emotional response to and subjective experience of a situation or place*

Anemoia – *the longing for a time one has never quite known*

Attribute – *defining qualities of experience, can be specific physical characteristics of the spiritual wellness dimension*

Awe – *a feeling of reverential respect mixed with fear or wonder*

Awe-absorption – *the tendency to be fully immersed in internal and external stimuli during an awe experience*

Awe physiology – *the effects of an awe experience resulting in goosebumps, chills, and changes in facial expression*

Awe-spotting – *the ability to discover and utilize moments of pause to become more present and mindful experiencing awe*

Awe walk – *a stroll in which you intentionally shift your attention outward instead of inward*

Axioms of sacred places – *from the publications of Belden Lane, these describe four pre-existing patterns of sacred places including: they are not chosen, they choose; they are ritually made extraordinary; they can be trod upon but not entered; and they are both centripetal and centrifugal*

Axis mundi – the vertical axis between celestial poles and Heaven and Earth

Background buildings – *often overlooked, can play spiritual and sustainable roles by providing a sense of continuity, connection to history, and grounding within a community*

Bioinspiration – *a biophilic design approach that seeks innovative solutions by emulating the strategies, mechanisms, and processes found in nature*

Biomorphism – *design and art utilizing organic, flowing forms and patterns derived from living organisms, often evoking a sense of naturalism and fluidity*

Bounding – *a placemaking attribute defined by different meanings, orientations, edge-markers, and bounding forms*

Brill, Michael – *studied charged places, embraced places, and sacred place patterns*

Celestial moment – *a feeling of connectedness to the larger expansive universe*

Charged places – *places creating an ancient stirring within us, where there is a wave of sensory unity*

Clairsentience – *"clear feeling," mystical perception or knowing*

Clairvoyance – *"clear vision," perception beyond normal sensory content*

Climax community – *borrowed from ecology, it is a relatively stable and self-sustaining community that represents the final stage of sustainable succession in a given urban environment*

Contemplative environment – *a space, either physical or mental, that fosters quiet reflection, introspection, and a sense of inner peace, often characterized by minimal distractions and an atmosphere conducive to focused thought and spiritual awareness*

Connectedness – *awe-inspired state of relationships and affinities between other people, places, and the world as a whole*

Consecration – *the action of completion and making or declaring something sacred*

Core affect – *a causal, central, inner, and often foundational, heartfelt experience of the sacred*

Crepuscular light – *light and skies experienced at dawn and dusk*

Cross-state retention – *the ability to remember experiences between secular and sacred transcendent episodes*

De-materialization – *reducing the amount of physical material used in building forms while maintaining or enhancing functionality and often focusing on the interplay of light and space*

Eden Project – *located in Cornwall, United Kingdom, designed by Nicholas Grimshaw, and completed in 2000. It features two large biomes that cluster with smaller domes*

Elaborated awe – *awe experiences altered by culture-specific norms, meanings, and practices*

Elicitors – *general features of stimuli that evoke the experience of awe*

Embraced places – *place experiences of intimacy, affection, and humble in character*

Emotions – *distinct feelings that are associated with non-verbal expressions, subjective experiences, and neural and physiological responses*

Emotional intelligence – *the ability to understand, use, and manage emotions in positive ways to relieve stress, communicate effectively, empathize with others, overcome challenges, and defuse conflict*

Emplacement – *the act or experience of situating and locating within a place (thin place)*

Enchantment – *charmed feeling of fascination, attraction, pleasure, and recognition of the world's spirituality*

Enhanced perception – *where all senses are functioning, activated, and focused with an increase of attention*

Enlivening – *a quality or energy that is life-giving, vital, and animate, contributing to the process of transformation*

Ephemeral – *a transitory numinous experience lasting for a short period of time*

Epiphany – *the awareness and experience of something extraordinary, supernatural, or divine*

Ethereality – *a place or experience that is born from ether and the otherworldly, celestial, and light-filled*

Euphoria – *feeling of intense well-being and happiness*

Everyday sacred – *heightened and numinous experiences that occur within ordinary places and architecture*

Existential questions – *issues of uncertainty, human beginnings, future existence, carrying capacity of the Earth*

Extraordinary experiences – *astonishing encounters that are remarkable, memorable, and unusual*

Fascination – *the power, charm, unusual nature, or attraction of an object, place, or experience*

Florence Nightingale – *influential during the Crimean War of 1853–1856, recognizing the need for clean hospital wards*

Flourishing – *a state of optimal human functioning characterized by positive emotions, engagement, relationships, meaning, and accomplishment*

Forest bathing – *contemplative practice of all-senses emersion into a forest atmosphere*

Geomancy – *the art of placing or arranging buildings or other sites auspiciously*

Geomantic amnesia – *a partial or total loss of memory, forgetting our connections to the Earth, Earth energy, and wholeness*

Global Wellness Institute – *a non-profit organization with the mission to empower wellness worldwide by educating the public and private sectors about preventative health and wellness*

Golden mean geometry – *phi geometry utilizing the golden ratio (approximately 1.618) in its proportions and spatial arrangements to create a certain resonance and aesthetically pleasing and often naturally harmonious designs*

Golden thread – *a seamless sacred connection from source to ideation, to manifestation, to experience*

Grace – *the unconditional and intrinsic quality of elegance and beauty of form and nature*

Haptic experiences – *perceptions of texture, shape, temperature, and movement through touch, contributing significantly to our understanding of and interaction with the physical world*

Harmony – *the balance, consonance, and proportion of parts*

Health – *a state of complete physical, mental, and social well-being and not merely the absence of disease or infirmity*

Heterotopia – *Foucault's "other place" that is disturbing, intense, incompatible, contradictory, or transforming*

Hettler, William – *originally defined six approaches constituting a hexagonal model of wellness pillars in 1976*

Imago mundi – the terrestrial model of the world emerging from a point or the axis mundi

Immaterial – the state or quality of the non-physical without matter, such as spirit, soul, or life force

Inclusive – *including and encompassing all ideas, belief systems, and people*

Incorporeal – *insubstantial, having no material existence (body or form)*

Inspiration – *an inward experience of a charged, stirring, and extraordinary external cause or source*

Life purpose – *finding meaning that makes a positive impact through one's unique existence and actions*

Light – *the radiant source of truth, goodness, and beauty emanating from the divine, quality of sacred architecture*

Liminal space – *a transitional threshold and crossing-over to where something is nearing to unfold and be explained*

Lived space – *one of Lefebvre's triad of perceived, conceived, and "othering," all-embracing, and never fully knowable spatiality*

Lived spiritual experience – *the notion that numinous experiences occur naturally and everyday*

Living color – *experience of natural colors found in nature, flowers, animals, sunsets, rainbows, blue skies, the Northern Lights, and natural pigments*

Lodestar – *like the North Star, a guiding light for intentionality*

Luminosity – *the outward magnitude and emanation of a light-emitting source, divine apparition*

Materiality – *the material organization and expression that is honest and must not erode, deteriorate, or fall into disrepair*

Mesmeric places – *spaces that become a fascinating and profound power that is transfixed and spellbound*

Multiplication – *achieving urban growth by developing urban form to an optimal size and then multiplying by creating new forms*

Mystery – a profound enigma that perplexes and is not fully known, understood, or solved

Mystic state – *an experience that is ineffable, having noetic quality, is transitory, and facilitates passivity*

Nearness – *a close and intimate proximity to "the Other" in both space and time*

Nested domains – *the hierarchical organization of spaces or systems where smaller, more specific areas or functions are contained within larger, more encompassing ones*

Noetic – *mental or cognitive activity related to numinous experiences, revelations, and gained knowledge*

Nones – *non-religious, atheist, agnostic, or spiritual affiliations*

Non-material – *not matter, physical or substantive, but rather intellectual, abstract, conceptual, or spiritual in nature*

Nudge design – *involves subtly altering the environment or choices available to individuals in a predictable way, without forbidding any options, influencing their behavior and decisions particularly toward wellness*

Numinous – *Rudolf Otto's experiences of fascination, mystery, and terror, in the presence of divinity*

Otherly – *experiences that are different, occurring outside of the self and the ordinary*

Orientation – *siting with focus on the Sun, sky, land contours, geomantic fields, cardinal directions, landmarks, views, natural or urban features*

Passage – *a distinct neutral space of pause, clearing, and awakening*

Passive survivability – *coined by Alex Wilson in 2005 in the wake of Hurricane Katrina, promoting design features that include cooling-load avoidance strategies, capabilities for natural ventilation, a highly efficient thermal envelope, passive solar gain, and natural daylighting*

Pathways to Wellness Architecture and Design – *a Global Wellness Institute white paper designed to guide investors, developers, architects, and project stakeholders, this paper presents a new paradigm of wellness architecture and design aimed to promote health and wellness outcomes for people, the built environment, and nature*

Peak experience – *Abraham Maslow's concept of an altered state of consciousness and elevated form of perception*

Perceived vastness – *observing something physically larger than oneself or a grand idea*

Pedestrianization – *urban circulation places that integrate natural, mixed-use, and transportation functions into human scale*

Peer support – *spiritual wellness through prosocial interactions*

Phenomenal unity – *the experience of wholeness, especially as time is perceived to stand still*

Plurilocality – *Edward Soja's concept of the existence of differences and complexities of multiple dimensions of space*

Positive emotions – *markers of flourishing or optimal and enduring well-being*

Postsecularism – *the re-emergence and coexistence of both religion and non-faith-based social, political, and cultural impulses*

Prayer – *an invocation, process, or ceremonial participation directed to a deity or universal quality/energy through deliberate communication or direct devotional action*

Presence – *the state of being in a place (human, Earth, and cosmic) or the existence of unseen forces or spirit*

Prosocial – *positive awe behavior promoting social acceptance that is friendly and helpful*

Pro-environmentalism – *behaviors that support biospheric values, place identity, and climate change awareness*

Proxemic – *Edward T. Hall's behavioral concept of the hidden organization, interactions, and use of space*

Psychic amphibians – *have the ability to retain memories between secular and transcendent experiences*

Quadrivium – *the fourfold of study of sacred number, geometry, music, and astronomy*

Qualitative architecture – *emphasizes the subjective experiences, sensory perceptions, and emotional responses to built spaces, prioritizing the quality of human experience over purely quantitative, formal or functional considerations*

Quiet awe – *transcendent experiences derived from less grand elicitors occurring on a more intimate scale*

Rapt attention – *complete focus, interest, fascination, and deep absorption*
Rescaling – *Process of changing the scale and proportion of our circumstances*
Resonance – *intentional proportions that resonate with natural frequencies, fostering a sense of harmony and connection within the built environment*
Reverence – *deep respect or regard for someone, something, or some place*
Ritual spaces – *designated areas, either physical or conceptual, that are intentionally set apart and imbued with meaning for the purpose of conducting rituals, ceremonies, or practices that hold symbolic or spiritual significance*
Sacred geometry – *ascribes symbolic meanings and resonances to certain geometric shapes, forms, and proportions*
Sacred places – *non-secular places of renewal, healing, meditation, historic significance, and religious experiences*
Sanctuary – *a safe place for sacred experiences; in religious architecture, place containing the high altar*
Scale – *measures relativity between participant and place; scale varies from vastness to intimacy*
Secular spirituality – *refers to the cultivation of inner peace, meaning, high-level wellness, and connection to something larger than oneself without reliance on traditional religious doctrines or institutions*
Self-transcendent experience – *altered state and feeling of diminished self (small self) relative to one's surroundings (thin place)*
Sensory unity – *a confluence of sensual experiences (visual, auditory, haptic, olfactory, and somatosensory)*
Serenity – *an emotion where behavioral and cognitive responses are associated with feeling calm, peaceful, and untroubled*
Small self – *an awe-stimulated diminishment of the self due to a vastness of experience and surroundings*
Spatial generosity – *the design principle of providing more space and a quality of space that are beyond those strictly necessary for the intended function*
Spirit – *the breath of life in one's heavenly being or the inspiring character of an extraordinary building*
Spirit of place – *gives meaning, value, emotion, identity, and mystery to place*
Spirituality – *gives meaning to existence and subsequently allows one to transcend beyond the present context*
Soul – *the ineffable essence and life force of one's earthly being, or the endearing character of a loved building*
Soundscape – *produces decreased stress annoyance and improved health outcomes*
Source experience – *the feeling of nearness and unity in proximity to the extraordinary, sacred, or divine*
Stewardship – *an ethical value and conduct that embody nurturing, care of, and responsibility for resources and places*
Sticky urbanism – *streetscapes with enticing street fronts, colorful façades, pedestrian activity*
Still point – *a location with no size or dimensional attribute, where time stands still*

Surrender – *diffusing temporal density, letting go, and being open to uncertainty and the unknown*

Sympathetic resonance – *phenomenon where a vibratory body responds to vibrations having a harmonic likeness*

Synchronicity and coincidences – *where circumstances and personal experiences have meaning connections*

Temporal density – *where too many activities, tasks, ideas, and feelings occupy a given time frame*

Terror – *the feeling induced by danger, threat, and where the overwhelming aspect of the numinous appears*

The Other – *Rudolf Otto's concept of the non-rational mystery and absolute existence without relating to any other*

Thin place – *spatial threshold where a svelte veil exists between our secular realms and the sacred world; a holy bridge*

Third place – *developed by Ray Oldenburg, a special place away from home where one can feel safe, comfortable, playful, and social*

Third space – *Edward Soja's concept of real and imagined, and knowable and unknowable, qualities of lived space*

Thomas Moore – *author of* The Re-enchantment of Everyday Life *which describes enchantment as the inflow of spirituality in everyday activities*

Transcendence – *experiences that climb and occur beyond the normal and physical realms*

Unity experience – *a subjective sensory experience where parts and fragments amalgamate into a single whole*

Value–action gap – *the inconsistency between what people say they value or believe and how they actually behave in real-life situations*

Wholly Other – *Rudolf Otto's concept of psychic states with certitude of the transcendent otherworldliness, completely different than and separate from all other things that exist*

Wild awe – *heightened awareness of the vastness and power of nature, awakening instincts and often evoking terror*

Well-being – *having positive emotions, engaged activities, good relationships, meaningful life, and a sense of accomplishment in the pursuit of one's goals*

Wellness pillars – *wellness directed toward physical, mental, emotional, social, financial, environmental, and spiritual well-being*

Wonder – *perceiving something rare or unexpected but not threatening*

Suggested Reading

Baum, Fran, & Matthew Fisher, Critical Public Health, https://www.tandfonline.com/doi/abs/10.1080/09581596.2010.503266.

Balboni, Tracy A., Tyler J. VanderWheele, & Stephenie Doan-Soares, Spirituality in Serious Illness and Health, https://jamanetwork.com/journals/jama/article-abstract/2794049.

Brill, Michael, Using the Place-Creation Myth to Develop Design Guidelines for Sacred Space, 1985, https://oaktrust.library.tamu.edu/handle/1969.1/ETD-TAMU-3103?show=full.

Buettner, Dan, Blue Zones: 9 Lessons for Living Longer From the People Who've Lived the Longest, *National Geographic*, 2012.

Carrol, John E. *Sustainability and Spirituality* (Albany, NY: State University of New York Press, 2004).

Casement, Ann, & David Tacey, Eds., *The Idea of the Numinous: Contemporary Jungian and Psychoanalytic Perspectives* (London, UK: Routledge, 2006).

Dunn, Halbert, *High Level Wellness* (Pitman, NJ: Charles B. Slack, 1977).

Ehrenfeld, John R., *Sustainability by Design* (New Haven, CT: Yale University Press, 2008).

Eliade, Mircea, *The Sacred & The Profane: The Nature of Religion* (Orlando, FL: Harcourt Brace, 1959).

Global Wellness Institute, Wellness Architecture and Design Initiative 2023 Trends, https://globalwellnessinstitute.org/global-wellness-institute-blog/2023/08/07/wellnessarchitecture-design-initiative-2023-trends/.

Global Wellness Institute, What Is Wellness? https://globalwellnessinstitute.org/what-is-wellness/.

Heschong, Lisa, *Visual Delight in Architecture: Daylight, Vision, and View* (London, UK: Routledge, 2021).

Ichioka, Sarah, & Michael Pawlyn, *Flourish: Design Paradigms for Our Planetary Emergency* (Axminster, UK: Triarchy Press, 2021).

James, William, *The Varieties of Religious Experience* (Whitefish, MT: Kissinger, 2010).

Kellert, Stephen R., *Biophilic Design: The Theory Science and Practice of Bringing Buildings to Life* (Hoboken, NJ: Wiley, 2008).

Keltner, Dacher, *Awe: The New Science of Everyday Wonder and How It Can Transform Our Lives* (New York, NY: Penguin Press, 2023).

Kopec, Dac, *Person-Centered Health Care Design* (New York, NY: Routledge, 2021).

Lawlor, Robert, *Sacred Geometry: Philosophy and Practice*. (Crossroad, 1982).

Louv, Richard, *Last Child in the Woods: Saving Our Children from Nature-Deficit Disorder* (Chapel Hill, NC: Algonquin Books, 2008).

McEwen, Bruce, Stress and Your Body, https://www.youtube.com/watch?v=0TUDwXPq67k.

Olszewske-Guizzo, Agnieszka, *Neuroscience for Designing Green Spaces: Contemplative Landscapes* (London, UK: Routledge, 2023).

Otto, Rudolf, *The Idea of the Holy* (London, UK: Oxford University Press, 1923).

Ramirez-Duran, Daniela, Positive Psychology, What Is Social Wellbeing? 12+ Activities for Social Wellness (accessed June 1, 2023), https://positivepsychology.com/social-wellbeing/.

Roberts, Kay, & Cheryl Aspy, Development of a Serenity Scale, https://www.researchgate.net/publication/15347724_Development_of_the_Serenity_Scale.

Soja, Edward, *Thirdspace: Journeys to Los Angeles and Other Real-and-Imagined Places* (Malden, MA: Blackwell, 1996).

Spiegel, Ross, & Dru Meadows, *Green Building Materials: A Guide to Product Selection and Specification* (New York, NY: Wiley, 1999).

Tabb, Phillip James, Thin Place Design: Architecture of the Numinous, https://www.annuity.org/personalfinance/financial-wellness/

Tabb, Phillip James, & Lahra Tatriele, *Wellness Architecture and Urban Design* (New York, NY: Routledge, 2025).

Travis, John, Illness and Wellness Continuum, 1972, https://www.houseofhealth.co.nz/wellnesscontinuum-blog-1-physical-health/

Tuan, Yi-Fu, *Space and Place: The Perspective of Experience* (Minneapolis, MN: University of Minnesota Press, 1977).

Wilson, Alex, Passive Survivability (accessed July 11, 2013), https://www.buildinggreen.com/oped/passive-survivability.

Wilson, Edward O., *Biophilia: The Human Bond with Other Species* (Cambridge, MA: Harvard University Press, 1984).

VanderWeele, Tyler, Spirituality Linked with Better Health Outcomes, Patient Care, https://www.hsph.harvard.edu/news/press-releases/spirituality-better-health-outcomes-patientcare/

Zorn, Justin, & Leigh Marz, *Golden: The Power of Silence in a World of Noise* (New York, NY: Harper Wave, 2022).

Index

For Product Safety Concerns and Information,
please contact our EU representative GPSR@taylorandfrancis.com
Taylor & Francis Verlag GmbH, Kaufingerstraße 24,
80331 München, Germany

Printed by Integrated Books International,
United States of America